PAGANISM

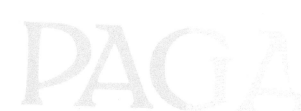

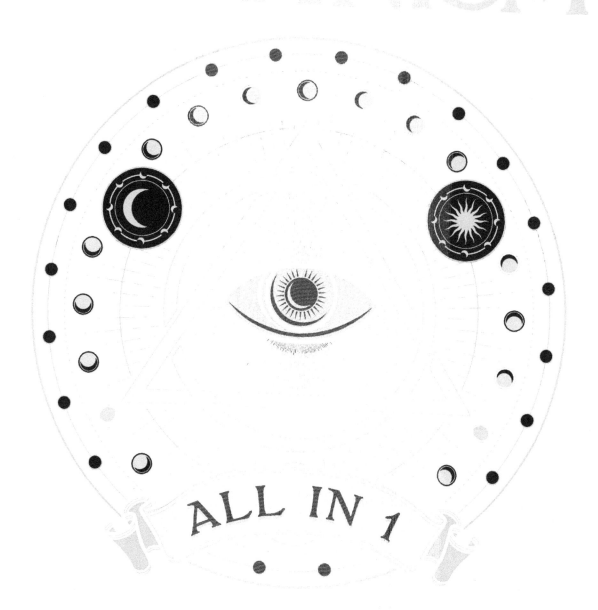

ALL IN 1

575 TECHNIQUES & INSIGHTS
for Inner Balance through Magic Practices

Find Spiritual Growth & Personal Transformation through
RUNES • WICCA • HERBALISM • SHAMANISM • MANIFESTATION

INGRID CLARKE

© Copyright 2023 - All rights reserved.

The content contained within this book may not be reproduced, duplicated, or transmitted without direct written permission from the author or the publisher.

Under no circumstances will any blame or legal responsibility be held against the publisher, or author, for any damages, reparation, or monetary loss due to the information contained within this book, either directly or indirectly.

Legal Notice:

This book is copyright protected. It is only for personal use. You cannot amend, distribute, sell, use, quote, or paraphrase any part, or the content within this book, without the author's or publisher's consent.

Disclaimer Notice:

Please note that the information contained within this document is for educational and entertainment purposes only. All effort has been executed to present accurate, up-to-date, reliable, and complete information. No warranties of any kind are declared or implied. Readers acknowledge that the author does not render legal, financial, medical, or professional advice. The content within this book has been derived from various sources. Please consult a licensed professional before attempting any techniques outlined in this book.

By reading this document, the reader agrees that under no circumstances is the author responsible for any direct or indirect losses incurred as a result of the use of the information contained within this document, including, but not limited to, errors, omissions, or inaccuracies.

Table of Contents

The 5 Pillars of Runes...1

The 4 Pillars of Herbalism..95

The 5 Pillars of Wicca..201

The 4 Pillars of Shamanism...301

The 7 Pillars of Manifestation...387

THE 5 PILLARS OF RUNES

FOUNDATION   LAYOUTS AND SPREADS   SENSE OF RUNES   CASTING   READING

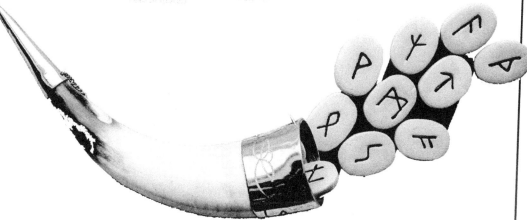

97 TECHNIQUES & INSIGHTS

to Connect to Your Higher Self Through the Magic and Rituals of Runelore. Tap Into Your Intuition by Harnessing the Power and Wisdom of Runic Symbols

INGRID CLARKE

Table of Contents

Introduction 5

Pillar 1: Foundation 7

Chapter 1: Foundation 9
    Defining Runes 9
    Using the Runes 13

Pillar 2: Runic Scripts 15

Chapter 2: Different Runic Scripts 17
    Early Germanic 17
    Anglo-Saxon 18
    Nordic 19
    Medieval 19

Chapter 3: Elder Futhark 21
    The Aetts of the Elder Futhark 21

Chapter 4: Younger Futhark 31
    History of the Younger Futhark 31
    The Runes of the Younger Futhark 32

Chapter 5: Anglo-Saxon Futhorc 41
    History of the Anglo-Saxon Futhorc 41
    The Runes of the Futhorc 42

Pillar 3: Casting 57

Chapter 6: What You Need to Know About Rune Casting 59
    History of Rune Casting 59
    How to Cast Runes 60
    Tools of the Trade 63

Pillar 4: Layouts and Spreads 65

Chapter 7: Layouts and Spreads List **67**
    Runic Layouts and Spreads 67

Pillar 5: Reading **73**

Chapter 8: Interpreting Runes **75**
    Casting and Interpreting Runes 75

Conclusion **87**

References **89**

Introduction

Are you struggling to make sense of a meaningful life event? Do you feel like the universe is trying to tell you something, but you cannot understand what it is saying? Runes could be the answer. These ancient symbols hold the power of the cosmos and offer insights, protection, and divine knowledge that can unlock the answers to some of life's most difficult questions. Unlike many forms of divination, rune reading has been around for centuries and was used by our ancestors to seek guidance. They believe runes have a unique ability to tap into unseen forces and energies that provide a deeper understanding of ourselves and our place in the world. With their help, you can gain clarity in any situation, find direction when lost, and discover a new purpose in life.

Likewise, runes can give us a glimpse into deeper truths hidden from our everyday view. By understanding how to use and solve them, you can learn how to read unseen threads of fate and even rewrite your destiny. This book provides a comprehensive guide on runecraft, exploring the five pillars of runology: rune scripts, spreads and layouts, interpretation based on questions asked, and more. As you journey through this initiatory process into the world of runology, you will gain an insightful new lens through which to view life's complexities. The information in this book will give you a firm footing in recognizing when life calls for you to invoke the wisdom of runes, unlocking their language and your potential.

Everyone faces trials and tribulations that can be hard to bear. But true strength lies in those who strive to overcome these difficulties and learn more about themselves and our world. Our modern society is saturated with technology, making it easy to become disconnected from our environment. Also, it leads us to lose not only sight of nature but also the spiritual power within ourselves. Engaging with our natural surroundings can reconnect with life's mysteries and foster greater well-being.

Having endured burnout in the past and coming from a Scandinavian family with Pagan roots, I have dedicated my life to exploring different healing practices. I have gained incredible insight into metaphysical practices and occult traditions from all over the world. Likewise, I feel a unique connection to the runes, those magnificent cosmic symbols so beloved by my ancestors. As an empath, it is my role to pass on the extensive knowledge and wisdom I have acquired through my long years of research on bringing relief to those who need it. Furthering this quest is my deep appreciation for herbalism, crystal healing, astrology, and spiritual philosophies.

This book delves deep into the study of runes, providing insightful knowledge into where they come from and how to use them. You will find 97 techniques, tips, and strategies on how to explore the transformative world of runecraft, offering a journey of self-discovery and spiritual enlightenment, peppered throughout the entire book. It's intentionally designed this way to serve as your guide along each step of the process.

Uncover the history of runes, including the Elder Futhark and Younger Futhark as well as the Anglo-Saxon futhorc. That said, you will gain a thorough understanding of these ancient symbols. Yet, not only will this book educate readers in casting and interpreting runes based on whatever question is asked or layout is chosen. As such, it also offers detailed knowledge about various spreads and layouts. Hence, this book gives insight into this powerful yet simple approach to uncovering the truth.

Unraveling the secrets of our fate can be daunting, especially when life's obstacles seem to stand in our way. But with the use of runes, we can gain insight into our future and uncover the mysteries that are hidden from us. Through my research and publishing of the techniques I share in this book, I have better understood myself and aligned with a path forward. Utilizing these special symbols has allowed me to strengthen my awareness. Likewise, I have become more prepared to decipher life's cosmic puzzles.

The end goal of this book is to help you on a journey of spiritual enlightenment and awakening. Also, it will guide you in tapping into your intuition, understanding your motivation, building self-confidence, and making decisions that will lead you to a better tomorrow. Embark on a voyage of self-discovery by unlocking the runes' secrets and uncovering the divine power within us all. Through rune wisdom and reading, you will be given an insight into life's complexities that can open your eyes to new perspectives. Furthermore, this knowledge can provide practical advice on how to apply them in real-life situations. Plus, guide you toward attaining personal growth and clarity. Let us begin this fantastic journey.

Pillar 1
Foundation

Crafting a solid foundation is an essential part of any learning journey. An apt analogy to this process is building a house. The structure must be sound before anything else can be constructed. In this chapter, we will ensure that your fundamental understanding is adequately cemented in place. This foundational knowledge will act as the base upon which more complex topics can be developed, helping to ensure that you build your understanding logically and systematically. Additionally, having real-world relevant facts or examples connected to this information can help strengthen your grasp of the subject.

1

What you need to know about Runes

There is much mystery surrounding the origins of the runic symbols. Tales from Norse mythology tell of how Odin, ruler in chief of Asgard and a most revered god among the Norse Pantheon, sacrificed himself on Yggdrasil, the cosmic tree connecting Nine Worlds. Hanging for nine days and nine nights, he was able to unlock the mysteries of the universe symbolized by runes. By definition, runes are inscribed characters or symbols believed to have magical properties. It was through his immense sacrifice that Odin revealed their hidden meaning. Such stories perpetuate the mythos associated with runes, which embed themselves in our collective imaginations as we explore their history and purpose.

Defining Runes

The runes are not just used for divination and magic, but they also carry much historical significance. Used by many Germanic societies from the 1st to 2nd century AD, these runes have been adopted into various languages that use the Latin alphabet. Unlike today's Latin alphabet, each rune is an ideogram representing sounds, objects, or ideas. Thinking about it, they are much like Egyptian hieroglyphs or Ancient Chinese characters. This uniqueness makes them invaluable tools for divination, fortune-telling, and advice-seeking. Furthermore, many medieval scholars believed runes could be used as powerful talismans to protect oneself from misfortunes. All these make runes a fascinating part of history.

Definition

Learning about something new can be an exciting journey, especially regarding runes. As the Merriam-Webster Dictionary outlines, runes have three distinct meanings. As such, these three are the characters used by early Germanic people, mystery and magic, and Old Norse poetry or songs. Moreover, another interpretation of this ancient alphabet is *"secret conversation"* or *" something hidden."* Hence, a concept that carries a certain degree of power. This power is further emphasized with reference to Norse mythology, which tells of an origin story for runes where each letter holds both a sound and a concept. Through this lens, it becomes clear why rune-speaking people believed in the strength of words so strongly that they embedded symbols of power in their letters.

Linguistic History

From ancient Nordic tribes to modern-day esoteric practitioners, runes have been used across time and cultures as a written form of communication. Three of the most renowned alphabets crafted from runes are—

Elder Futhark

The Germanic runic alphabet, also known as Elder Futhark, was an ancient script used by Germanic tribes in Northwest Germany during the Migration Period. Made up of 24 runes, it got its name from its first six letters *(F, U, Þ, A, R, and K)*, which spelled out 'futhark.' An example of one of these tribes was the Goths, who are believed to be among the first to have adopted this writing system. Despite being labeled as *'barbarians,'* they defeated the Roman empire. Also, they gained recognition for their powerful alphabetic system that held many esoteric meanings. In addition, some early Christian missionaries used these runes as a tool to spread their message, providing further evidence of their importance throughout history.

As we have mentioned before, using runes for magic or divination purposes predates the creation of the alphabet itself. During the time the Elder Futhark was created, writing was considered to be a tool for magic. There were only a select few in each tribe who had the skill to write and read these magical signs known as runes. Spells were cast using the runes, fortunes told, and secret messages. The Elder Futhark writing system itself is considered to have been a *"secret"* language of symbols. Through its hidden lore, the power of the gods could be brought into the physical world, and the will of the inscriber made manifest.

Anglo-Saxon Futhorc

The second prominent runic alphabet used by the Anglo-Saxons was the 'Futhorc,' derived from earlier Germanic runes. It was brought to Britain when three powerful Germanic tribes, the Angles, Saxons, and Jutes, invaded in the 5th century AD. Each tribe had its language. As such, Old English for the Angles, Old Saxon for the Saxons, and Old Jute for the Jutes were written using Futhorc. After conquering Britain, Anglo-Saxons brought their culture and traditions to their new lands. They also brought Norse mythology and beliefs, which blended into local Celtic folklore. Subsequently, it gave rise to a unique culture that can still be seen today in British customs and traditions.

For half a millennium, the Anglo-Saxons developed their version of the popular Germanic writing system known as runes. Adapting the Elder Futhark alphabet, they utilized new symbols and amassed 33 characters. Then, nine more than its parent and 17 more than the Younger Futhark. In doing so, they could transpose their language, Old English, onto stone and parchment for future generations to study. This adaptation of an ancient script is a testament to the Anglo-Saxon's dedication to preserving their culture and history.

Younger Futhark

The Younger Futhark, or Scandinavian Runes, was used by the Vikings from 793 to 1066 A.D. as a form of communication and record-keeping. This writing system had only 16 runes compared to the 24 that its predecessor, the Elder Futhark, had. The main reason for simplifying the runic alphabet is to increase literacy levels among the Germanic tribe. Plus, there is a growing need for writing down more complex information. As a result, it has become an essential part of Viking history and culture, with many rune stones still standing today.

Besides, the Elder Futhark was an ancient writing system used mainly by the elite for divination or other magical purposes. Meanwhile, Younger Futhark was widely used and adopted by people of all social classes across Scandinavia. Consequently, it was simplified to make carving messages on stones, making it a valuable communication tool. Even though the 350 existing inscriptions of Elder Futhark are scarce compared to the more than 3000 runestones written in Younger Futhark, they cover a broad spectrum. As such, they include prophecies, everyday conversations, and even humorous remarks. Evidently, its success lies in its ability to enable ordinary people to leave behind a tangible trace of their culture, ideas, and thoughts.

Medieval Runes

Emerging from the Younger Futhark of the 13th century, Medieval Runes, or Futhork, consisted of 27 characters and were used across Scandinavia in the Middle Ages. This script also served as the basis for the highly popular runology of the 16th century, with many runes modified or taken directly from existing symbols in the Younger Futhark. Tracing back further, these runes originated from the Older Futhark. While the meanings of these runes stayed largely unaltered, their sound representation and physical shape varied considerably between different alphabets. To highlight this development even more, it is believed that some runes were explicitly developed to represent new sounds that arose during this period.

Latin Writing Invades

In the late 11th century, the Latin alphabet became a competitor to the Futhork in Scandinavia. However, since it was still expensive to write with a quill and ink on parchment, essential for Latin writing, the clergy mainly used it. Meanwhile, the Old Norse language continued to be written down using runes carved on wood, stone, or other hard surfaces using sharp objects. Likewise, Latin prayers and many Medieval church objects display rune engravings. These include medieval runes engraved on church bells, baptismal fonts, and relic containers carved on church doors, walls, and front porches.

During the 13th century, Latin writing began supplanting runes and was used to write down medieval Scandinavian laws. This transition quickly led to Latin becoming the dominant writing system among politicians and clergypersons. Although the public transitioned from using runes to Latin letters, some still maintained the usage of runes for various esoteric purposes such as divination, magic, and secret messages. The study of runology eventually rose after rune scholars in the 16th century started studying their history and using it academically. Additionally, several manuscripts documenting Nordic mysteries and spells were composed during this period, testifying how runes were kept alive in Nordic culture even when Latin had become popularized.

The Birth of Runology

Runology is an ancient and powerful field of study that traces back to Johannes Bureus in the 16th century. He was the royal librarian for the King of Sweden and believed that the runes had a practical use and held mystical and holy properties. This spiritual belief has been strengthened recently due to archaeological evidence, such as rare runestones, linking it to prosperity, longevity, and protection. Bureus' larger contribution to Swedish culture included being a tutor and advisor to King Gustavus Adolphus. Likewise, he was considered the *"father of Swedish grammar."* As such, his work can be seen throughout Scandinavian culture today. This commitment to preserving Old Norse culture earned him recognition as a proponent of Gothicism with solid ties to the Geats. Besides, he claimed they were direct descendants of those who conquered the Roman Empire. Likewise, he believed that runes, the Old Norse tribe's writing system, were not just letters like those in Latin. Yet, they were something extraordinary and even sacred.

Mythological Origins

I know I hung on that windswept tree,
Swung there for nine long nights,
Wounded by my own blade,
Bloodied for Odin,
Myself an offering to myself:
Bound to the tree
That no man knows
Whither the roots of it run.

None gave me bread,
None gave me drink.
Down to the deepest depths, I peered.
Until I spied the Runes.
With a roaring cry, I seized them up,
Then dizzy and fainting, I fell.

Well-being, I won.
And wisdom too.
From a word to a word
I was led to a word,
From a deed to another deed.

(Poetic Edda, ca.1200 AD, The Speech of the High One)

The poem above tells the tale of Odin All-father, the chief of Norse mythology. He acquired knowledge of runes by performing a ritualistic sacrifice, suspending himself from Yggdrasil for nine nights and days. Known as a source of great wisdom, Urd's Well lies directly below Yggdrasil's branches, where Odin saw symbols of the universe encoded within it. This divine insight likely made him the most powerful god among Germanic tribes. To commemorate his achievement, *Wednesday, or "Woden's Day,"* is still named after him. Moreover, many attribute Odin with abilities such as wisdom, knowledge, sorcery, and poetry, all governed by the runic alphabet.

Meanwhile, stories involving Odin are often associated with his deepened knowledge of the universe's mysteries. He famously drank from the Mead of Poetry, an enchanted elixir that granted him the power to become a *'skald'* or scholar. Its ability allowed him to remember and recite any information learned and to solve any problem he set his mind to. As a result, he was revered as the great magician and All-father of the Norse Pantheon. With this knowledge and power, Odin was also seen as the perfect being to understand runes and teach others how to read them.

The Germanic tribes did not believe these symbols had been invented or created. Instead, they saw them as pre-existing forces of the cosmos which Odin imparted upon certain people, known as runemasters. As such, this way allows them to interpret their powerful meanings for divination purposes or engrave them for protection and magic spells. Additionally, these runes were considered a source of wisdom that could connect one with spiritual guidance or ancestral knowledge.

Using the Runes

Now that we know more about their linguistic history and mythological origins, it is time to explore the uses of runes. Not only were they used as a writing system, but they also served as a tool for magic or divination. Runes were inscribed in places of importance and even within Christian churches, calling upon the gods for protection and blessing. Furthermore, runes were found engraved on swords, ceremonial and used in battle, carved onto wooden strips, or painted on pebbles or stones for divination. With this new knowledge, runes can be seen as symbols of communication and conduits of spiritual power with various applications in both protective and predictive realms.

The first historical record we have of Germanic peoples using the runes for divine or occult purposes comes from Tacitus, the renowned Roman historian, and politician, who wrote a detailed account of it in his book *Germania 10* (98AD):

> *"They attach the highest importance to taking auspices and casting lots. Their usual procedure with the lot is simple. They cut off a branch from a nut or seed-bearing tree and slice it into strips; they mark it with different signs and throw them randomly onto a white cloth. Then the state's priest, if it is an official consultation, or the father of the family, in a private one, offers prayer to the gods and, looking up towards heaven, picks up three strips, one at a time, and, according to which sign they have previously been marked with, makes his interpretation."*

Ancient runes have been around for centuries, having been discovered and decoded by multiple civilizations. Odin was believed to be the god of prophecy, who gifted our species with his powerful symbols. As we delve into these symbols and the practice of rune reading, it is essential to remember that they have been used as a form of divination and magic for more than two millennia. This ancient insight can be applied to this day to bring new clarity and understanding into our lives.

Casting and Drawing Runes

Uncovering further knowledge and insights lies at the heart of rune casting. Each rune is a double-edged sword, containing both an *'external'* and *'internal'* meaning. Its main purpose is as a pictogram to tap into cosmic powers for divination. After preparing the space for your runes, place them onto a flat surface to protect them from sliding and bouncing around too much. Once cast, they are interpreted in terms of where they lay relative to the caster and how they are arranged compared to other runes used in that casting session. Learn more about unlocking these mysteries in chapter six of runelore: casting. Commit to learning more about runes and rune casting to get the most out of your readings. Their secrets are waiting for you to uncover.

Another way to practice divination with runes is called 'drawing runes.' This is similar to drawing a card from a tarot deck. The diviner can lay the runes face-down on a flat surface or pull them out of an opaque bag. In one method, the diviner passes their non-dominant hand over the face-down runes until they feel attracted to one that stands out, then flips it and interprets its meaning. In the second method, three runes are drawn from the bag, one at a time. These individual rune readings are then interpreted as part of a larger reading according to what was asked when starting the divination process. Some believe that which rune is chosen or drawn is determined by the spiritual energies present in their environment at that moment.

Runecraft and Runic Magic

"Beer, I bring thee, tree of battle,
Mingled of strength and mighty fame.
Charms it holds and healing signs,
Spells full good, and gladness-runes."
(Burrows, 2007, p.139)

Runes are sacred symbols in Norse mythology inscribed on stones, wood, and objects to divine the future or call upon supernatural powers. These same runes can be used to cast spells as they were believed to have a connection with the gods. In the poem *Sigrdrífumál*, *Brynhildr* bestows a beer blessed with runes of joy and gladness upon Sigurd. The Poetic Edda is a legendary collection of Old Norse poems thought to have been written between 800-1150 AD. This work of literature is an integral part of Norse folklore and provides an insight into how pre-Christian Scandinavians viewed their world.

Brynhildr then explains the various magical uses of the runes for the following seven stanzas. Here is an overview of the different uses Brynhildr mentions.

- **Victory Runes.** Carved and used on sword hilts to ensure victorious combat.
- **Ale Runes (ølrunar).** Used as a protective charm against being bewitched through ale served by a host's wife.
- **Birth Runes (biargrunar).** Utilized in childbirth to help aid safe delivery.
- **Wave Runes (brimrunar).** Incanted and carved on the stem and rudder of ships for protection from sea dangers.
- **Branch Runes (limrunar).** Scribed onto east-facing trees for healing purposes.
- **Speech Runes (malrunar).** Inscribed to enhance one's rhetoric skills.
- **Thought Runes (hugrunar).** Engraved to sharpen the mind.

Knowledge of rune magic and divination has been around for centuries, tracing its roots back to the Middle Ages. Runes have a rich history with many cultures and languages, containing immense power and potential in their use. With this foundational understanding of runes, you can now begin to explore the possibilities their symbols can bring to your life. In the next chapter, we will dive into Runic Scripts to understand how different languages use these runic alphabets. To make sure you get as much out of runes as possible, it is essential to research their origin before using them. As such, some have been known to have strong ties with ancient Norse mythology. With that in mind, may you soon enjoy the fortuitousness that casting and reading runes can bring.

Pillar 2
Runic Scripts

With our understanding of runology as a foundation, it is time to explore the next pillar: runic scripts. Runes were used for many purposes, including divination and magic, but their primary use was as letters of the alphabet. Ancient runic artifacts, such as rune staffs carved with symbols, provide us with tangible evidence that runes were used to form written language. It is possible to organize your knowledge of runes by viewing them through the lens of the three main runic alphabets: *Elder Futhark, Younger Futhark, and Anglo-Saxon Futhorc.* Understanding these alphabets requires an overview of the runic script, what it is, and how it functions within its given context.

2

Different Runic Scripts

From the 3rd century to the 16th or 17th century, Germanic people in northern Europe, Britain, Scandinavia, and Iceland used runes as a writing system. A late arrival in the history of writing systems, these pictographs are far older than the alphabets they were incorporated into. This chapter will explore the three early runic scripts. As such, it will trace their spread and evolution and delve into the tribes and cultures that harnessed them. Let us step towards mastering runelore as we discover more about their past. Connecting with a mythical past filled with power and depth, runes can bring wisdom and insight to our lives today.

Early Germanic

The Elder Futhark is an ancient runic alphabet combining elements from Proto-Indo-European and indigenous Northern European cultures. It was in use until the 8th century AD, after which other variations of Runic alphabets, like Anglo-Saxon Futhorc, emerged. This script was inscribed on objects ranging from jewelry to weapons, indicating its widespread usage in Northern Europe during this period.

At the time of Elder Futhark's emergence, the world was experiencing a period known as Late Antiquity. New technology, including iron weapons and tools, replaced bronze during this transitional period, marking a dramatic shift in many cultures' practices. This shift set into motion the Migration Period (300–800 AD), where Early Germanic tribes invaded and settled in areas formerly occupied by the Western Roman Empire, an event now affectionately referred to as *"Barbarian Invasions."* The early Germanic tribes brought their writing system, Elder Futhark, with them as they spread through Europe over five centuries.

The Runic Script Heads Abroad

The Migration Period was a time of immense cultural change in Europe, and with it came the spread of the Elder Futhark script. This ancient Germanic alphabet was widely adopted from Germany throughout Scandinavia, western Europe, and even as far east as Poland, Ukraine, and Romania. During this period, the Elder Futhark was a source of stability for new settlers across many nations, providing a common language to trade goods and express ideas. In addition, it also provided an invaluable link to their shared cultural past by connecting pre-Christian Germanic mythology with local Pagan practices throughout Europe.

Scholars trace the beginnings of the Elder Futhark, a runic alphabet that originated in a fusion of Roman and Gothic culture, to an uncertain date between 1 BC and 5 AD. This belief is contested by some who believe that it was first developed as early as 27 BC. The oldest surviving example of this writing system is an ancient runestone in Sweden that dates back to the 5th century AD. Aside from providing insight into their origin, this script has long been used as a form of communication and divination by many cultures worldwide, including Scandinavia, Britain, and Germany.

Moreover, ancient runes serve as a relic of the past and contain much history. One such artifact is the *Spearhead of Kovel*, discovered 30km outside of Kovel, Ukraine, in the early 3rd century. The runes inscribed on it are believed to be *"thither rider"* in Danish translation. This victory rune was not meant as a boast but as an offering to Odin himself. The immense spiritual significance of spears at that time had been deeply embedded in Germanic culture, particularly among the Goths, who treated these weapons with magical reverence. Through these artifacts, we can better understand the rich mythology and beliefs held by our ancestors.

Likewise, from the mysticism and mythology of Early Germanic people, runes have long held special meaning and purpose. During the 7th to 9th centuries AD, the Elder Futhark underwent a transfiguration, resulting in two distinct runic alphabets. This period marked the Viking Age's start, characterized by European exploration and colonization. Plus, it was indicated the time when runes began to be used for political means, personal reflections, and stories of everyday life.

Anglo-Saxon

During the Viking Age, the Norsemen pillaged, plundered, conquered, and colonized much of Europe. In addition to their settlements in the British Isles and Ireland, Greenland, and Normandy, they even reached eastern Europe. One of the most daring Vikings set foot in North America when they landed in Newfoundland, making them the first Europeans to do so. The Norse Peoples also established formidable kingdoms and earldoms across Europe and Britain. As such, it includes York *(Jórvík)* in northern Northumbria and Dublin *(Dyflin)* in Ireland. Along with their culture and traditions, they brought their distinctive runic writing system with them as they spread across northern Europe and the British Isles.

The Celts, originating from the Germanic region, made their way to Britain as early as 500 BC. Yet, there is no surviving evidence of them using runes or any writing system. This may be attributed to their quick conquest and colonization by the Romans, who viewed anyone outside Rome as 'barbarians' rather than preserving their history. During this period, Latin reigned as the predominant writing system of the British Isles. Despite that, its use was limited due to a lack of literacy.

However, during the invasion of Britain in the 5th century AD by the Angles, Saxons, and Jutes, the runes are believed to have been documented in history books. After winning over the Romans, the Anglo-Saxons stayed primarily in England. They also evolved into what is now known as the English race, while Ireland, Scotland, and Wales retained more Celtic influence. The areas controlled by the Anglo-Saxons contained abundant evidence of rune usage.

Nordic

As the Elder Futhark evolved into the Anglo-Saxon Futhorc in Britain, a transformation occurred on the European continent. Coinciding with the Viking Age came the onset of the Younger Futhark. Although these two runic scripts derived from the Elder Futhark, they had some critical differences. The primary distinction is that while extra runes were added to the Futhorc, eight were removed from the Younger Futhark, leaving only 16 characters. This notion of simplification started in the late 7th century and was finalized around the 9th century when Vikings held sway over much of Europe. This period created the shapes and styles we commonly associate with runes today and their most renowned wielders: *The Norsemen or the Vikings.*

Younger Futhark and the Viking Age

The Younger Futhark is believed to have been in use since around 800 AD, and its arrival changed the history of writing as we know it. As it spread rapidly across Scandinavia and Viking Age settlements, these runes were used by kings, warriors, traders, and citizens. As such, they use runes for various reasons when documenting, creating a love letter, or invoking the gods. Subsequently, the rune alphabet was versatile enough to be used for anything a person desired.

Compared to its predecessor, the Elder Futhark, a *"secret"* script solely known and used by the literate elites for religious purposes. Yet, this Younger Futhark opened up literacy and writing to all levels of society. Old Norse continued as mainly a spoken language. However, writing increased drastically due to the introduction of these versatile runes that could do just about anything.

As the Younger Futhark arose, it was divided into two dialects. These two are the Danish long-branch runes and Swedish or Norwegian short-twig runes. The former was used for inscriptions on stone. Meanwhile, the latter was for everyday purposes. Yet, both are private and official carved into the wood. Over time, the short-twig runes evolved into a simpler version of their long-branch counterparts. In the 10th century AD, these further simplified runes took form in a dialect called *"Hälsinge"* or *" staveless runes."* This dialect originated in Hälsingland, Sweden. Also, it was the culmination of a gradual process that began with Elder Futhark giving way to its younger variation. These staveless runes are so named because they typically omit their stave (vertical line), making it easier to write longer texts.

However, attempts to adapt the Younger Futhark runes for everyday use failed, with Latin eventually becoming the preferred writing system throughout Scandinavia as the region became increasingly Christianized. By the 12th century, Latin was overwhelmingly used for writing in Scandinavia, and the runes reverted to their original purpose as a 'secret' script.

Medieval

As the Viking Age neared its close, the invention of dotted runes, known as stung, ushered in the Futhork, or *"Medieval Runes."* This new set of runes added a dot or bar accent marker to simplify the Younger Futhark's issue of one rune representing more than one sound. The various accents distinguished between *'i,' 'e,'* and *'j'* runes depending on whether a dot, bar, or nothing was present.

By the early 13th century, the medieval runic alphabet had been fully formed. This alphabet expanded the 16 characters in the Younger Futhark, eventually reaching 27. Those who carved runes, known as runemasters, often chose to use and modify existing runes rather than make new ones. In this way, many of the runes featured in the Futhark were directly derived from those in the Elder Futhark. Although there may be subtle differences between versions of these ancient symbols, their esoteric meanings remain primarily unchanged throughout each script.

Runes Return to Their Original Use

When the runic alphabet moved to its final form of 27 characters in the Middle Ages, Latin was also introduced in Scandinavia. Yet it remained a foreign writing practice until the 16th century. This meant runic script remained popular for official memorials and records of important occurrences. Likewise, it was widely used for writing diaries and practicing magic or divination. This was especially true in Iceland, with its Rune Poems and manuscripts written in Medieval runes up to the 19th century. Moreover, Sweden mostly used runic calendars until that same period. Additionally, knowledge of their magical and divinatory uses has been preserved throughout history due to the 16th century's development of Runology.

Runology

The runes have been used and studied for divination purposes for a far longer time than the tarot has. Their use tracks back at least 2,000 years. The study of the runes began in the 16th century with the specialized branch of German linguistics known as runology. As mentioned in the previous chapter, the academic study of the runes started with the Swedish polymath JohannesBureus. Bureus considered the runes as tools for magic and divination handed down the generations from his Old Norse ancestors. He even went on to create his esoteric interpretation of the runes. While Bureus may have been the first runologist, he was not the last. This way, the runic script and the hidden meaning of the runes have carried on to the modern day.

Now that you understand the history and application of runes, it is time to infuse the magic, rituals, and wisdom of Runelore into your life. Subsequent chapters will teach you to use these timeless symbols' legendary might and wisdom to access your intuition.

3

Elder Futhark

As the oldest known runic alphabet, the Elder Futhark is a powerful source of knowledge and understanding. It forms the basis for all other runic scripts and contains 24 unique characters with distinct meanings. Ages-old runes were used by cultures worldwide to communicate with each other and access divine knowledge. This chapter explains their meanings and guides how to interpret them in your rune casts. Furthermore, these symbols may still help connect you to universal energies for spiritual growth and insight.

The Ætts of the Elder Futhark

The ancient Elder Futhark alphabet is divided into three distinct groups of eight runes, collectively known as ættir or "clans" in Old Norse. These clans have strong linkages to each other and can be used to form connections between past and present. Each group is rich in symbolic meaning, depicting ancient Norse gods, concepts, and beliefs. As such, the three ættir of the Elder Futhark includes the following:

- Freyr/Freyja's Ætt
- Heimdall's Ætt
- Týr's Ætt

Per ætt, which translates to 'family,' is a group of runes assigned to a specific god from the Norse pantheon. Fascinatingly, the name of each god matches the first letter of their corresponding set of runes—the Elder Futhark. Learn more about this magical language by exploring its different ættir and their divine rulers.

Freyr/Freyja's Ætt

The two powerful twins of Norse mythology, Freyr and Freyja, rule the first eight runes of the Elder Futhark. Freyr and Freyja, children of Njord, belong to the Vanir pantheon. This class of Norse gods is associated with wisdom, fertility, and the ability to see into the future.

Freyr means "Lord" in Old Norse and is the god of fertility. He was one of the most revered gods among both the Norse and Germanic people. As the god of fertility, Freyr had power over anything that grew, which is why he was so revered and prayed to by the Norse and Germanic peoples. Meanwhile, Freyja means "Lady" in Old Norse and is the goddess of love and beauty, sex and war, gold and fertility. She is also the goddess of seiðr *(seidr)*, the Old Norse word for a type of magic that could see into the future and influence it.

Freyr and Freyja's set of runes is known as the ætt of the nurturer - a representation of life, love, happiness, and joy. Like tarot cards, runes also have corresponding meanings. Yet, their connotations depend on whether upright or merkstave (reversed). Merkstave meaning is not the exact opposite of the original interpretation; think of it as a shadow to its light. Not all runes carry a merkstave, though, since some are impossible to tell if they are right side up or upside down. For rune casting, we will explore the eight runes of Freyr/Freyja's Ætt and discuss their light and dark meanings. Additionally, most Norse religions view divination as acquiring insight into one's personal growth rather than trying to predict future events. As such, knowledge about Norse mythology can help parse these runes better.

Fehu (ᚠ)

The rune fehu is connected to the Norse god Freyr and the goddess Freyja. Also, it serves as a reminder that success can be achieved through hard work and effort rather than solely relying on luck. It also symbolizes abundance, good fortune, and the potential for growth in various areas of life. Furthermore, numerous interpretations of fehu involve energy, foresight, creation, and destruction. In other words, it represents the power to transform a present situation into something greater. Ultimately, fehu stands for hope, wealth, and joy that can be attained when we take the necessary steps toward prosperity.

Fehu, when reversed in casting, indicates a loss due to one's actions or behavior. It can refer to losing material possessions, assets, or self-esteem interpreted as greed, discord among relationships, and burnout. In addition, fehu's negative form could symbolize poverty, cowardice, or being bound by obligations. All this serves as a reminder to take caution in life and our decisions, which could have greater implications than intended.

Ūruz (ᚢ)

The rune ūruz is the second in Freyr/Freyja's Ætt and dates back to the Proto-Germanic language. This form symbolizes physical strength and untamed potential. When appearing face-up in a divinatory casting, it signifies tremendous energy and hidden power. Conversely, its merkstave form carries implications of weakness, misdirection, obsession, lust, and violence. Depending on where it appears with other runes, ūruz may signify understanding, wisdom, sexuality, sexual desire, or maleness. When interpreted through these various lenses, ūruz suggests positivity. Yet, unexpected changes are coming into your life due to self-formation and a need for mindful actions.

Thurisaz (ᚦ)

The 'th' of the Futhark, Thurisaz, is believed to mean 'giant,' as in the mythical creature. Norse gods were often embroiled in a war with these powerful beings. Ragnarök was sparked by fire giants siding with Loki and Surtr against Odin and the Æsir at the apocalyptic battle. Interestingly, not all deities shared this hostility; Thor was half-giant and Odin's eldest son. Furthermore, giants have often been associated with wisdom, strength, and hidden knowledge, symbols of divine power that could explain why gods so fiercely regarded them.

Moreover, the rune Thurisaz is steeped in history and speaks to the power of duality. It is strongly associated with magical symbolism, representing the forces of connection and opposition within the universe. These opposing forces can be used for constructive purposes. However, they can lead to conflict, defensiveness, or destruction if unchecked. As a representation of vitality and sexual energy, Thurisaz is believed to symbolize fertility and uncontrolled aspirations. Understanding this intricate relationship between positive and negative points can unlock more powerful aspects of their own will.

On merkstave meaning, its presence in a reading can be seen as a warning of the potential for betrayal, malice, hatred, or lies to enter one's life. As such, it is associated with feelings of vulnerability. Likewise, it could be interpreted as a sign that something is amiss in one's environment or with a relationship.

Those looking for further insight might use it to evaluate if there are any negative influences present in their lives that need to be addressed. Additionally, the rune has been used for centuries by those seeking guidance about their future and possible outcomes. Thus, providing yet another layer of significance when it appears in readings.

Ansuz (ᚠ)

Represented by the letter 'a', Ansuz is the rune signifying insight and connection to one's spiritual self. It can be interpreted as a blessing bestowed upon you or an indication to accept divine advice. Commonly thought to refer to Odin himself, this symbol of knowledge and wisdom carries omens of good health, truth, and harmony. Additionally, this ancient symbol is known for its spiritual guidance, symbolizing that one should heed the advice bestowed upon them by the gods. Ansuz has also been connected to creative communication, indicating that it may benefit those looking to create or engage with their audience meaningfully. Yet, when its interpretation is reversed, it may warn of misunderstanding, manipulation, and negative feelings such as vanity and arrogance.

Raidho (ᚱ)

The 'r' of the Futhark, Raidho, symbolizes a journey of physical travel and transformation. It indicates that you are about to embark on a journey leading to personal growth and evolution. This rune encourages decisive action toward making the best next move. Also, it relates to the rhythms of life and how your rhythm can fit within them. Furthermore, tracing this rune in grounding rituals is believed to help clear away any negative energy preventing you from furthering your journey. Ultimately, raidho speaks to the beauty of discovery and changing perspectives that comes with traveling life's path.

For its merkstave interpretation, raidho suggests a time of disruption and impending crisis. This could be interpreted as a warning that something is about to disturb or halt your progress or journey in life or even foreshadow death itself. In Norse mythology, raidho was associated with journeys, communication, and traveling great distances. It was also seen as being related to death and the afterlife. This connection to fate and destiny makes this rune important in divination and understanding life events.

Kaunan (ᚲ)

Kaunan, the 'k' rune of the Elder Futhark, is closely associated with healing. This interpretation of the rune emerged during a period of magical and spiritual practices in Scandinavia. The rune was believed to give strength and courage to those who sought its aid in recovering from sickness or injury. By looking more deeply into its meaning, kaunan can be interpreted as an invitation to boldly move toward physical and mental health. Much like the Kenaz (torch), which many prefer, this original k-rune signifies new possibilities and a rediscovery of inner strength.

The appearance of Kaunan in reading or interaction can bring about profound shifts in energy and decisions. As such, it can signify both positive and negative outcomes. Likewise, it is associated with revelation, knowledge, creativity, clearing vision, and new energy sources, allowing you to create the life you want. On the shadow side, however, Kaunan signifies false hope, instability, loss of illusion, lack of creativity, and coming disease or illness. It could also portend a breakup or feeling exposed. Considering this symbol's aspects can help interpret your readings and uncover potential personal changes ahead.

Gebo (X)

First rune on the runic alphabet symbol after 'futhark,' Gebo, is derived from the 'g' phoneme and is translated to 'gift.' This rune signifies an equilibrium between giving and receiving. Yet, it is not limited to material things. Instead, it includes emotional and spiritual gifts exchanged in relationships and business contracts. Moreover, it stands for a transfer of energy which can be beneficial or detrimental depending on how it is used. Thus, gebo symbolizes the significance of balancing generosity with assertiveness.

In the context of divination, Gebo can denote an offer or gift-giving, with an expectation of something in return. It may also suggest that an individual has given too much, leading to feelings of loneliness, greed, or obligation. However, when lying in opposition to other runes, Gebo changes its meaning to indicate a loss of equilibrium. As such, it can be either self-sacrificing oneself excessively or having to make payments through no fault of your own. In these cases, it can be viewed as a sign of bribery.

Wunjo (ᚹ)

Wunjo is the 24th rune in the Elder Futhark. It has been used to represent both the letters 'w' and 'v,' with its meaning connected to joy, love, fertility, spiritual reward, and community. Likewise, it brings comfort, pleasure, success, harmony, and prosperity. But it is also important to remember that too much of a good thing can be bad. Hence, avoid becoming overly excessive when interpreting wunjo.

Aside from that, Wunjo is believed to originate in Viking culture, which associated it with the god Odin and his infamous rage. Subsequently, its merkstave version of this rune is a sign of despair. Likewise, it is related to misguided decisions or alienation from others. In extreme cases, it can represent uncontrolled anger, an out-of-control frenzy, and even intoxication or possession. This rune is said to indicate a state of confusion and mindlessness. It can also signify a lack of control over one's actions and a disconnection from reality.

With Wunjo, we come to the end of the ætt of the first degree, ruled over by the "Lord" Frey and the "Lady" Freyja. Like the two gods who rule over it, this ætt is composed of opposites. In fact, three pairs represent each rune in the word Futhark. Fehu and Ūruz, the domesticated and the wild. Then, Thurisaz and Ansuz, the giants and the gods. Meanwhile, Raidho and Kaunan, the journey (experience) and the sickness (knowledge). Moving on to the next aett of the Elder Futhark, let us explore more aspects this ancient alphabet has to offer.

Heimdall's Ætt

Heimdall is described in Norse mythology as the watchman of Asgard, the realm of the gods and its guardian. Odin gave Heimdall the task, the chief god he served faithfully, to sound a horn known as Gjallarhorn when Ragnarök begins. This serves as an alert that Ragnarök is starting and a warning to all beings in Asgard. Along with his role as watchman of Asgard, Heimdall also guards Bifröst, an enchanted rainbow bridge connecting Midgard (the realm of mortal men) and Asgard. To counterbalance, Heimdall's role in guarding heaven's entrance is Móðguðr (Mordgud). As such, Móðguðr is a maiden etin who stands guard over Gjallarbrú. This is a bridge crossing the river Gjöll which leads to hell in Norse mythology. Ergo, Móðguðr tasked with guiding those who have recently died across it so they cannot return to the land of the living.

The guardian of heaven and the guardian of hell ruling over this ætt symbolizes change, growth, and transformation. These runes can help clarify your purpose and strength to overcome life's challenges. Through these eight runes, you can decipher deeper meanings in your surroundings and use them to guide and inform your decisions. Learning to read and interpret these symbols allows you to uncover hidden layers of understanding that provide insight into our lives. Thus, this set of runes is much more than a simple divinatory tool; it is a gateway to self-discovery and enlightenment.

Hagalaz (H)

The first rune in this set is Hagalaz (h), which means 'hail.' This rune symbolizes nature's destructive, creative force and things outside our control. The way to think of the three ættir is as three 'levels' of a life's journey. The first ætt deals with the external and internal influences that create the individual. This second set, sometimes called Hell's Ætt, is about testing and challenging to help further the individual grow and develop. This is captured from the first rune—Hagalaz—which symbolizes tempering, testing, or enduring a trial leading to heightened inner harmony if the storm can be weathered first.

Hagalaz is the second rune that does not have a merkstave form. As with Gebo, this does not mean that Hagalaz cannot be interpreted in a 'dark' way, but that it is another rune that lies in opposition (if it falls with the rune skew or sideways in a casting). If it lies in opposition, Hagalaz warns of an impending natural disaster or catastrophe of some kind or form. It can also mean losing power or feeling powerless to control the pain and suffering in your life.

Naudiz (†)

The 'n' of the Elder Futhark, Naudiz, signifies a time of need and distress. It is an obstacle to success, prompting you to tap into your inner strength and show greater resolve. Naudiz challenges you to control your emotions and act with poise during strife. These traits define endurance and determination in life. This powerful symbol implies survival and provides a unique opportunity to hone patience in challenging moments. With its origins firmly planted in Norse mythology, naudiz stands out as a representation of the journey towards triumph.

On the other hand, Naudiz suggests confinement and a lack of autonomy. It can come in various forms, from arduous labor to deprivation and deprivation of essential things. This could also be interpreted as unfulfilled needs, financial instability, and almost unbearable hunger. In extreme cases, Naudiz merkstave can even signify death from starvation or poverty. To further explain this concept, in Icelandic culture, it was believed that when someone had surpassed their limits or faced mortifying conditions, their spirit would turn into a wraith known as a 'naudhiz.' As such, they will be forced to live out the remainder of their existence in hideous poverty and deprivation.

Isaz (I)

With the meaning of "ice," Isaz (i) is the rune of challenge, frustration, and seeking a way to overcome them. The imagery of freezing is the best way to interpret this rune. As such, Isaz indicates that you are physically or psychologically in a state of frozen action, a block. To rectify this, take some time out to seek clarity from within and prepare for what is to come as you get *'unstuck.'* Isaz is a rune that reinforces the meaning or interpretation of the other runes connected to it in the cast. Also, Isaz has no merkstave form. Yet, if lying in opposition, it can be interpreted as selfish behavior or an over-indulgence in sensual pleasures. Likewise, it can be a forewarning of a possible betrayal of trust or treachery or that plots are afoot against you.

Jēran (⟨)

The J-rune, or *"Jēran,"* symbolizes reaping the rewards of your efforts. Likewise, it can be interpreted to mean peace, prosperity, happiness, hope, and success. Sometimes, it is referred to as "jera" and represents the continuous cycle of life in the universe. As a positive omen, it is believed that when this rune appears, it honors good fortune and could bring abundance in all areas of life. Additionally, Jēran carries with it the meaning of a *"good harvest"* or *" good year."* Hence, it signifies greater assurance for those around them that their future will be filled with plenty.

Aside from that, Jēran has no merkstave version. Yet, this rune is often seen as a sign of misfortune and can portend delays or plan disruptions. Those with this rune in opposition can expect their good fortune to be unceremoniously reversed without warning. It also shows that timing is everything when making meaningful changes. Also, it emphasizes the importance of being prepared for the unexpected.

Eihwaz (ʃ)

Representing *'y'*, Eihwaz stands for *'yew tree'* and is the start of the second half of the Elder Futhark. Symbolically, it represents Yggdrasil, the world tree. As such, it symbolizes strength, dependability, trustworthiness, and reliability. In Norse mythology, this rune is associated with enlightenment and protection. Eihwaz is a sign that you are on the right path to achieving your goals and can attain them with effort. Then, in its inverted form (merkstave), Eihwaz can indicate confusion or weakness. Subsequently, it signifies a need to seek clarity and gain inner strength. Ultimately, this rune serves as a reminder of humankind's potential for self-discovery and growth.

Perthro (⌐)

Although the precise meaning of Perthro, represented by the *'p'* of the Elder Futhark, is unknown, its significance is known to be a lot cup. Warriors used this ancient dice box to cast lots to determine their fate before a battle. Perthro is associated with Orlog, an old Norse term for *"fate"* or the fundamental principles of the universe. It represents secrecy, hidden knowledge, and understanding of our destiny. Some interpret it as determining one's path, while others consider it a sign of uncertainty. In addition, it is said that casting lots with this rune served as a way for Northern Europeans to communicate with their gods during times of crisis and upheaval. Yet, in merkstave readings, perthro suggests the feeling of addiction and loneliness. For instance, it can be seen as a sign of a lack of progress, deep unhappiness, or emotional malaise.

Algiz (ᛉ)

In the ancient runic alphabet, Algiz or *'z,'* symbolizes protection and stands for the spiritual bond between mortals and deities. It serves as a shield to ward off evil forces and assists in connecting to one's higher self. Likewise, it may point out an awakening or divine favor in one's life. Furthermore, it denotes the importance of controlling energy to avoid potential pitfalls. Conversely, when its inverted form appears in a cast, it indicates hidden dangers or losing access to the spiritual realm. Thus, it is a sign of rejection, suggesting something should be changed soon.

Sowilō (ᛋ)

Heimdall's Ætt's final rune, sowilō, means *'sun'* and signifies success, accomplishment, and honor. It also speaks to wholeness, positive transformation, and the power to realize ambitions. Connecting your higher self to your innermost thoughts and feelings, this rune stands as a reminder that the sun's energy can be used to clear away negative influences. As such, it is an emblem of spiritual cleansing and renewal. Furthermore, sowilō is believed to grant access to greater awareness and intuition, allowing for a deeper understanding of one's existence.

Sowilō, in merkstave, suggests a lack of connection with our spiritual selves. It could signify delusions, misguidedness, and actions resulting from bad counsel or advice. When interpreted as an omen, it could mean that one will face failure in achieving their goals if they are not well thought out. Further, this rune also signifies a disconnection from nature. As such, it is a blockage to our inherent natural wisdom and connection to the energetic powers within us.

As we have seen, the second set of the Elder Futhark, known as Heimdall's Ætt, delves into the *"Great Trials of Life."* These runes bear the weighty truth of self-development and our connection to destiny. They speak of a journey that culminates in sowilō, an inner strength that grants us the ability to choose our path. With this knowledge, we can become fully formed, successful individuals, conquering life's great trials.

Týr's Ætt

Týr, the god of war and sacrifice, justice and order, and patron of warriors, governs the final set of runes in the Elder Futhark. He was revered for his cosmic judgment and moral values and encouraged spiritual achievement. Connected to this is the belief that he had a hand in the mythical heroes from legends or myths. In fact, he is remembered as a symbol of established order and atonement. As such, it makes sense why these eight runes have been placed under his protection, for they represent some form of struggle, resolution, or peacekeeping within society. Thus concludes our journey into defining the great symbols that make up the Elder Futhark.

Tiwaz (↑)

Tiwaz, also known as the rune of Tyr, is a symbol of justice and honor. It stands for a victory achieved through taking the right course of action. Also, it encourages its followers to take time for self-reflection. Likewise, to analyze and identify their strengths and weaknesses. The courage this rune highlights means making difficult decisions with the potential for personal sacrifice to win and reach success. With perseverance and dedication, its followers will eventually emerge victorious.

For the merkstave of Tiwaz, it signifies difficulty in progress and stagnation. Often, it is characterized by an imbalance between thought and action. It is also a warning sign of blocked creativity, paralyzing self-sacrificing, or over-analysis. Additionally, it can be interpreted as the diminishing of passion due to a lack of communication or injustice that leads to separation. Understanding this rune can greatly help personal growth. For instance, it reveals blind spots and shows how one's life may need adjustment to restore harmony and balance.

Berkanen (ᛒ)

The second rune in Týr's Ætt is berkanen. Representing the letter 'b,' this rune means 'birch' and signifies fertility, birth, and growth. It is a rune of liberation or regeneration, renewal, and the start of something new. Plus, it could also mean that new love is about to come into your life, romantic or otherwise, and that prosperous times are ahead. Berkanen merkstave is a sign of problems, especially those related to family or domestic issues. Likewise, it is a sign of anxiety or carelessness, abandonment, or losing control. Finally, berkanen merkstave warns of stagnation, being sterile (infertile), or deception.

Ehwaz (ᛖ)

Carrying the meaning of 'horse,' Ewhaz is the 'e' of the Elder Futhark. Symbolizing movement, progress, and development achieved, it inspires collaboration and trusts in relationships. It also represents a strong connection to those around it. Whether for marriage or partnership, loyalty and faithfulness are associated with this rune. Additionally, ehwaz is a sign of good fortune and freedom, as it could symbolize success after a journey or a change in direction. This rune, therefore, serves as an affirmation that all changes are positive ones.

On the merkstave side, ehwaz signifies restlessness or unease that must be addressed. This rune symbolizes the need for balance and careful consideration when changing one's life. The so-called merkstave is seen as a cautionary note. As such, it can portend unhappiness caused by hastily made choices or betrayals of trust. The key with this rune is to ensure that any changes are done slowly, thoughtfully, and in a way that honors both the past and future.

Mannaz (ᛗ)

One of the few runes where you can immediately recognize the English word derived from it is mannaz. The 'm' phoneme means 'man' or 'humankind.' It symbolizes the self, your perception and treatment of others, and their views of you. Mannaz is a sign of friendship and hostility, depicting order in society and structure in the divine. As well as being associated with intelligence and creativity, this rune indicates that aid or assistance will soon enter your life. Additionally, mannaz has traditionally been used as a talisman to bring luck to its wearer. Its connection with humanity affords it extra spiritual power when used to invoke good fortune and protection.

As for the merkstave interpretation of mannaz, it implies mortality and human frailties like depression, delusion, and blindness. This symbol speaks to the darker nature of our thoughts. As such, these thoughts include manipulation, deceit, or cunning with malicious purpose. If this rune appears in your casting, it could represent a warning not to expect any help or guidance in what you seek to know.

Laguz (ᛚ)

The letter *'l,'* laguz, means *'lake'* or *'water'* and signifies healing, fertility, and renewal. It captures the flow of water, such as with the tides of the sea, and symbolizes the energy of life and growth in an organic way. Laguz represents the power of imagination, dreams, and fantastic mysteries. Likewise, it shows the hidden depths of this world and the one below it (the underworld). Finally, it can be seen as a sign of success or of acquiring something you have been seeking, but with the equivalent exchange of a price paid.

In terms of its merkstave form, laguz indicates impending changes, often of uncertain nature. It can manifest as an unwise decision, stagnancy in life, or even a mental disorder. Though not consistently negative, it may indicate an approaching period of difficulty. Yet, it may represent an opportunity to confront fears and take risks that could lead to personal growth and transformation.

Inguz (ᛜ)

Inguz, the *'ŋ'* phoneme, is the rune representing the god Ing. This is an older name for Freyr, the god of Earth. Inguz is a sign of fertility for men, of growing internally, or of a time for rest and recovery. It represents shared virtues or common sense, family bonds, and the warmth of humankind. If inguz appears in your casting, this is a sign that you should listen to your inner self and are ready to close off loose ends and head in a new life direction. However, unlike other runes, inguz has no merkstave form when lying in opposition. Instead, if interpreted, it suggests the idea of effort without any apparent change or tangible reward.

Dagaz (ᛞ)

With dagaz or *'d'*, it carries the meaning of *'day'* and symbolizes a time of awakening, heightened awareness, or an upcoming breakthrough. It is a sign of clarity that breaks through the uncertainty of the night that came before. Dagaz indicates that it is time for you to get planning for your next adventure or get ready to embark on one. Plus, it is a sign that you have the willpower to enforce the change or transformation you want to see in your life. Likewise, dagaz is the rune of hope and happiness, living your ideal life and being secure and confident of your path forward. If this rune appears in your casting, interpret it as meaning that a time of growing and releasing or balancing opposite forces is upon you.

Like ingaz before it, dagaz also signals the end of a chapter by reaching your limits or being blind to something that influences you. Sometimes, dagaz also points to being in an entirely helpless position. Connected to this idea is the Norse concept of wyrd. As such, it is a belief that fates beyond their control predetermine one's destiny. Whatever actions are taken will shape the outcome, but ultimately, one's ultimate path is out of their hands.

Othala (ᛟ)

Othala is the 24th rune of the Elder Futhark rune system. This rune holds great significance for those who practice Nordic spirituality. The symbol of othala is associated with prosperity, wealth, and inheritance. It represents a connection to one's past and family legacy. For this reason, othala often acts as a reminder to stay grounded in traditional values while embarking on new experiences. Besides that, it is seen as a protector during the transition, providing stability and security in times of change.

The card of othala, when reversed, is associated with being out of touch with one's culture and customs. This may lead to feeling disconnected or a sense of loss. It may also signify difficulties finding success due to bad luck or unfair discrimination. Lastly, othala could point to poverty, displacement, slavery, or feeling held captive by something.

4

Younger Futhark

The Younger Futhark, also known as *"Viking Runes" or* the *" Scandinavian Runes,"* was the successor to the Elder Futhark alphabet. This transition was seen in Scandinavia during the 7th to 8th centuries AD, with the Elder Futhark slowly being replaced by its successor in the 9th century. During this same period, Proto-Norse gave way to Old Norse. As such, it provided an opportunity for further linguistic and literary development. Subsequently, it has strongly influenced Scandinavian culture. As well as serving as an essential writing system, runes were used for magic purposes and are still respected and valued today.

Moreover, the Younger Futhark was a more condensed form of the Elder Futhark. As such, it consists of only 16 runes as opposed to its predecessor's 24. This reduction in characters was concurrent with an increase in the number of phonemes used by the Scandinavian people. Used throughout the Viking Age (793-1066 AD), it experienced a steady decline. That is due to Scandinavia integrating Christian ideologies alongside the Latin script. Despite this waning usage, Young Futhark runes were still employed in an auxiliary capacity. Usually, they are utilized for magical and divinatory practices or secret messages inscribed as memorials. With its decline came a shift away from runes as the central writing system of Germanic and Scandinavian peoples, heralding a new era within these societies.

Tracing its roots back to the Elder Futhark, the Younger Futhark runes were used in divination and rune casting. Likewise, it served as a written language for ancient northern European societies. There are two main branches of the Younger Futhark. These two include the Danish long-branch and Swedish or Norwegian short-twig runes, further divided into Hälsinge Runes. This chapter outlines the Younger Futhark's origins, history, and evolution from its earliest beginnings. Plus, it will provide invaluable insight into how this powerful symbolic system can be used to divine our future.

History of the Younger Futhark

Late in 700 AD, the Viking Age began. During this time, there was a mass change in the world. For instance, Scandinavian and Germanic people, or the Vikings, conquered much of Europe and Great Britain. With this age of expansion and exploration also came a change in the language of these raiders, pillagers, and conquerors from Proto-Norse to Old Norse. Also, ancient northern cultures shifted from the obscure Elder Futhark, used for personal runemasters, to the Younger Futhark, a much more widespread and accessible writing system.

As literacy flourished among the Norse people in the 9th century AD, so did the use of the Younger Futhark. Though there was some overlap between the Elder and Younger Futhark symbols from 650 to 800 AD, the Elder Futhark eventually succumbed to its successor. The Younger Futhark was better suited for the times. Also, the Vikings utilized it in matters both serious and light. As such, it was used in trade documents, diplomatic correspondences, poems, jests, and personal messages.

Long-Branch Runes

While the Younger Futhark is the name for the runic script, a few variations have been found. The oldest of these is known as the Danish long-branch runes. This branch-rune originated in and around modern-day Denmark, the ancestral home of the Danes. Primarily, they were carved on stone and are the more complicated versions of the Younger Futhark runes. Yet, they are still simpler than those of the Elder Futhark because they only have one vertical line known as a *'stave.'*

Short-Twig Runes

Developing after the Danish long-branch runes came to the short-twig version of the Younger Futhark runic script. Primarily used in Sweden and Norway, these runes were easier to carve. Also, compared to their long-branch counterparts, they were formed without a full vertical stave. During the end of the Viking Age, short-twig runes became more popular, continuing in use even into medieval times. Besides that, they can be considered the short-hand or cursive version of the runes. Due to that, scribes and traders favored them, as they were easier and quicker to carve. Moreover, they are also known as the Rök runes. As such, they are named after the Rök runestone, the longest runic inscription engraved on the stone.

The Runes of the Younger Futhark

Runes were used to cast spells and were believed to represent power, protection, and good luck. These runes were inscribed on amulets and jewelry the Viking people wore. Furthermore, Norse mythology often describes the runes as a language the gods gave to humanity. The Codex Sangallensis 878 is an illustrated manuscript estimated to date back to around 830 AD. As such, it contains 24 stanzas related to the runes of the Younger Futhark.

This codex, recorded in a monastery in Switzerland, contains many alphabets of the ancient world. On page 321 is the Abecedarium Nordmannicum, three lines presenting the runes of the Younger Futhark. On the same page are the runes of the Anglo-Saxon Futhorc. However, this recording does not give us an explanation of the meanings of the runes. For that, we looked to the Icelandic Rune Poem recorded in the 15th century and translated into English by B. Dickens in 1915.

Let us delve deeper into the runes and the messages they hold. The Icelandic Rune Poem offers excellent insight into the meaning of each rune in the Younger Futhark. Also, it provides an interpretation for us to ponder and orient our castings. Taking the time to contemplate their meanings can open new perspectives on life's questions.

Freyr/Freyja's Ætt

As we mentioned earlier, the ætt ruled over by Freyr and Freyja lost its final two members as the runic alphabet transformed from the Elder to the Younger Futhark. Two runes, ansuz and kaunan changed in shape. Meanwhile, the rest remained the same, although their pronunciation differed from their counterparts. This is because the spoken language of the Elder Futhark was Proto-Norse. In contrast, the language of the Younger Futhark, the Scandinavian Runes, was Old Norse, the language of the Vikings.

Fé (ᚠ)

> *"Source of discord among kinsmen*
> *and fire of the sea*
> *and path of the serpent."*
> **(Icelandic Rune Poem Verse 1)**

Younger Futhark's *'f'* and *'v,'* fé represents wealth and abundance. During the Viking Age, *'cattle'* and *'wealth'* were considered the same, so this sign was highly regarded. Fé remained intact with its original meaning throughout both Elder and Younger Futhark eras. Forging a link between physical and spiritual well-being, it also has strong ties to potential success or happiness if cast upright. However, if reversed, it can represent a failure or significant loss. Yet, it still offers wisdom on preventing disaster in this context. In addition to this significance, fé is often connected with spiritual growth and prosperity, signifying the reaping of the rewards for hard work and dedication.

Úr (ᚢ)

> *"Lamentation of the clouds*
> *and ruin the hay-harvest*
> *and abomination of the shepherd."*
> **(Icelandic Rune Poem Verse 2)**

The Younger Futhark rune ᚢ, also known as úr, holds a spectrum of meanings from *'shower'* to *'iron'* and even *'rain.'* Yet, it contrasts with its elder version, ūruz, which means *'wild ox.'* There have been two widely accepted interpretations of ᚢ in the Elder Futhark. One is ūruz *(aurochs)*, and the other is ūrą *(water)*. Old English and the Anglo-Saxon futhorc stay true to its úr rune's meaning of *'auroch.'* But when considering Old Norse and the Younger Futhark, ᚢ takes on a new interpretation of úr *(denoting 'rain')*. If you want to explore this rune's significance in more detail, let us unpack its enigmatic úr form. Likewise, let us learn how it can influence your divination readings.

Upright Úr is often seen as a symbol of new beginnings and potential. When upright, it signs fertility and signals that blessings may come your way or something unexpected could arise. On the other hand, in its reversed form, úr conveys misguided force or energy and serves as a reminder to stay vigilant. Those bearing this rune are cautioned to take heed of their surroundings to protect themselves from sudden danger.

Þhurs (þ)

> *"Torture of women*
> *and cliff-dweller*
> *and husband of a giantess."*
> **(Icelandic Rune Poem Verse 3)**

Thurs *(Þhurs)* is the Younger Futhark equivalent of Thurisaz *(þ)*. It carries the meaning of *'giant,'* representing the main opposition to the gods in Norse mythology. The interpretation of þhurs is similar to the Thurisaz of the Elder Futhark. This is the rune of brute strength and signifies conflict and vitality. If reversed in its merkstave form, it is a warning sign of impending danger or malice.

Óss (ᚯ)

> *"Aged Gautr*
> *and prince of Ásgarðr*
> *and lord of Vallhalla."*
> **(Icelandic Rune Poem Verse 4)**

Óss (ᚯ) is the Younger Futhark equivalent of the a-rune from the Elder Futhark, ansuz (ᚨ). They may look and sound different, but both are believed to represent Odin, or *'God'* in Norse mythology. As such, the óss rune is associated with communication, the ability to convey insight, wisdom, and good advice. In contrast, its merkstave is linked to deceit and manipulation through miscommunication or misunderstanding.

Reið (ᚱ)

> *"Joy of the horsemen*
> *and speedy journey*
> *and toil of the steed."*
> **(Icelandic Rune Poem Verse 5)**

Reið, or ræið in Old Norse, is the Younger Futhark's version of raidō. It carries the same runic shape, sound, and meaning as its Elder Futhark version. This is the rune of the journey or the quest for enlightenment, and it means *'riding'* in both the physical and metaphorical sense of movement. On its good side lies personal evolution through experience, while on its bad is a dislocation from the world's rhythm.

Kaun (ᚴ)

> *"Disease fatal to children*
> *and painful spot*
> *and abode of mortification."*
> **(Icelandic Rune Poem Verse 6)**

Replacing kaunan, the '*k*' rune of the Elder Futhark, is kaun, the '*k*,' '*g*,' and '*ŋ*' of the Younger Futhark. Carrying the exact meaning of 'ulcer' and representing sickness and disease or the curing or avoidance thereof, Kaun is the rune of wisdom achieved through suffering. Though it is known for hardship, the rune Kaun also represents positive transformation and clarity of vision. When reversed in a casting, however, its meanings become more ominous. As such, it can be a warning of illness, feeling exposed to vulnerability, or lack of learning from suffering.

Heimdall's Ætt

As discussed in the preceding chapter, Heimdall's Ætt concerns beginnings and endings, transformation, and chaos. This second set of runes infers an entranceway to heaven, the underworld, and even other realms. Like the first ætt, two runes had been removed in the Younger Futhark. As such, these two are eihwaz (yew tree) and perthro (lot cup). Then, one rune from this ætt, Algiz (z-rune), was relocated to Týr's Ætt, being changed into its new R-rune form. Thus, the remaining five runes further explain the spiritual journey associated with this ætt.

Hagall (ᚼ)

"Cold grain
and a shower of sleet
and sickness of serpents."
(Icelandic Rune Poem Verse 7)

Hagall, formerly known as hagalaz (H) of the Elder Futhark, is a rune that symbolizes sudden change. It emphasizes the importance of learning from hardships. Likewise, it highlights accepting the tests and challenges that accompany personal growth. There is no negative interpretation associated with this rune. However, it can sometimes be interpreted as an omen of a pending disaster. The long-branch version of Hagall is 'ᚼ,' while its short-twig variant is 'ᚽ.' Lastly, its meaning remains unchanged, as it translates to '*hail.*'

Nauðr (ᚾ)

"Grief of the bondmaid
and state of oppression
and toilsome work."
(Icelandic Rune Poem Verse 8)

Keeping the same runic shape as naudiz and the meaning of '*need*' or '*constraint*,' nauðr is much the same as its Elder Futhark equivalent. This includes the way to interpret it in your castings. It is the rune of necessity and difficulty. In its upright form, nauðr represents inner strength amidst distress or confusion. On the contrary, its merkstave form signifies want, poverty, or unmet emotional needs. Finally, the long-branch form of nauðr is 'ᚾ,' while the short-twig version is 'ᚿ.'

Íss (ᛁ)

"Bark of rivers
and roof of the wave
and destruction of the doomed."
(Icelandic Rune Poem Verse 9)

The single-stave rune of isaz remained unchanged in its evolution into íss. However, it did pick up another phoneme to represent along the way, standing for both the sounds *'i'* and *'e'* in the runic script of the Younger Futhark. Meaning *'ice'* is the rune of self-control and signifies seeking a way to overcome challenges and frustrations. As a single stave, íss has no merkstave form. Yet, if it lies in opposition, it could be a sign of betrayal, self-centered behavior, or over-indulgence in the world's pleasures.

Ár (ᛅ)

"Boon to men
and good summer
and thriving crops."
(Icelandic Rune Poem Verse 10)

Jēran (ᛃ), the j-rune of the Elder Futhark, has a fascinating past. Once meaning *'good harvest,'* it evolved into ár (ᛅ), which stands for *'plenty.'* Even more remarkable is its shift in pronunciation from representing the *'j'* sound to *'a,' 'æ,'* and *'e.'* This transition from Proto-Germanic to Old Norse was likely the cause of this dramatic change. Additionally, the rune served several purposes throughout ancient history. For instance, it can mark important milestones by symbolizing natural elements.

While the rune shape and associated sounds might have undergone an evolution, the meaning of the rune remained the same. Like jēran before it, ár is the rune of good results from skill, knowledge, hard work, and good timing. In other words, it is the rune of reaping what you sow. In its upright form, ár represents success, happiness, or prosperity. With no merkstave form, ár is a sign of a possible setback, bad timing, or a reversal of luck or fortune when in opposition. Also, the long-branch form of ár is 'ᛅ,' while the short-twig version is 'ᛆ.'

Sól (ᛋ)

"Shield of the clouds
and shining ray
and destroyer of ice."
(Icelandic Rune Poem Verse 11)

As the Elder Futhark had sowilō (ᛋ) to represent the 's' sound, so does the Younger Futhark have sól (ᛋ). Both mean 'sun,' but the younger version had an added meaning. In comparison, sowilō represents the elemental force of the sun's energy. Then, sól is the personification of the sun in the form of the goddess Sól. Regardless, it does not change how it is interpreted in your castings but adds to its meaning, as the sun goddess resides in this rune.

Moreover, sól is the rune of success, achievement, and wholeness. In its upright form, this rune indicates positive change and that you are on track to achieving your life goals. Yet, in opposition, as it has no merkstave form, sól indicates a disconnection from your purpose or a risk of losing sight of your goals. This rune's short-twig version is ' ∤.'

With the rune of the sun comes the end of the second ætt. Now that Heimdall's five runes are covered, it is time to turn to the final set of the Younger Futhark.

Týr's Ætt

Losing the most runes out of the three, Týr's Ætt gained one back as the z-rune transformed and moved from Heimdall's Ætt to the end of the alphabet. From that, Týr's Ætt in the Younger Futhark consists of five runes. Ruled over by Týr, the one-handed god of cosmic judgment and moral values, this ætt deals with the forces of the cosmos. As the final part of the runic alphabet's magical journey, Týr's Ætt symbolizes the knowledge gained from the trials of the previous ætt. Aside from that, it also represents this knowledge being put to use beyond the self to better the family, the community, or even human society at large. Through this, one may become in tune with the cosmic laws of love, collaboration, responsibility, and contribution to the future of our planet. While on this journey, the individual becomes enlightened and reaches spiritual fulfillment.

Týr (↑)

"God, with one hand
and leavings of the wolf
and prince of temples."
(Icelandic Rune Poem Verse 12)

Týr (↑) serves as a reminder of the Norse god, Týr, the patron god of justice and heroic glory. It denotes victory, honors, and a need to define strengths and refine intentions. Its merkstave meaning warns against over-analyzing, sacrificing too much of oneself, or being out of touch with one's purpose. A long-branch version, '↑,' and a short-twig variant, '↑,' exist for this rune. Additionally, Týr is similar in shape and meaning to its equivalent in the Elder Futhark, tiwaz (↑). This ancient symbol is a powerful reminder to stay true to one's course, no matter the outcome.

Björk (ᛒ)

"Leafy twig
and little tree
and fresh young shrub."
(Icelandic Rune Poem Verse 13)

The second rune of Týr's Ætt is björk (ᛒ). Likewise, it is called bjarkan or bjarken and is the evolution of the Elder Futhark's berkanen (ᛒ). Having the same rune shape, it also carries the same meaning as its descendant in the Younger Futhark. Björk represents the voiced 'b' and unvoiced 'p' while berkanen only stands for 'b.' This rune means *'birch,'* a tree that symbolizes spring and rebirth. As such, björk is the rune of conception, gestation, and birth. Plus, it is the rune of feminine energy and divinity. When upright, it is a sign of renewal or the start of something new. However, lying in opposition is a sign of problems ahead or stagnation. Aside from that, björk does not have a short-twig version.

Maðr (ᛉ)

> *"Delight of man*
> *and augmentation of the earth*
> *and adorner of ships."*
> **(Icelandic Rune Poem Verse 14)**

With the removal of ehwaz, the e-rune of the Elder Futhark, maðr (ᛉ) is next in Týr's Ætt. Evolving from the Elder Futhark's mannaz (ᛗ), the meaning and the sound represented remained the same. Then, only the word and the runic shape change. With the meaning of *'man'* or *'human,'* maðr is the rune of human life and intelligence. It not only refers to humankind as a whole but also to the first man from Norse and Germanic creation myths, mannus. Our main source for mannus comes from Tacitus, one of Rome's historians who included the myth of mannus. This mannus is a Latinization of *'mannaz'* in his book Germania 10, published in 98 AD.

According to Tacitus, Mannus was the son of Tuisto, the divine ancestor of the Germanic peoples, who was the son of Earth. The children of Mannus are recorded in ancient songs of the Germanic people as the original ancestors of many early Germanic tribes. It is in the light of the original families of humanity with which you should view this rune as a symbol of the human family.

The runic symbol for maðr, ᛉ, is derived from algiz, ᛉ, the z- rune of the Elder Futhark. Algiz connotes *'protection,'* signifying a spiritual bond between humans and the gods. An upright appearance of maðr in your castings points to awareness, capability, support, or help. On the other hand, an inverted rendering of this symbol alludes to mortality or the difficulties faced by humankind. Moreover, maðr does not have a short-twig variant.

Lögr (ᛚ)

> *"Eddying stream*
> *and broad Geysir*
> *and the land of the fish."*
> **(Icelandic Rune Poem Verse 15)**

The evolution of laguz (ᛚ) from the Elder Futhark finds a similar form in lögr (ᛚ) of the Younger runic alphabet. Both runes carry the meaning of *'lake,'* *'sea,'* or *'water,'* with the same runic shape and representing the same phoneme *(l)*. Lögr is the rune of life energy and purification. It symbolizes the washing away of unwanted or no longer-needed parts of ourselves as we *'cleanse'* the energy of our lives.

When cast in an upright form, it symbolizes that you are on the right path to reaching your goals. Akin to nature's equilibrium, this calls for a cost, a price to pay for the success you wish to gain. Conversely, if cast in a reversed or 'merkstave' form, it implies difficulties and uncertainty lie ahead. No short-twig version of lögr was indicated.

Yr (ᛦ)

> *"Bent bow*
> *and brittle iron*
> *and giant of the arrow."*
> ***(Icelandic Rune Poem Verse 16)***

With the meaning of *'yew'* or, more specifically, *'bow made from a yew tree,'* yr (ᛦ) carries the same meaning as eihwaz (ᛇ) of the Elder. They are, however, different in their runic shape and the sounds they represent. Also, it is the recreation of the Elder Futhark's z-rune, algiz (ᛉ). Yr captures the change in how *'z'* was pronounced as Proto-Germanic evolved into Old Norse. The z phoneme became more of an *'r'* sound known as a voiced uvular trill, a hard, guttural *'r'* sound rolled with the back of the tongue. As such, it is written as *'R.'* Finally, yr (ᛦ) is an inversion of maðr (ᛘ), the life rune, often called the *'death rune.'* Besides that, this rune marks the only change of letter order the Futhark experienced as it evolved out of its elder form.

The Elder Futhark ends with the rune othala (ᛟ), the symbol of heritage or inheritance. It is a reminder to honor our ancestors by returning what was given to us and, in turn, passing it on. On the other hand, the Younger Futhark concludes its runes with Yr (ᛦ), a symbol representing death and rebirth. ᛦ is etched onto gravestones because this rune is thought to aid souls in their journey beyond the physical world. In addition, yr also signifies embarking on life's goals and gaining inner strength. Unlike the other runes, there is no 'merkstave' meaning associated with yr, nor does it boast any short-twig variant.

With the ancient rune of yr, representing death and resurrection, we complete Týr's Ætt and the Younger Futhark. This chapter detailed our knowledge of the Elder and Younger Futharks and how to interpret each rune in your readings. Now it is up to you to decide which version you prefer. The upcoming chapter will explore the fascinating Anglo-Saxon Futhorc and one of its main works, the *'Anglo-Saxon Rune Poem.'*

5

Anglo-Saxon Futhorc

The Elder Futhark was the original runic alphabet, representing Germanic languages in Northern Europe. Its evolution into the Younger Futhark around 200 AD marked the beginning of its use on the Scandinavian and European mainland, where Old Norse reigned supreme. A sister system to the Younger Futhark emerged to fit a foreign language in the British Isles. This system, known as the futhorc, comprises 33 runes used for Old English.

From the 5th to 12th centuries, Anglo-Saxon runes were ubiquitous and served as the main writing system for Old English. However, with Latin's dominance in the 7th century AD, runes gave way to their alphabetical counterpart. Nevertheless, futhorc remained popular for divination and protective spells until the 12th century.

The futhorc was more developed than its sister system, taking after its parent script by extending from 24 to 33 runes. In this chapter, readers will journey through this final main runic system. Plus, we will understand how it differs from its predecessor and sister alphabets.

History of the Anglo-Saxon Futhorc

In the mid-5th century, the Anglo-Saxon Migration marked a turning point in British history. The end of Roman rule over the British Isles in 410 AD and the emergence of the Anglo-Saxon culture and people were significant events in this period. As Rome's grip on Britain faltered, England was among the first regions to suffer its weakening influence. Without Roman protection, local tribes such as Britons and Celts rose against Roman provinces held in England. This led to a decline in Roman military presence on British soil until their departure.

On the arrival of the Angles, Saxons, and Jutes, they changed Britain's leadership landscape. As such, they swiftly claimed power by establishing kingdoms of their own. Before this power shift, British Celtic and Latin were widely spoken, with Latin alphabets used for writing. By the time several centuries had passed, Old English was established as England's primary language, accompanied by its distinct writing system known as Anglo-Saxon Futhorc. These developments positioned England at a significant crossroads of history, culture, and language.

Originating from West Germanic tribes, the Old English language had a variety of influences influencing its development. The Angles, Saxons, Jutes, and Frisians all contributed to what later became Old English. A version of the runic alphabet known as 'Anglo-Frisian' runes was also heavily influenced by the languages spoken in the areas mentioned.

The Latin alphabet eventually supplanted Old English and runic script towards the end of the 7th century. As Christianity spread throughout England, Latin soon replaced both as the language of written communication during this period. Even so, runes continued to be used for divination until the 11th century.

Various texts note how these modified runic alphabets were interpreted differently across cultures. For example, Anglo-Saxon runes were used differently than their Nordic variants. Some sources indicate they were even employed in anti-witchcraft spells and magical incantations. This further highlights how diverse yet nuanced rune symbols can become when adapted across varying contexts and geographical locations.

The Runes of the Futhorc

Like the other two runic scripts, futhorc split into three sets of runes known as ættir. Each set consists of eight runes governed by a god or goddess. In addition to being used for traditional divination purposes, these runes can also be used in protective spells and other magical practices. Furthermore, nine new runes were added to the back of the futhorc. As such, these provide insights into magical powers and their meanings, which can be explored further. Consequently, this section offers the opportunity to delve deeper into all three ættir and examine what the new runes offer.

Freyr/Freyja's Ætt

From ancient times, runes have been used to convey wisdom and teach lessons. The first set of runes in the journey of the runic alphabet, Freyr and Freyja's Ætt, is composed of opposing forces we encounter while growing up. It symbolizes the challenges a student has to endure when they begin their esoteric studies into runology. This cluster of runes reflects conflicts between domestication and freedom, gods versus demons, and light and darkness. Moreover, the " *Gift Rune*" and " *Glory Rune*" at the end of this ætt are not juxtapositions but rewards for hard work given to an initiate. A gift for the trials faced, and ultimately glory for the prize won (wisdom).

When it comes to understanding how futhorc differs from Elder Futhark or Younger Futhark, there is an Anglo-Saxon rune poem that provides explanations of each rune's meaning as our basis. This poem was written by Christian monk Ælfric, also known as " *Ælfric the Grammarian,*" in his manuscript *Cotton Otho B.x fol. 165a – 165b* around 8th or 9th century.

The knowledge within these runes can be used to educate us on how different symbols represent different stages of growth in life; it is an invaluable resource that can guide us through our initiation into life. With the runes showing our way, we can use them as tools to master life's challenges on our journey for wisdom and glory.

Feoh (ᚠ)

"Wealth is a comfort to all men;
yet must every man bestow it freely,
if he wishes to gain honor in the sight of the Lord."
(Old English Rune Poem Verse 1)

From the earliest days of our journey with the futhorc, there is a definite difference in the mood that comes through its poem compared to those crafted for the Younger Futhark. While Icelandic and Norwegian rune poems depict fé (ᚠ) as a "*cause of strife among men,*" its Old English counterpart interprets it as an equal comfort to all so long as they share it. This concept of mutual exchange presents a notable contrast with the idea of sacrifice conveyed by the previous runic poem.

Feoh (ᚠ) signifies its sister rune in the Younger Futhark and its ancestor in Elder Futhark while maintaining a similar form. It is also associated with 'f' and 'v' sounds, which can be heard from its earliest incarnation as fehu (ᚠ). Representing wealth, this rune symbolizes family support during our developmental years, reminding us that we eventually have to go forth and strive for our prosperity. To clarify this point, feoh represents our ambitions despite hardships and adversities.

Ur (ᚢ)

"The aurochs is proud and has great horns;
it is a very savage beast and fights with its horns;
a great ranger of the moors, it is a creature of mettle."
(Old English Rune Poem Verse 2)

The rune úr (ᚢ) of the Younger Futhark has roots in Norse mythology, signifying the power of self-formation and transformation. It speaks to the ability to use one's inner strength and change the course of life, providing an energizing potential when cast upright. Meanwhile, a merkstave reading denotes domination by external forces blocking growth. Connected to '*aurochs,*' an extinct wild ox species known for its strength and unpredictable nature, this rune provides a potent reminder that with self-determination comes great power.

Þorn (Þ)

"The thorn is exceedingly sharp,
an evil thing for any knight to touch,
uncommonly severe on all who sit among them."
(Old English Rune Poem Verse 3)

A place where the futhorc differs from both versions of the futhark is in the meaning of the Þ rune of the alphabet. Although it keeps the same sound and shape, Þ means '*thorn*' in Old English, whereas it means '*giant*' in Old Norse and Proto-Germanic. The runes thurisaz (Elder Futhark) and þurs (Younger Futhark) were the runes of brute strength, as well as the connection and opposition between the giants (demons) and the gods. Þorn, however, is a rune of destruction and defense. It represents the sharp *"thorns in your side"* that serve as obstacles for you to overcome and grow stronger from.

The ancient rune þorn has many interpretations. For instance, it could signify strength and hardiness gained through harrowing experiences. Likewise, it foretells a warning of dangers and betrayal on the path ahead. However, some have theorized that its meaning '*thorn*' is a metaphor for Thor. He is the powerful half-giant son of Odin associated with thunder. This interpretation casts þorn as the rune of opposites and brute strength, reinforcing a complex and potent symbolism.

Þorn is a symbol and an example of wisdom from Norse mythology that can be applied to life today. Its relevance has endured through centuries, offering guidance for seekers who wish to grasp its symbolic and practical meanings.

Ōs (ᚩ)

"The mouth is the source of all language,
a pillar of wisdom and a comfort to wise men,
a blessing and a joy to every knight."
(Old English Rune Poem Verse 4)

The rune of truth and justice, ōs, has two different meanings in the futhorc. The first meaning is *'god,'* which refers to Odin specifically. This meaning mirrors ansuz (ᚨ) in the Elder Futhark and ós (ᚬ) in the Younger Futhark. Then, the second interpretation of ōs is as meaning *'mouth.'* Such interpretation is another reference to Odin, who has the *"breath of life,"* according to the Poetic Edda. Odin is also the master communicator able to inspire one and all. As such, ōs is the rune of the gods, inspiration, and communication with others and your higher self. Regarding our journey through the runic alphabet, ōs *(motivation and communication with the gods)* is the balance to þorn *(obstacles and the danger of demons)*. Similarly, this is the same as ós was to þhurs in the Younger Futhark and as ansuz is to thurisaz in the Elder Futhark.

When cast upright, ōs signifies that knowledge or communication with your higher self or other powers is incoming. As the rune of inspiration, ōs is a sign that divine energies are interested in you and your life's journey. Yet, if cast reversed, ōs is interpreted as a sign of miscommunication, misdirection through manipulation, or delusion about your goals or life's purpose.

Rād (ᚱ)

"Riding seems easy to every warrior while he is indoors
and very courageous to him who traverses the high-roads
on the back of a stout horse."
(Old English Rune Poem Verse 5)

Another rune that remains unchanged in the different runic scripts is rād (ᚱ). This rune is raidho (ᚱ) in the Elder Futhark and reið (ᚱ) in the Younger. Representing the journey, it sees us set out on our path of initiation into the greater mysteries of life and living. Cast upright, this rune is a sign that you are going through a time of personal evolution. It shows you are on the path to having the experiences you need to become the person you want to be. However, in merkstave, rād signifies you are becoming disconnected from your life's journey or purpose. Likewise, it tells that you must get back on track as soon as possible or risk facing unnecessary hardships.

Cēn (ᚳ)

"The torch is known to every living man by its pale, bright flame;
it always burns where princes sit within."
(Old English Rune Poem Verse 6)

Another place where the futhorc differs from the other two runic scripts is the inclusion of the 'c' character of the alphabet. Where kaunan (ᚲ), meaning *'ulcer,'* represents the *'k'* sound alone. Then kaun (ᚴ), the Younger Futhark equivalent with the same meaning, represents the *'k,' 'g,'* and *'ŋ'* sounds, and cēn (ᚳ) stands for k and tʃ *(a strong 'ch' sound)*. Meaning *'torch,'* this is the rune of enlightenment. It represents the gaining of knowledge through learning and experience. Likewise, it means having the ability to improve our skill sets and begin to apply what we have learned back into the world.

Cēn, when cast upright, symbolizes gaining newfound knowledge and undergoing a process of personal development and growth. It is the essence of directed energy and indicates expertise in honing one's craft. On the other hand, if cēn appears reversed, it can reflect being out of sync with your inner guidance or having misplaced priorities. Additionally, reversed cēn may warn of an impersonal attitude, lack of awareness, or superiority complex.

Gyfu (ᚷ)

> *"Generosity brings credit and honor, which support one's dignity;*
> *it furnishes help and subsistence*
> *to all broken men who are devoid of aught else."*
> **(Old English Rune Poem Verse 7)**

While Freyr and Freyja's Ætt ends with kaun, the k-rune of the word futhark, the futhorc follows the ways of its parent script and includes two more runes in its first ætt. The first is gyfu (ᚷ), the evolution of gebo (ᚷ), which stands for *'gift.'* This is the rune of generosity and stands for equivalent exchange, in terms of what you put in is what you get out. As such, it is the 'gift' of improving yourself, enhancing your skills, and experiencing the world to the fullest.

When upright, gyfu shows that you are about to receive a *'gift'* of equivalent size to the sacrifice you have made to earn it. It can also mean that your vision is about to clear and that you have the divine blessing to continue. Yet, gyfu does not have a merkstave form. Nevertheless, if lying in opposition, it signifies over-dependence or greediness. Also, it is a sign of overly sacrificing oneself for no equivalent gain.

Wynn (ᚹ)

> *"Bliss, he enjoys who knows not suffering, sorrow nor anxiety,*
> *and has prosperity and happiness and a good enough house."*
> **(Old English Rune Poem Verse 8)**

The rune wynn (ᚹ) is one of the oldest runes in the futhorc, and its evolution from wunjo (ᚹ) is traced to the Elder Futhark alphabet. When read upright, this rune represents hope and harmony, symbolizing glory or spiritual rewards. Alternatively, if cast in merkstave, it is a sign of alienation, ignorance, and potential danger.

Throughout history, wynn has been associated with feelings of contentment stemming from correctly utilizing one's will or mastering a skill. It can also be interpreted as promoting accomplishment, prosperity, or fellowship. To further illustrate its significance, it may be helpful to mention that many Norse tribes would inscribe this rune on their weapons before heading into battle for protection from harm.

Heimdall's Ætt

Once the initiate has passed the tests and choices of Freyr or Freyja's Ætt, they receive the gift of wisdom and the reward earned for their sacrifices. When they realize this wisdom's glory and come to terms with their reward, the initiate is ready to move on to Heimdall's Ætt, the ætt of becoming a warrior.

Hægl (ᚻ)

"Hail is the whitest of grain;
it is whirled from the vault of heaven
and is tossed about by gusts of wind
and then it melts into water."
(Old English Rune Poem Verse 9)

The rune *'hail'* stands for life's unpredictable twists and turns. Think of it like preparing to move to a new city and encountering unexpected obstacles and opportunities. Turning to the rune shape, we see that it is a close copy of its parent rune, hagalaz (ᚺ), which was also drawn with a double-barred variant in some dialects of the Elder Futhark. Moreover, the h-rune of the Younger Futhark, hagall (ᚼ), looks quite different but carries the same meaning.

Hægl symbolizes the struggles needed to become resilient. As such, it is the rune of casting, tempering, testing, and enduring. Likewise, it is like forging a blade that requires constant patience and effort, and growing strong requires facing hardships and continuing. So, with the arrival of hægl, the first rune in Heimdall's Ætt, we are challenged to show our strength.

When hægl appears upright in your cast, it signifies growth and balance. However, it can also be an ominous sign pointing to danger or loss. For example, you could be preparing for a big move, and the rune warns you must prepare for any potential problems.

Nȳd (ᚾ)

"Trouble is oppressive to the heart;
yet often, it proves a source of help and salvation
to the children of men, to everyone who heeds it betimes."
(Old English Rune Poem Verse 10)

Next, we have nȳd, the futhorcian variant of naudiz and sibling to the Younger Futhark's nauðr. The runic shape (ᚾ), meaning *"need,"* and sound value (n) of this rune have remained the same since the Elder Futhark days. This is the rune of hardships and strength-building. It involves agreeing with Orlog (your destiny) and making it your own. While hægl pushes us with unexpected events, nȳd shapes us into our destined selves.

When cast upright, nȳd signifies an understanding of the fundamental truths of life. It is the drive of innovation and becoming more self-reliant. Conversely, it can be a warning of lack or difficulty when it appears reversed. For instance, if you want to achieve your dream career but keep finding nȳd in your readings, it may indicate that you need to reassess your plan and make some changes to get closer to your goal.

Īs (I)

"Ice is very cold and immeasurably slippery;
it glistens as clear as glass and is most like to gem;
it is a floor wrought by the frost, fair to look upon."
(Old English Rune Poem Verse 11)

Another rune that has not changed much in the main runic alphabets is the i-rune of isaz from the Elder Futhark, íss from the Younger Futhark, and īs from the futhorc. All three mean *'ice'* and represent the rune of self-control and focus. On our runic journey, īs symbolizes the stillness and fortitude of mind we must develop to keep our egos in check. After the tempering and molding the last two runes, īs deals with cooling and solidifying. As we gain more spiritual knowledge and greater spiritual awareness through the tests and trials we face and overcome, we become more headstrong. As such, our egos will inevitably grow to match our new strengths. Īs serves as a reminder to develop the self-control and the stillness of mind necessary to keep this strengthening ego in check.

When cast upright, īs is a sign of growing clarity or developing self-awareness. With no merkstave form, it indicates self-aggrandizement, egoistic behavior, over-indulgence, or other forms of losing self-control.

Gēr (♦)

"Summer is a joy to men when God, the holy King of Heaven,
suffers the earth to bring forth shining fruits
for rich and poor alike."
(Old English Rune Poem Verse 12)

The Anglo-Saxon symbol of jēran (♦), otherwise known as the j-rune from the Elder Futhark, is also known as gēr (♦). This rune has a double meaning, with both interpretations being *'good harvest'* or *'good year.'* Cast upright, gēr represents an acknowledgment for all the hard work and positive actions undertaken. It suggests that reaping the rewards of your journey is just around the corner. Additionally, it stands tall as a sign of peace and prosperity.

Unfortunately, being cast in opposition can signify poor timing, stagnation, and regression. Gēr does not have a merkstave form, which could represent an inability to progress due to inconvenient timing opportunities. It comprises two parts; a spearhead pointing upwards to embody success and an arrow pointing downward to characterize a lack of momentum.

Ēoh (ʃ)

"The yew is a tree with rough bark,
hard and fast in the earth, supported by its roots,
a guardian of flame and a joy upon an estate."
(Old English Rune Poem Verse 13)

The representation of Yggdrasil in the runic alphabet, ēoh (ᛇ), is the evolution of eihwaz (ᛇ) from the Elder Futhark. This is a rune that was cut from the Younger Futhark. Meaning *'yew tree,'* ēoh is the rune of life, death, and renewal. It is the rune of the world tree, the tree of life. By life and death, ēoh does not only means the coming and leaving from this mortal coil. Yet, it signifies the life of new habits or the end of unwanted personality traits. In our journey through the runic alphabet, ēoh represents the growth of the individual over the years. Like a tree sheds its leaves in the winter before growing new ones in the spring, we leave parts of ourselves behind and develop new skills as we continue down the path of life.

If cast upright, ēoh foretells making moves toward achieving enlightenment or that you are on the right path to obtaining what you seek. But cast merkstave is a sign of dissatisfaction, weakness, or confusion.

Peorð (ᛈ)

"Peorth is a source of recreation and amusement to the great,
where warriors sit blithely together in the banqueting hall."
(Old English Rune Poem Verse 14)

The p-rune of the Futhorc is Peorð (ᛈ), which evolved from its precursor, perthro (ᛈ), a rune that does not appear in the Younger Futhark. As such, its closest modern English translation is an equivalent phrase for *'lot cup,'* used by Vikings to play a game of fate. This special rune encompasses the potential, chances, and luck that each person experiences on their life journey. If peorð appears right side up, it forecasts good fortune and success. However, when reversed, it signals hardships beyond our control.

Eolh (ᛉ)

"The eolh-sedge is mostly to be found in a marsh;
it grows in the water and makes a ghastly wound,
covering with blood every warrior who touches it."
(Old English Rune Poem Verse 15)

After the peorð rune comes the x-rune of the futhorc, eolh (ᛉ). This symbol carries a deeply spiritual and protective meaning. It is the Anglo-Saxon equivalent of the Elder Futhark's z-rune, algiz (ᛉ), while its younger counterpart is the R-rune, yr (ᛦ). These three runes have different names and meanings: algiz and eolh being *'elk,'* while yr translates to *'yew.'* While this rune can be seen as a sign of death in the Younger Futhark, it signifies rebirth and protection in Elder and Anglo-Saxon runic scripts.

The deeper spiritual significance behind casting eolh includes the growth of personal strength and protection from danger. When cast upright, it indicates a blooming connection with your higher self by allowing yourself to be open to messages from above. However, the reverse side of this same rune portrays separation from this connection or danger that may arise on your path. As such, it may suggest caution rather than joyous celebration during its interpretation.

Sigel (ᛋ)

"The sun is ever a joy in the hopes of seafarers
when they journey away over the fish's bath,
until the courser of the deep bears them to land."
(Old English Rune Poem Verse 16)

The final rune of Heimdall's Ætt, the ætt of the warrior, is sigel (ᛋ). Meaning *'sun,'* this is the evolution of sowilō (ᛋ) from the Elder Futhark and sibling to sól (ᛋ) from the Younger Futhark. All carry the same meaning, with sigel and sól identical in their runic shape. Sigel is the rune of success. Like Freyr and Freyja's Ætt ends positively with gyfu *(gift)* and wynn *(joy or bliss)*, so does Heimdall's. With eolh, we connect to the divine and with our higher selves. With sigel, we reach the success and wholeness that comes from achieving victory in battle or mastery of a skill.

Sigel appearing upright in your casting is a sign of guidance or hope. It signifies that you are on track to achieving your goals and are living your life's purpose. However, sigel does not have a merkstave form. Lying in opposition means false success, bad advice, or losing sight of your goals or purpose.

Týr's Ætt

Týr, the God of Justice and heroic patron, presides over the final ætt of the runic alphabet. This ætt is associated with being a skilled warrior, embodying all the necessary traits to excel in their chosen field. Unlike Heimdall's Ætt, which covers trials and tests to become a warrior, this is the stage where one becomes one, completing the third stage of life and our journey through rune lore. This stage marks an initiation into understanding divinity and its profound meanings.

Tīr (ᛏ)

"Tiw is a guiding star; well, does it keep faith with princes;
it is ever on its course over the mists of night and never fails."
(Old English Rune Poem Verse 17)

The first rune in the futhork's third ætt is tīr (ᛏ), the evolution of tiwaz (ᛏ) from the Elder Futhark, with its sister being týr (ᛏ). All three refer to the enigmatic god of the Germanic peoples, Tyr. This is the rune of justice and sacrifice. In the Anglo-Saxon Rune Poem, tīr represents the *"guiding star"* (North Star). Used by sailors in ancient times to navigate the seas in the northern hemisphere, this star came to symbolize a moral compass and a physical one. A spark of order and control in the cosmos, Tyr is the god of order, control, and justice. On our runic journey, tīr represents the building of our willpower and developing our moral compasses as we become spiritually awakened humans.

Cast upright, tīr is a sign of honesty, justice, and victory achieved through faith in the divine, loyalty to your moral compass, or self-sacrifice. The merkstave of tīr warns of mental paralysis, overanalyzing, or overly sacrificing yourself. It can also indicate injustice or some other kind of imbalance.

Beorc (ᛒ)

*"The poplar bears no fruit; yet without seed, it brings forth suckers,
for it is generated from its leaves.
Splendid are its branches and gloriously adorned
its lofty crown which reaches to the skies."*
(Old English Rune Poem Verse 18)

Beorc is another rune that mostly stays the same between the different runic alphabets. The runic shape (ᛒ), meaning (birch), and sound value [b] remain the same in all three, except the Younger Futhark adds the *'p'* sound to its version of ᛒ, björk. In the Elder Futhark, it goes by the name *'berkanen.'* This is the rune of the Birch Goddess, birth, and sanctuary. As the first tree to come back to life as winter changes to spring, the birch symbolizes the cycle of life: *birth, death, and rebirth*. With ēoh, this cycle is not just about the birth or death of a person. Yet, more to do with the birth, death, and rebirth that happens as the seasons change and we grow into different versions of ourselves. Likewise, Beorc is the rune of female fertility and the fruition of ideas and goals.

In its upright position is a sign of becoming, a changing lifestyle, or sanctuary through divine protection and healing. Although it cannot be cast merkstave, beorc is a sign of sterility, stagnation, blurred vision, or conspiring forces when lying in opposition.

Eh (ᛖ)

*"The horse is a joy to princes in the presence of warriors.
A steed in the pride of its hoofs
when rich men on horseback bandy words about it;
and it is ever a source of comfort to the restless."*
(Old English Rune Poem Verse 19)

Next is the e-rune of the futhorc and the evolution of ehwaz (ᛖ) from the Elder Futhark, eh (ᛖ). This rune does not appear in the Younger Futhark. Meaning *'horse,'* eh is the rune of travel and progress. It symbolizes the outer and inner journeys we take in life and the trust we must have in the *'vehicle'* or *'steed'* that is our body. Like a horse with a skilled rider, eh represents the symbiotic relationship we must have with ourselves and others.

If cast upright, eh signifies harmony, loyalty, or friendship. It can also be a sign of collaboration and trust. In merkstave form, eh is a sign of disharmony, betrayal, or an enemy acting against you. Finally, it can also indicate indecisiveness or mistrust of your path.

Mann (ᛗ)

*"The joyous man is dear to his kinsmen;
yet every man is doomed to fail his fellow,
since the Lord, by his decree, will commit the vile
carrion to the earth."*

(Old English Rune Poem Verse 20)

With the meaning of *'man'* or *'humankind,'* mann is a rune that embodies intelligence, planning, and increased awareness. It is featured in the Elder Futhark and Younger Futhark runes, mannaz (ᛗ) in the former and maðr (ᛘ) in the latter. When we progress on our runic journey, mann symbolizes our ambition to reach out for self-discovery, to be closer to what resides inside us. This rune also speaks of humanity's capability to shape reality with otherworldly forces and natural elements.

Having it cast upright, mann carries energies invigorating intelligence and awakened understanding and realization of one's inner potential. In contrast, when presented in merkstave mode, it may induce depressive states or unrealistic feelings of superiority, a manifestation of mortals' emotional hurdles.

Lagu (ᛚ)

"The ocean seems interminable to men,
if they venture on the rolling bark
and the waves of the sea terrify them
and the courser of the deep heed, not its bridle."
(Old English Rune Poem Verse 21)

The rune lagu is believed to be one of the oldest runes in practice. It originates from the Proto-Germanic language and has been used in different runic alphabets for centuries. Although it keeps a similar shape and sound, the interpretations vary slightly between cultures.

From the Elder Futhark, laguz refers to *'lake,'* while in Younger Futhark, it could symbolize *'water'* or *'waterfall.'* In the Anglo-Frissian period, lagu was known as the *'ocean'* or *'sea.'* Moreover, it stands for life energy and intuition powering any evolutionary process.

In divination, this rune gave a positive connotation when appearing upright: *passing tests and achieving growth.* On the other hand, its reversed position could indicate that someone might be lost in fantasies or controlled by manipulative forces.

Ing (ᛝ)

"Ing was first seen by men among the East Danes,
till followed by his chariot,
he departed eastwards over the waves.
So, the Heardingas named the hero."
(Old English Rune Poem Verse 22)

The ŋ-rune of the futhorc, ing (ᛝ), is found in the Elder Futhark as inguz (ᛜ) but is not included in the Younger Futhark. Ing's shape changed from the parent alphabet to the child, but the meaning remained. They represent the Proto-Germanic god Ing or Inwi. This god was known as Yngvi in Old Norse and Ingƿine in Old English and is an earlier name for Freyr.

Before he became known by the moniker 'Lord,' Freyr was known as Ing. Freyr is the god of fertility, peace, and good weather. As such, ing is associated with the meaning *'seed.'* This is the rune of earth, agriculture, male fertility, and sexuality. On our runic journey, ing represents the act or process of creation. The best way to think of this rune is like the way we use the suffix -ing at the end of verbs to add action to it. Doing, being, creating; the process of activity and creation.

When cast upright, ing is a sign of gestation, growth, or spending time to improve oneself. Ing cannot be reversed, but lying in opposition is a sign of frivolous behavior, immaturity, taking action, or putting in effort without gaining positive change.

Ēðel (✧)

"An estate is very dear to every man,
if he can enjoy there in his house
whatever is right and proper in constant prosperity."
(Old English Rune Poem Verse 23)

With the meaning of *'heritage'* or *'inheritance,'* ēðel (✧) is the futhorc's version of the o-rune from the Elder Futhark, othala (✧). This is the rune of home, connecting with your ancestors and drawing on and adding to the spiritual power from your ancestral land. Ēðel provides a link to the rune feoh (wealth), the first letter of the runic alphabet.

In the Elder Futhark, othala is the 24th and final rune that symbolizes inheritance, home, and land. Meanwhile, in the Younger Futhark, it is moved to become second last. This switch in position suggests the importance of taking a moment to reflect on how you use your wealth before embarking on a journey to come full circle. Furthermore, this spiritual journey is only possible when understanding the meaning behind each rune and how each relates to one other. Such knowledge can help us expand our understanding of our past, present, and future and live consciously as part of a greater cycle.

Upright, ēðel means prosperity, freedom, and the betterment of your group. Reversed, ēðel speaks of poverty, homelessness, or losing touch with one's ancestral land. Likewise, it is a sign of mistreatment, such as racism or xenophobia.

Dæg (ᛞ)

"Day, the glorious light of the Creator, is sent by the Lord;
it is beloved of men, a source of hope and happiness
for the rich and poor,
and of service to all."
(Old English Rune Poem Verse 24)

For the final runic symbol of Týr's Ætt, the futhorc rune dæg (ᛞ) is derived from the Elder Futhark's dagaz (ᛞ). Both runes hold a similar meaning of *'day'* or *'dawn'* and share the same shape. It marks the end of a journey depicting the life and purpose of human life. Likewise, it represents the unity of one's self, synthesis with the environment, and connecting opposites to gain enlightenment.

When cast upright, dæg symbolizes an awakening, alertness, or an upcoming positive shift. On the contrary, if it lies in opposition, then it means someone is blind to their predicament or that an unfavorable situation is likely to arise. This highlights how important it is for people to consider their pasts and futures, living in the moment while being aware of what may come next.

Other Runes

Although the journey may be over for the three ættir of the runic script, this is not the end of the futhorc's extended alphabet. There are still five more runes in the Anglo-Saxon rune poem, totaling 29. In some dialects of the futhorc, it was then further extended by four more runes to reach a total of 33 characters in its runic alphabet. The futhorc can be used either in its 24 runes version derived from the Elder Futhark or in its 26-rune version where āc (ᚫ), 'oak,' and æsc (ᚫ), 'ash' are included. Along with ōs (ᚫ), 'god,' these runes are the evolution of the a-rune from the Elder Futhark. Ansuz (ᚫ), split into three different sounds, accommodates Old English's developing vowels and other Anglo-Frissian languages. After that comes the runes that were added later, as Old English and the futhorc developed, and have no connection to the runes of the Elder Futhark. Let us go through these final runes of the Anglo-Saxon futhorc.

Āc (ᚫ)

"The oak fattens the flesh of pigs for the children of men.
Often it traverses the gannet's bath,
and the ocean proves whether the oak keeps faith
in an honorable fashion."
(Old English Rune Poem Verse 25)

Āc, one of the runes of Elder Futhark, is derived from its parent rune ansuz (ᚫ), which translates to *'god.'* This symbolizes the potential for small beginnings to blossom into something greater with continuous growth and progress. Represented by an acorn growing into a mighty oak tree, it reflects the power of potentiality. It stands for strength and endurance, used to build ships due to its incredible ability to withstand storms and strong winds.

When cast upright, āc indicates that you have all the resources required to succeed; if these are not present, they shall soon be acquired. There is also an indication of making good use of one's potential. Conversely, when cast merkstave, it speaks of a hindering obstacle that could threaten your growth and warns against not utilizing one's potential fully.

Æsc (ᚫ)

"The ash is exceedingly high and precious to men.
With its sturdy trunk, it offers a stubborn resistance,
though attacked by many a man."
(Old English Rune Poem Verse 26)

The third child of ansuz (ᚫ) is the æ-rune, æsc (ᚫ), from the futhorc. This runic symbol is closely related to the ash tree. Like its elder sibling, the oak is a dependable and vitally important resource for weapon manufacture and crafting. Instilled with stability and resilience in times of hardship, upright æsc serves as a beacon of protection, hope, and healing for those who bear it. Conversely, when reversed, this rune denotes a period of difficulty where one may feel overpowered by external stubbornness or other obstacles.

With this symbolism, there are plenty more fascinating facts surrounding ash trees and their uses throughout history. Not only have they been integral to Norse mythology as sacred places of worship. Yet, they have also been used to create tools such as mallets and axes since ancient times. Furthermore, both their wood and bark were integral components in various medications due to the antiseptic properties discovered in them. Altogether these qualities make the runes associated with the ash tree some of the most reliable symbols for safety and security, according to Futharks lore.

Ȳr (ᛦ)

"Yr is a source of joy and honor to every prince and knight;
it looks well on a horse and is reliable equipment for a journey."
(Old English Rune Poem Verse 27)

Associated with the yew tree, the y-rune of mastery, ȳr (ᛦ), is the second rune in the Futhorc. This symbolizes the longbow, an iconic and powerful weapon used throughout history. It calls for dedication to art, sport, or any skill you master. Furthermore, if upright, it promises capability and potential success in what you set out to do. However, if reversed, it warns against a lack of required skills, laziness, or inertia hindering progress.

To use this power effectively, one must understand its deep cultural roots. According to Norse mythology, the first longbow was created by Ullr (Oller), a skilled master archer who lived alongside Odin in Asgard. Before his death, he also tutored his beloved son Baldr using bows and arrows. This connection between Ullr and ȳr brings a reverence for a craft that has been central throughout time.

Ior (ᛡ)

"Iar is a river fish, and yet it always feeds on land;
it has a fair abode encompassed by water, where
it lives in happiness."
Old English Rune Poem Verse 28)

Ior (ᛡ) is the io-rune (yo) of the futhorc carrying the meaning of *'eel.'* This is a variant of the j-rune, gēr (ᛄ), which means *'year'* or *'harvest.'* Ior, on the other hand, represents Jörmungandr, the World Serpent. Along with Fenrir and Hel, Jörmungandr is a child of Loki and the giantess Angrboða, who were all foretold to be the ones to bring about Ragnarök. As such, the three children were separated; Hel was sent to the underworld, Fenrir remained under watch in Asgard, and Jörmungandr, the middle child, was thrown into the oceans of Midgard (Earth). In the depths of the oceans, the World Serpent grew to encircle the globe and then bit down on its tail, representing the ouroboros. When Jörmungandr releases its tail once more, Ragnarök will commence.

As such, ior is a protective or binding rune. More than that, this rune represents a snake. As a serpent can live both in water and on land, this is the rune of the duality of life. When ior appears upright, it signifies the death of something old, the birth of something new, or a combination of both. However, ior cannot be cast merkstave, but when in opposition, unavoidable hardships or danger are coming up.

Ēar (ᛠ)

"The grave is horrible to every knight,
when the corpse quickly begins to cool
and is laid in the bosom of the dark earth.
Prosperity declines and happiness passes away
and covenants are broken."
(Old English Rune Poem Verse 29)

The last character in the Anglo-Saxon Rune Poem is ēar (ᛠ), the ea-rune of the futhorc. With the meaning of *'grave,'* this is the rune of the past, ending, or death. This rune was a late addition to the futhorc, with its first use recorded in the 9th century. While other runes dealing with death did so in a way that captured the growth that occurs through the ending of one thing and the beginning of another, ēar is death personified or symbolized. Upright, ēar speaks of a happy ending or the completion of some goal or task. Merkstave, ēar is an omen of death or loss and sadness.

Northumbrian Runes

Rune diviners and enthusiasts discovered the Northumbrian Runes in the 8th century AD as an addition to the Anglo-Saxon futhorc. Some individuals have adopted these runes to supplement their divination practices, providing a more comprehensive range of symbols. The interpretation of these four characters can be personalized for the individual user based on what resonates with them naturally. Although the Latin script replaced the futhorc for Old English writing, these runes can still be used to benefit from their full potential in spells and other forms of magick.

Cweorð (ᛢ)

As an iconic symbol of transformation in the Anglo-Saxon rune, cweorð or cpeorð (ᛢ) reflects the use of flames in a myriad of ways. As such, it is a source of heat and light, a method to purify the deceased and their souls, or an emblem of strength. It has roots in peorð (ᛈ), the p-rune of the futhorc. In addition, it is the second fire rune in the futhorc, preceded by cēn (ᚳ), which denotes 'torch' and stands for enlightenment.

When upright, this rune stands for courage and endurance in overcoming life's challenges, with transformation being its primary connotation. On the other hand, if it appears reversed, it signals potential destructive forces at work that may prevent you from achieving your goal. Its associated meanings can be further contextualized through a closer look at how the fire was viewed by Anglo-Saxons, providing them with security and sanctity in their homes and offering liberation during funeral pyres.

Calc (ᛣ)

The next Northumbrian rune is calc, another form of k-rune that means *'chalice'* (calic) or *'chalk'* (cealc). What calc refers to is unknown, but the 'chalice' definition fits better for divination purposes. Under this meaning, 'calc' refers to a ritual cup or goblet and invokes the legend of the Holy Grail from the tales of King Arthur and the Knights of Camelot. Calc is the rune of offerings, as a chalice is used to drink from during a ceremony. It also symbolizes the death and rebirth that an individual goes through during a ceremony and the natural ending of things that inevitably must happen. When cast upright, calc is a sign of something coming to a positive conclusion or an upcoming spiritual transformation. Then, if cast merkstave, calc warns of an untimely termination of something or an unexpected sacrifice.

Stan (ᛥ)

With the meaning of *'stone'* and the sound value of *'st,'* stan symbolizes not only the immovable obstruction that stone can be. Yet, it can also be the little game pieces made of stone. Stan is the rune of material obstacles and the unavoidable difficulties we face. It also symbolizes the link between our divine souls and earthly bodies. Stan appearing upright signifies strength, achievement, and the skill and ability to overcome obstructions in your path. Meanwhile, stan does not have a merkstave form but means a blockage, obstacle, or other upcoming hardships and difficulties.

Gar (ᚷ)

The futhorc is an alphabet of 33 runes believed to possess immense power, covering three pillars of runology: Runic Scripts, Casting, and Divination. Gar, or ḡ, is the final rune in the extended Anglo-Saxon futhorc. It symbolizes success in battle and carries the meaning of *'spear,'* a reference to Odin's Gungnir, which never missed its target. In terms of sound, it is similar to gyfu (gift), but a victory from gar comes from more hard work than from receiving a gift. When upright, it represents a reward for hard work or suspicion of success. However, lying in opposition can be interpreted as a loss or hindrance to achieving your goals.

Pillar 3
Casting

Now is the time to take your understanding of runes and the varying runic scripts to the next level by divining your future. The Elder Futhark, Viking runes from the Younger Futhark, and Old English from the Anglo-Saxon futhorc, each of these runic alphabets offers something different. Before you begin casting, consider which best resonates with your inner self, as it can become a powerful vehicle for exploring your fate.

Unlocking a deeper understanding of runology will give you all you need to interpret and synthesize information through rune casting. Visualization, meditation, and reflection create an environment conducive to exploring higher knowledge. This allows us to connect deeply with symbolism and its meaning, uncovering our destinies.

6

What You Need to Know About Rune Casting

Rune casting has helped to guide people through life and all its big decisions since before. The runes were formed into the alphabet known as the Elder Futhark. This makes divination and magic the original uses of the runes. Their use as a writing system comes in a distant second. As with reading Tarot cards, casting runes is not a form of fortune telling or some ineffable way of predicting the future. Instead, the runes provide insights into specific questions that you ask. They do this by delivering our influential subconscious minds with a potent medium to solve the *'problem'* of the question asked. Our brains are massive problem-solving machines; all they need is the right key to unlock the true potential of the human mind. The runes were initially recorded by Odin the Allfather as he sought to understand the mysteries of life and the cosmos. For instance, they are the perfect key for unlocking the divine within us all, guiding you to the answer you seek, but your higher self already knows.

In this chapter, we will talk about everything rune casting, from the history of rune casting, to how to make your own rune sets, before ending with how to cast runes.

History of Rune Casting

By the nature of runes, mystery and secrecy surround their earliest use. The word *'rune'* means *'secret message,'* after all. Rock carvings found in Northern Europe and throughout Scandinavia from the Bronze and early Iron Ages are believed to be the earliest incarnation of runic writing. As we said in Chapter 1, the first mention of the runes being used for divination and magical purposes is from *Germania 10,* written by the Roman historian Tacitus in the 1st century AD. Tacitus describes the classical way of making runes (cutting a branch from a nut-bearing tree and slicing it into strips before carving runes on each) and casting them.

As the prolific historian explains, the runes were randomly thrown onto a white cloth, as you would shuffle the Tarot deck before laying out the cards. Then, a priest or the family's father would say a prayer to the gods in which they would invoke the blessings of specific deities. After doing so, they would then ask their question and, staring up at the heavens, move their hand over the cast as they pick the first of three runes. After being drawn to a specific rune, the caster would pick it up and interpret it in terms of the meaning of the rune and how it was positioned compared to the caster (upright, merkstave, or lying in opposition). Once the first rune has been selected and interpreted, the caster repeats the process for the remaining two runes of the cast, analyzing each as they are chosen before giving an overall divination for the three runes cast and how they relate to the question asked.

And so finishes Tacitus' historical account of the use of runes for divination. Interestingly, while this account comes from the first century, it is only around the fourth century AD that the alphabet known as the Elder Futhark became commonly used throughout Scandinavia and northern Europe.

How to Cast Runes

Now that we know more about the history of rune casting, it is time to turn to the runes themselves. This section will cover how to make your own rune sets and what materials to make them from. After that, we will dive deeper into the world of rune casting and how you can best draw on the magic and divine energies of these ancient and timeless symbols to enhance your daily life.

Making Your Own Rune Set

The first thing you will need after knowledge to cast runes is the rune set itself. You can buy a set of runes; there is nothing wrong with doing so. Search *"rune sets"* on your chosen browser or Amazon, and you will get a miasma of great options for masterful craftsmanship. Make sure to read the customer reviews before selecting one, and you are onto a winner of having your rune set in no time. If you are wondering whether you should buy a wood, stone, metal, glass, or crystal rune set, we will get to that next up in this section.

For the more crafty people who prefer the hands-on approach of making their own rune sets, let us go through the steps you will need to follow and the things you need to know to do so.

1. Choose Your Materials

As we saw in Tacitus' account, the primary material used to make a rune set in ancient times was wood, preferably from a nut-bearing tree, but this is not the only option out there, and you are more than free to choose a different one if it resonates with your energy more. In fact, this is crucial. Here are the most commonly used materials that runes are made out of:

Wood

The favored material for making runes throughout history has been wood. As we saw in the breakdown of the rune meanings, some runes directly symbolize trees. Trees were an integral part of Norse mythology, with the runes appearing to Odin on the bark of Yggdrasil, the world tree. Yggdrasil is considered an ash tree, so this is often the wood chosen for making runes. However, any nut or seed (fruit) bearing tree will serve fine. You could use yew, birch, or oak, for example. Before cutting the branch off your chosen tree, ask permission beforehand to ensure the right energy is stored in the wood you will use to make your runes. Also, leave an offering of water for the tree after chopping off the branch to complete the ceremony.

If you want to make your runes out of wood but do not have access to the right kind of trees or do not want to cut them, you can buy blank wooden rune sets online. Once you have your slices or blocks of wood, then comes the time to either paint, carve, or pyrograph (burn into the wood) the runes onto them, but more on this later.

Pebbles or Stones

If you live near a beach, river, or mountain, you could create your rune set out of the pebbles or small stones you collect from there. It is not just about the power of the runic symbols but also the energy you put into them that matters, and connecting your rune set to the land you live in is always a great idea. Remember that engraving runes in stone is much harder than carving them on wood. You could opt to paint your pebble rune set, but this will fade over time unless properly cared for.

Bones

A more controversial material to use for your rune set is bone. Some people enjoy the more shamanistic image of casting bones, and since it is all about the energy you put into making and using them, there is nothing wrong with that. Just try to ensure that the bones come from an animal that died of natural causes or, if hunted, a similar prayer and offers were made to honor the animal's sacrifice as would be made for cutting a branch from a tree.

Clay

From the macabre to the mundane, clay is our final common material to make your rune set. Clay is easy to work with and easy to engrave runes on. Just make sure to bake and seal your clay runes properly to ensure they remain chip-free for as long as possible.

Whichever material you use to make your rune set, the key is consistency in size and shape. Also, ensure your runes are small enough to cast in your hands. Once you have chosen your material and have a strip of wood, pebble, or clay piece ready for each rune, the time to begin creating a rune set comes.

2. Begin the Ritual

First, you will need to select a sacred space or a place where you feel most comfortable and have room to work. If you have not sanctified a place in your house for such things before, you can perform the Hammer Rite or Hammarsetning to do so. This space protection rite draws on Mjolnir, Thor's hammer's power to protect and consecrate a specific area around you. Thor is the protector of Asgard and Midgard; with his mighty hammer, he separates order and chaos. To perform the Hammer Rite, stand up straight in your workspace and visualize yourself holding Mjolnir out. Invoke Thor's name in sanctifying and protecting your space as you hold Mjolnir in the four cardinal directions, beginning with the north. Then, hold the hammer up to the sky above you before facing it below you to complete the sphere of protection. Once this is done, your space is ready to begin working on your runes.

Think over the mystical history of the runes and invite the gods or goddesses who rule over them into your space as you consecrate it for the inscription of your runes. Odin, Freyja and Freyr, Heimdall, and Týr; invite these deities to add their energies to the creation of your rune set. Pour a symbolic tot of wine, apple juice, or milk for the gods as you ask them to steady and guide your hand in the task. Invoke the blessings of your ancestors and invite any other wights (spirits or supernatural beings) you feel connected to or wish to have around. With your materials laid out in front of you, dedicate this moment to the creation of runes, and when you are ready, pick up your first strip, tablet, or pebble, and call on Freyja and Freyr as you inscribe the runes of their ætt.

Say the rune out loud once you are done painting or carving it, and remind yourself of its meaning and interpretations as you do so. Hold the rune up to your mouth as you name it, visualizing what most reminds you of that specific rune. Let us take fehu, for example. Visualize what you most strongly associate with *'wealth,'* concentrate on this as you carve or paint, and imbue the rune with this energy, as you name it. Once you inscribe the rune, place it on a white cloth or napkin.

Traditionally, runes would also be made yours completely by tracing the runic symbol with your blood. This stains the runes with your unique *"fluid of life."* This is by no means compulsory. If you stain your runes, you could mix a few drops of blood into red paint or prick your finger and trace the lines. As for the paint, you could use red acrylic paint, or a mixture of red ochre and linseed oil works just as well.

3. Consecrate Your Rune Set

After allowing your runes to dry, sit back down and re-invite the gods into your space. Meditate for a bit on the purpose of the runes and their powerful potential to help you achieve what you seek. Concentrate on the magical nature of the runes, ruminate on the magic that exists all around us just beyond sight. Accept the divine gift of these symbols that allow us to comprehend the mysteries of the cosmos through runology. Then, if you have not done so already, arrange your runes in order and separate them into the ættir so that you have three rows of eight runes each on your white casting cloth.

Go through each rune once more, tracing the symbol with your eyes, visualizing that which you most associate with its esoteric meaning as you name it. Take your time to intensely focus on each rune in your set, thinking over the runic journey we discussed in the previous paragraph as you do so. Then, when you are done, thank the gods, goddesses, ancestors, and wights for their participation in the creation of the runes. Your runes are now sealed and ready for use!

Using Your Runes

With your freshly made or bought rune set, you can begin casting and reading these timeless signs of cosmic forces. In other words, it is time to learn about the process of rune casting.

Prepare Your Space

One thing that will get you in the right headspace for casting runes is to begin each time in the same way and place. This ritual could include placing your runes out in front of you on a white cloth before meditating on them for a while. You could also light candles or set out crystals to help create the right ambiance or vibe. After that, ensure that you are facing north and get comfortable. Then, invite the gods and ask them for their blessing and energy in the reading to come. If you are in a new place, conduct the Hammer Rite to sanctify the space before laying out your runes.

Form Your Question

To tap into the runes' divine powers, you need to have a specific question to ask them. Think carefully about what you seek to ask and how best to word it. *"Yes-No"* questions do not work for rune casting, so express your question in a more general, open-ended way. Rather than *"Will I get this job?"* you could say, *"What are the chances that I will get this job?"* for example. Or, better yet, *"How will it feel once I have this job?"* You must focus on your feelings behind the question and use this energy to guide your reading.

Cast the Runes

With your question in mind, pick up your runes and shake them in your hands. Hold them up to your lips as you speak your question before casting them out onto your casting cloth. The best way for beginners to go from here is to remove all the runes that fell face-down and set them aside. Then, gather the remaining runes, repeat your question, and cast them out again. Remove any face-down runes and continue this until you have five or fewer left in the cast. Once you do, leave these runes as they fall on your casting cloth.

Read their Meaning

With five or fewer runes remaining, it is time to read their meanings. It is best to write down the runes and their positions in a journal before interpreting how they answer your question. Record the runes from left to right. Also, note if the rune was cast upright, merkstave (upside down), or in opposition (sideways). Then, work on divining what these specific runes and their position mean for you and your question. Refer to the earlier chapters of this book as and when you need to review how to interpret the different runes.

Tools of the Trade

Now that we know how to make our runes and the basics of rune casting, it is time to go over the different tools of the trade for runology. These are the things, besides this book and your rune set, that you will want to get to enhance your casting and make divining simpler and more efficient.

Rune Pouch

The first thing you want to get to protect your runes is a rune pouch. This is the bag you keep your runes in to keep them from getting damaged or lost and to make them easily transportable for when you are doing your rune casting on the move. If you prefer a wooden box or another container to keep your runes in, that is perfectly fine, too. Whatever you choose, pick something that aesthetically represents and protects your rune set.

Casting Cloth

As mentioned earlier in this chapter, we cast runes onto a white cloth called a 'casting cloth.' This is done to keep the runes from getting scuffed or damaged, as well as to enhance the energy of the reading. A casting cloth, called a *'rune cloth' or 'altar cloth,'* can be as plain or patterned as you want it to be. It can be as large or small as you like. Make sure you can cast all your runes onto it comfortably. It can also be any most appealing shape, with round and square being the usual choices. You could make your rune cloth or buy one online. Some people choose to have protective runes patterned on their casting cloth, while others prefer to use it as a *'map'* that serves as another layer to their readings. This is used for more advanced casting methods, as seen in Chapter 7.

The *'map'* of a rune cloth generally comprises a central circle encompassed by a larger circle divided into four sections. Then, four lines connect the outer circle to the four corners of your casting cloth. This design symbolizes the nine worlds. Midgard (Earth) in the central circle, with Asgard in the North-East quadrant of the outer circle. Below Asgard is Svartalfheim (the realm of the dark elves or dwarves), with Hel to the left of it. Making up the final of the four is Álfheim (the realm of the light elves). The outer North area belongs to Muspelheim (the realm of fire), the East to Vanaheimr (the realm of the Vanir), the South to Niflheim (the realm of ice), and Jötunheimr (the realm of the first giants). This makes up the nine realms of Norse mythology.

Casting Pillow

Known as a 'stol,' this is a pillow embroidered or painted with runes you sit on while casting runes. This is to increase your comfort (especially when casting outdoors) and call upon the rune's energies on your stol when casting. Sitting on a casting pillow also means you are raised a little higher above your casting cloth, allowing you to reign over your runes like a god looking down at another plane.

Mearmots

Mearmots are personal talismans or magical items that you use to focus your mind and add to the energy of the casting. These could include candles, crystals, precious stones, or other objects that get you in the zone for reading runes. Besides the talismans that you bring to each casting, you should also try to bring something with you related to the question you are going to be asking of the runes. For example, if you are asking a question related to someone in your family, bring a picture of them or something that belongs to them. If you are doing a casting for someone else, then ask them to bring along mearmots that are special to them and are related to the question they plan to ask of the runes.

Pen, Pencil, and Paper

The final tools you need for your rune castings are a pen or pencil and a journal to record yours. While it is not essential to write down your readings, it is beneficial, as new interpretations can arise as you write them down. Keeping a rune journal lets, you easily notice patterns and trends in your readings. It is also useful to keep a summary of the rune meanings written down at the front of your rune journal. Finally, it is also a good idea to write down your question before you begin the casting to cement it in your mind and help you focus on it.

With the tools of the runic trade, we have finished with another chapter and another pillar of runology! You are now ready to put the runes to use. We covered a basic casting method in this chapter, but in the next, we will go over some different kinds of runic spreads and more advanced layouts as we move onto the fourth pillar of Runology: Spreads and Layouts.

Pillar 4
Layouts and Spreads

With all the background knowledge you need to become a pro rune caster, you are ready to start using the runes. The first three pillars provided us with the foundational understanding of Runology. Now, it is time to put all that knowledge to use and start casting runes. In this fourth pillar of Runology, we will learn about the different spreads and layouts you can use in your readings. These spreads and layouts help us determine exactly what these powerful symbols are trying to tell us about our question. When interpreting runes, we look at the meaning of the runic symbol itself (depending on whether it's upright, in opposition, or merkstave) and how it is connected to other runes in the reading. It is this second point that spreads and layouts help us with. Let us get going with the next part of our journey into the world of Runology by learning about the different structures you can use to gain the clearest, most detailed answer from the runes you can.

7

Layouts and Spreads List

When using the runes for divination, it is important to note which runes are present and where they fall in the casting. The sequence in which the runes fall forms a pattern known as a *'spread.'* A spread helps to determine the significance and way to interpret a rune in your reading. For example, your first rune in a reading could represent the past, the second an obstacle, and the third your present situation. Spreads range from two runes to including the full 24 runes of the futhark. All the spreads and layouts we use to *'map'* out the answer we seek are modern inventions. This is because we know precious little about the divination rituals of the ancient people. As such, making the spread you use your own is fun. Some people use the same spread every time they consult their runes, while others like to mix and max depending on the setting, surrounding circumstances, or information sought.

There are many different ways to structure your rune casting. As with whether to use the Elder Futhark, Younger Futhark, or Anglo-Saxon futhorc for your rune set, the choice 0f how to structure your readings is up to you. The previous chapter covered a basic way to begin casting and reading runes. In this one, we will dive in deep, looking at the different kinds of spreads and layouts you can use to enhance and advance your ability to interpret what these symbols of the cosmos are trying to tell you about your question. The more detailed or specific you want your answer, the more complex your spread or layout will be. This is so that more runes are included in the reading.

In this chapter, we are going to cover a wide variety of different layouts and spreads. We will review the simple or smaller layouts or spreads to use for more general questions and those designed for precise, guided answers.

Runic Layouts and Spreads

What is the difference between a layout and a spread? Simply put, a layout was created specifically for rune casting. On the other hand, a spread refers to tarot card spreads adapted for rune readings. While some prefer to keep it traditional and only use layouts for their castings, others feel more connected with the structure of a certain spread. Most people use the terms layout and spread interchangeably in a rune casting. What matters more than this is choosing a layout or spread that best fits your question and your desired answer's details. Let us go through the main layouts and spreads for you to choose from when casting runes.

Single-Rune Layout

The single-rune layout is the simplest way to cast runes, as it involves drawing only one tile. You can draw this single rune from your rune pouch or cast the runes on your casting cloth before, eyes to the sky, picking one. This layout gets a general feeling toward your question rather than specific information. It is also used if you are seeking a quick bit of insight into the main driving force of a certain situation.

Three-Rune Layout

A three-rune layout, also known as the 'past, present, future' layout, is a great way to track the effects or progress of something over time. This layout allows you to structure your casting using time.

If you cast your runes out or draw them from your pouch, ask your question and pick the first tile. This represents the past and the influences and circumstances related to the question. Place this tile on the left and interpret its meaning. Then, ask your question again and draw the next tile. This represents the present and those factors currently affecting your question. Place this tile in the middle in front of you. Ask your question and draw the third tile. This represents the future and is your question's outcome or result.

Fork Spread

Another pattern of the three runes is the fork spread. Like a fork in the road, this spread is used to gain insights when making an important decision or during a great change in your life.

The first tile represents the first possible outcome of your question and is placed on the left. It can also mean one of two choices that you have to make. The second tile is placed right of the center and is the other possible choice or outcome. The final rune is located south of the center (closest to you) and is your question's determining factor or outcome.

Relationship Spread

If you seek insights into what certain people mean to you, this is the layout to use. A relationship spread is a three-rune cast that shows what role people play in our lives. It can also be used to determine what role people play in the lives of others. For example, if you are trying to figure out what your spouse's overly friendly colleague means to them. This layout can also help you to determine the direction of the relationship between people.

Draw the first tile and put it left of center on your casting cloth. This rune is the energy that you are sending out toward this relationship. Draw your next tile and place it next to the first. This rune is the energy your partner puts out regarding the relationship. Finally, draw the third tile and place it above the previous two, connecting them. This rune represents the health and purpose of the relationship.

Four Direction Layout

Norse mythology tells tales of four mighty dvärgar (dwarves) charged with holding up the very sky itself. The dwarves stood in four cardinal directions: *Norðri in the North, Suðri in the South, Austri in the East, and Vestri in the West.*

The first tile of a four-direction layout is Norðri (North). Representing the past, Norðri covers past influences and desires that have led to your present situation. The next tile is Vestri (West), which symbolizes the present situation. A rune in this position gives insights into your current path and the influences you are presently under. The third tile is Austri (East), which deals with the veiled future. It is veiled because a rune in this position only speaks of possible future influences or obstacles that should be watched out for. Finally, we end the four-direction layout with Suðri (South). A rune cast in Suðri represents the possible outcome from the reading. In other words, what could result from you creating a new future using the insights gained from this casting.

Remember, though, that rune casting is not a predictor of the future. It merely offers insights to help and guide you to a desired outcome.

Diamond Spread

The diamond spread uses the same shape as the four-direction layout but with a different order for laying the runes and a different meaning for each position. This is the spread used to divine the forces active and at work in a certain situation or to reveal a hidden conflict or obstacle in your way.

The first tile in this layout is placed south of the center. This rune symbolizes the foundational level of your question and the basic influences acting on it. The next tile goes left of center and tells of one force acting for or against your question. The third rune is placed right of center and represents another force acting for or against the reason for the casting. Finally, the fourth rune is placed north of the center and is the outcome of the casting.

Elemental Spread

Another four-rune reading that forms the same shape as the four-direction layout and diamond spread is the elemental spread. This spread draws on the power of the elements and the forces and qualities they embody. This makes it an excellent option for those who prefer to draw on elemental forces rather than invoke the gods in their casts.

The first tile is placed north of the center and represents Earth. A rune in this position is the lesson you must learn in the physical world. Place the next tile right of the center. This is the air rune, and it represents lessons to learn in the world within your head, your mind. The next element is fire, placed south of the center. These are lessons you need to know in spirit. Finally, the left-center is the water element, representing lessons to learn emotionally.

Five-Rune Cross

The following layout to use in your readings is the five-rune cross. This layout resembles the four-direction layout we covered above, with an extra rune in the middle. While the pattern may be similar, the meaning of each position is very different.

Place the first tile closest to you at the bottom of the cross. This rune will represent the base things influencing your question. The next tile is placed left of center and signifies any obstacles to your question that must be overcome. The third rune is placed at the top of the cross and represents factors that could prove beneficial to answering your question or solving your problem. The right of the cross is the fourth tile, showing a possible outcome to your question. Finally, the fifth rune goes in the middle and symbolizes elements that may influence the outcome in the future.

Medicine Wheel Spread

If you seek a solution to a problem but do not know what course of action to take, then the medicine wheel spread is the layout. This is a five-rune cast with the same pattern as the five-rune cross. The meaning of each position, however, is quite different.

Begin by placing the first tile left of the center. This represents past influences or the origins of the problem. Place the next tile right of the center. This position covers any influences presently affecting your problem. The third tile goes south of the center, closest to you, and shows how the energy of the problem and its solution changes or will change. After that, place your next tile north of the center, symbolizing the problem or challenge itself. Finally, draw the fifth tile and put it in the center to complete the pattern. This rune represents what you should do or the power you need to call on, to solve the problem.

Odin's Layout

Another five-rune cast, Odin's layout, is a more advanced form of the three-rune layout we looked at earlier. Like with its simpler form, Odin's layout is used to gain insights about a particular issue's past, present, and future.

Draw your first tile and place it on the far left of your casting cloth. This position represents the distant past. Your second tile goes next to this one, still left of center, and signifies the recent past. Place the third tile north of the center. This is the present. The last two tiles are placed on the right, with the near future nearest to the center and the distant future next to it on the far side of the pattern.

Grid of Nine

In the Grid of Nine, there are three columns with three runes in each of them. The numbering, however, is not as you would expect it to be. In this layout, you cast out the runes, ask your question, and then pick up nine tiles, selecting them all before interpreting them. The runes are placed in the following order:

$$
\begin{array}{ccc} 4 & 9 & 2 \\ 3 & 5 & 7 \\ 8 & 1 & 6 \end{array}
$$

When reading the runes using this layout, begin with the lowest line first. This line outlines past influences affecting the subject matter of your question. Start with the eighth rune, which represents hidden past influences to your question. Rune one is next, which shows the basic influences from the past. The final one for the first row is rune six. This tile deals with how you, as the rune caster, feel about these past influences.

Next is the middle row, which is about forces acting on your question. First up in the middle row is the third tile you cast. Like the eighth rune below it in the column, this tile represents hidden influences, but this time those acting on your question in the present. After that, in the middle of the pattern is the fifth rune, which shows the present situation. Last in the middle row is the seventh rune. This is your attitude toward the current state of things related to your question.

The top row covers the outcome of the question you asked. It starts with the fourth tile drawn, which once again represents hidden influences, but this time those related to any obstacles or possible hindrances to the question's positive outcome. Next is the ninth rune, which deals with the best outcome to the subject matter of your question. The final rune in the set is the second tile drawn and signifies your attitude or response to the result of the casting. An interesting note about the Grid of Nine layout is that every row, column, or diagonal line adds up to 15.

Celtic Cross Spread

The Celtic Cross involves a more advanced pattern to use for your readings. When used for a Tarot reading, the first card in this spread is chosen to represent the questioner. For rune casting, you can select a rune that has meaning to you or the person asking the question (if you are doing a reading for someone else). You could also draw this rune randomly from your rune pouch. Either way, this rune will represent the energy of the casting. Draw the symbol on a piece of paper to remember it, and then place the tile back in your pouch so that it can appear in your reading. Concentrate on this rune and how it relates to the clarity or information you seek as you progress through this 10-rune spread.

With your guiding rune chosen and made the focus of the reading, you are now ready to begin. Cast out the runes or draw them one at a time from your pouch. Place the first tile in the center. This rune symbolizes the current situation regarding your question. Draw your second tile and place it on the first rune (if possible). This rune represents the forces that could oppose or be an obstacle to the question. Place the third tile south, in-between you and the first and second runes in the pattern. The third rune tells the hidden or underlying factors influencing the subject matter of your question. The fourth one is placed to the left of the first and second and deals with past influences or those in the process of ending. The fifth is placed in the north, above one and two. This indicates anything that may influence the answer you seek in the future, specifically the medium- to long-term. The sixth tile in the pattern is placed to the right of the first two and shows any influences shortly.

The following four tiles are placed in a column to the left of the sixth, beginning with seven at the bottom and ending with ten at the top. The seventh tile denotes your fears or trepidations toward the question, while the eighth signifies the influences from friends and family. The ninth tile expresses your hopes and beliefs, while the tenth is the outcome of your question.

Celestial Spread

A celestial spread represents a year, beginning with whatever month you are presently in. This is a great layout if you want a month-by-month feel for your question or are looking for an overview of the upcoming year. A celestial spread consists of 13 runes, with the 13th representing the main influence of the year as a whole rather than for a particular month.

The first rune represents the month you are in when you ask your question. Place this rune right of the center and write down its meaning and your interpretation. Then, draw your next tile and place it south of the center. The third rune goes on the left, and the fourth goes north of the center. The fifth tile is placed next to the first on the right, and the pattern continues this way, ending with rune 12 north of the center. As mentioned above, the 13th rune represents the year's primary influence. This tile is placed in the center, completing the pattern.

Pillar 5
Reading

With your question asked, tiles cast, and runes placed in the spread or layout of your choice, there is only one thing left to do—interpret the reading. Welcome, divine rune caster, to the final pillar of runology! Reading runes is not a science but an art. The answer to your question is not going to come in some formulaic or precise manner that automatically solves your problem. However, it will provide insights that help guide your thoughts and consider things from a different (divine) perspective. Reading runes is the culmination of everything we have covered in this book so far and is why you set out on this magical journey to become a rune caster in the first place. Let us look at how to put the runes to work in guiding you to a better tomorrow.

8

Interpreting Runes

While casting runes is pretty simple, interpreting them can be quite tricky. This is because the runes do not give you a straightforward answer but provide insights that help you think through your problems. In this way, the runes guide us, hinting at a solution provided by the unseen powers of the universe and interpreted by the caster. Your intuition and gut feelings play an essential part in reading runes. As we saw in earlier chapters, each rune has a variety of meanings and several different ways that they can be interpreted. The purpose you give each rune needs to consider its inherent meaning, the context of your question, surrounding circumstances, and the other runes in the read. Also, if you are using a layout or a spread, then the position of the rune in the pattern also needs to be considered.

In this chapter, we will go over some final tips for you to use when interpreting the runes of your cast. We will review how to cast and interpret your runes and end by providing you with a summary of the runes and their meanings. Let us get this final part of your runic journey underway!

Casting and Interpreting Runes

When reading runes, focus on how they relate to your life and the question you are asking. Do not focus solely on the rune itself, but always think about how the cosmos' powerful principles and forces represent themselves in your lived experience. For example, Fehu merkstave could signify losses through gambling, or it could be interpreted as losing one's wealth of spirit or self-esteem.

This section summarizes the runic symbols, sounds, and meanings that we looked at in Pillar 2: Runic Scripts. Use this summary when reading the runes to help you interpret them quickly and efficiently. This will help to ensure you do not lose the flow of the moment during a casting. The more you cast and interpret runes, the more familiar you will get with them. Initially, it will require much checking up on the rune meanings. It will also take time to consider how that meaning fits in with your question and into the position it falls in the pattern.

This summary will focus on the 24 runes found in the Elder Futhark. This is because these are the runes usually used for casting runes. We will, however, also go through the Younger Futhark and Anglo-Saxon futhorc equivalents to these runes. Remember that the meanings of these powerful symbols of cosmic forces and universal principles are not set in stone. They should always be considered in the light of your own lived experience. The following summary merely serves as a guide to help you understand what the runes are trying to tell you in that casting.

Freyr/Freyja's Ætt

Fehu	
Rune	ᚠ
Meaning	Wealth (cattle)
Symbolizes	Possessions and values
Sound	/f/ , /v/
Younger Futhark	Fé (ᚠ)
Anglo-Saxon futhorc	Feoh (ᚠ)
Upright	Hope, abundance, and success
Merkstave	Loss of something you value

Ūruz	
Rune	ᚢ
Meaning	Aurochs (wild ox)
Symbolizes	Physical strength and untamed **potential**
Sound	/u/
Younger Futhark	Úr (ᚢ) 'rain'
Anglo-Saxon futhorc	Ur (ᚢ)
Upright	Shaping of power; positive changes
Merkstave	Misdirected efforts or ignorant **actions**

Thurisaz	
Rune	þ
Meaning	Giant
Symbolizes	Connection and opposition; brute strength
Sound	/þ/ (/th/)
Younger Futhark	Þurs (þ)

Anglo-Saxon futhorc	Þorn (Þ) 'thorn'
Upright	Reactive or directed force; vitality and instinct-based will-power
Merkstave	Danger, betrayal, malice

Ansuz	
Rune	ᚠ
Meaning	God (Odin)
Symbolizes	Insight and communication with your higher self
Sound	/a/
Younger Futhark	Óss (ᚫ)
Anglo-Saxon futhorc	Ōs (ᚠ) 'god'; Āc (ᚠ) 'oak'; Æsc (ᚠ) 'ash'
Upright	Insight, inspiration, wisdom, harmony
Merkstave	Misunderstanding, manipulation, delusion

Raidho	
Rune	ᚱ
Meaning	Ride
Symbolizes	Travel, movement, the journey of life
Sound	/r/
Younger Futhark	Reið (ᚱ)
Anglo-Saxon futhorc	Rād (ᚱ)
Upright	Personal evolution; a sign you are on the right path
Merkstave	Disruption or disconnection; an omen of death

Kaunan	
Rune	ᚲ
Meaning	ulcer

Symbolizes	Wisdom or enlightenment
Sound	/k/
Younger Futhark	Kaun (ᚴ)
Anglo-Saxon futhorc	Cēn/Kenaz (ᚳ) 'torch'
Upright	Revelation, positive transformation, revitalized energy
Merkstave	Sickness, stagnation, suffering; arrogance, ignorance, elitism

Gebo	
Rune	X
Meaning	gift
Symbolizes	The balance between give and take
Sound	/g/
Younger Futhark	
Anglo-Saxon futhorc	Gyfu (X)
Upright	Rewards for sacrifices made, clarity of vision, divine blessing
In opposition	Loneliness, greed, overdependence; over self-sacrificing, bribery

Wunjo	
Rune	ᚹ
Meaning	Joy or bliss
Symbolizes	Hope, harmony, love, togetherness
Sound	/w/; /v/
Younger Futhark	
Anglo-Saxon futhorc	Wynn (ᚹ)
Upright	Comfort, contentment, fellowship; glory and spiritual rewards
Merkstave	Alienation or possession; frenzy or berserker's rage

Heimdall's Ætt

Hagalaz	
Rune	ᚺ
Meaning	Hail
Symbolizes	Sudden change; creative and destructive forces
Sound	/h/
Younger Futhark	Hagall (ᚼ)
Anglo-Saxon futhorc	Hægl (ᚻ)
Upright	Resilience, tempering, inner strength and willpower; growth and balance
In opposition	Powerlessness, suffering, impending disaster

Naudiz	
Rune	ᚾ
Meaning	Need or constraint
Symbolizes	Necessity and difficulty; restrictions required to build inner strength
Sound	/n/
Younger Futhark	Nauðr (ᚾ)
Anglo-Saxon futhorc	Nȳd (ᚾ)
Upright	Endurance, determination, restraint, patience; coming to terms with orlog
Merkstave	Restriction or loss of freedom; want or unmet emotional needs

Isaz	
Rune	ᛁ
Meaning	ice
Symbolizes	Self-control; stillness and fortitude of mind

Sound	/i/
Younger Futhark	Íss (ᛁ)
Anglo-Saxon futhorc	Īs (ᛁ)
Upright	Overcoming challenges; developing self-awareness and clarity
In opposition	Egocentricity, loss of control, over-indulgence in sensory pleasures; betrayal or treachery

Jēran	
Rune	ᛃ
Meaning	Year or harvest
Symbolizes	Reward for hard work and positive actions
Sound	/j/
Younger Futhark	Ár (ᛏ)
Anglo-Saxon futhorc	Gēr (ᚷ)
Upright	Positive results for earlier efforts, peace, prosperity; success and happiness
In opposition	Poor timing or an unexpected setback; reversal of luck and fortune

Eihwaz	
Rune	ᛇ
Meaning	Yew tree; Yggdrasil
Symbolizes	Life, death, and renewal
Sound	/y/
Younger Futhark	
Anglo-Saxon futhorc	Ēoh (ᛇ)
Upright	Enlightenment, protection, are on the right path to achieving your goals
Merkstave	Distraction or dissatisfaction; weakness or confusion

Perthro	
Rune	⌶
Meaning	Lot cup
Symbolizes	Orlog, fate, and the game of life
Sound	/p/
Younger Futhark	
Anglo-Saxon futhorc	Peorð (⌶)
Upright	Good luck and success; determining your own destiny
Merkstave	Stagnation or unhappiness; circumstances beyond your control

Algiz	
Rune	ᛉ
Meaning	Elk or protection
Symbolizes	Spiritual connection with the divine
Sound	/z/
Younger Futhark	Yr (ᛦ) 'yew'
Anglo-Saxon futhorc	Eolh (ᛉ)
Upright	Divine protection, spiritual awakening, connection with your higher self
Merkstave	Weakening of your divine link or repelling; impending danger if things do not change

Sowilō	
Rune	ᛊ
Meaning	Sun
Symbolizes	Success, accomplishment, honor
Sound	/s/
Younger Futhark	Sól (ᛌ)

Anglo-Saxon futhorc	Sigel (ᛉ)
Upright	Guidance and hope; positive change and achieving victory
Merkstave	Disconnection, false success, bad advice; losing sight of goals and purpose

Týr's Ætt

Tiwaz	
Rune	↑
Meaning	Týr
Symbolizes	Honor, justice, leadership
Sound	/t/
Younger Futhark	Týr (↑)
Anglo-Saxon futhorc	Tīr (↑)
Upright	Justice, victory, coming to terms with the self-sacrifice required to succeed
Merkstave	Over-analyzing, injustice, failure; diminishing of purpose and passion

Berkanen	
Rune	ᛒ
Meaning	Birch tree
Symbolizes	Fertility, cycle of life and death, new growth, rebirth
Sound	/b/
Younger Futhark	Björk (ᛒ)
Anglo-Saxon futhorc	Beorc (ᛒ)
Upright	Renewal, positive change, the beginning of something new
In opposition	Anxiety, domestic problems, blurred vision; forces conspiring against you

Ehwaz	
Rune	ᛖ
Meaning	Horse
Symbolizes	Movement and progress
Sound	/e/
Younger Futhark	
Anglo-Saxon futhorc	Eh (ᛖ)
Upright	Harmony, steady progress, loyalty
Merkstave	Disharmony, indecisiveness, betrayal

Mannaz	
Rune	ᛗ
Meaning	Man or Humankind
Symbolizes	Intelligence, planning, heightened awareness
Sound	/m/
Younger Futhark	Maðr (ᛘ)
Anglo-Saxon futhorc	Mann (ᛗ)
Upright	Self-actualization, divine influence, creativity
Merkstave	Mortality, destructive emotions, shortcomings of humankind

Laguz	
Rune	ᛚ
Meaning	Lake or water
Symbolizes	Life energy, collective memory, purification
Sound	/l/
Younger Futhark	Lögr (ᛚ)
Anglo-Saxon futhorc	Lagu (ᛚ)

Upright	Imagination, dreams, balance, growth; on-track to achieving your goals
Merkstave	Tumult, confusion, poor judgment; stuck in a downward spiral

Inguz	
Rune	◊
Meaning	Ing (Freyr)
Symbolizes	Male fertility, internal growth, creation
Sound	/ŋ/
Younger Futhark	
Anglo-Saxon futhorc	Ing (ᛜ)
Upright	Self-improvement, gestation, growth
In opposition	Immaturity, frivolity, effort without gain

Dagaz	
Rune	ᛞ
Meaning	Day
Symbolizes	Awakening or enlightenment
Sound	/d/
Younger Futhark	
Anglo-Saxon futhorc	Dæg (ᛞ)
Upright	Hope, happiness, certainty; heightened awareness and positivity
In opposition	Lacking vision or hopelessness

Othala	
Rune	ᛟ
Meaning	Heritage or inheritance

Symbolizes	Home, connection with your ancestors, spiritual roots
Sound	/o/
Younger Futhark	
Anglo-Saxon futhorc	Ēðel (ᛟ)
Upright	Prosperity, freedom, safety, spiritual aid
Merkstave	Losing touch with heritage, poverty, mistreatment

Conclusion

Welcome, my freshly initiated runologist, to the end of this book! We have taken quite the learning journey together as we traversed our way through the five pillars of runology. By absorbing the knowledge, techniques, and strategies in this book, you have taken more than a few steps forward on your path toward enlightenment. That is the true glory of runelore; we discover more about ourselves as we learn about these powerful symbols of cosmic forces and universal principles.

Whether you use the Elder Futhark, Younger Futhark, or Anglo-Saxon futhorc for your castings or a spread or a layout, the result is the same. You will gain insights into the hidden workings of the world and guidance on how to deal with any problems or obstacles that arise on your life's journey.

Reading runes requires more feeling than thinking. It is about the energy you bring to the casting, the divine powers you invoke, and the emotions and intuitions you feel as you interpret the tiles. It is not a science, but it often offers insights that no scientific process could provide you with.

Because it is about feelings, you should make rune casting your own. Create your own ritual space for casting runes, using the Hammarsetning to sanctify the space. Select a material for your rune tiles that resonates most with your psyche and design your casting cloth, rune pouch, and stol in a way that best captures what these ancient magical symbols mean to you. Finally, choose mearmots (personal talismans) that get you in the right frame of mind and emotional state for reading and interpreting runes, using a spread or layout that best maps out the answer you seek.

It is as simple as that! You are ready to use the runes to improve your life and those around you. Get in touch with your inner Viking and call on the wisdom of the runes to enhance your life's story. The world is full of mystery and wonder. Learn how to read these signs and tap into the wisdom of the divine through the power of the runes.

References List

A Little Sparkle of Joy. (2022). *The 24 Runes Meanings and How to Access Their Magic.* Www.alittlesparkofjoy.com. https://www.alittlesparkofjoy.com/runes/

Bellows, H. A. (2007). *The poetic Edda : the heroic poems.* Dover Publications.

Beltane, C. (2021a). *Anglo-Saxon and Frisian Rune.* Witches of the Craft®. https://witchesofthecraft.com/tag/anglo-saxon-and-frisian-rune/

Beltane, C. (2021b). *Norse Runes: Viking Runes, Norse Symbols & Much More to Know!* Witches of the Craft®. https://witchesofthecraft.com/2021/11/03/norse-runes-viking-runes-norse-symbols-much-more-to-know/

Caro, T. (2020). *What Does the Othala Rune Mean? [Upright, Reversed & Uses].* Magickalspot.com. https://magickalspot.com/othala-rune/

Connolly, L. (2021). *The Younger Futhark.* The Spells8 Forum. https://forum.spells8.com/t/the-younger-futhark/10365

Forefathers Art. (2019a). *Anglo-Saxon Runes - Futhorc of the Anglo-Saxons.* Forefathers-Art.com. https://forefathers-art.com/anglo-saxon-runes-futhorc-of-the-anglo-saxons

Forefathers Art. (2019b). *Younger Futhark - The Meanings of the Runes.* Forefathers-Art.com. https://forefathers-art.com/younger-futhark-the-meanings-of-the-runes

Gronitz, D. (2010). *Younger Futhork – Rune Meanings.* Www.therunesite.com. http://www.therunesite.com/younger-futhork-rune-meanings/#:~:text=The%20Younger%20Futhork%20consists%20of%2016%20runes%20and

Guido. (2022). *Tyr's Ætt.* Mind Unfolded. https://sites.google.com/site/mindunfolded/chapter-6/tyr-s-aett-1

Harris, J. (2022). *Runemarks: Using Runes | Joanne Harris.* Joanneharris.co.uk. http://www.joanne-harris.co.uk/books/runemarks/runemarks-using-runes/

Hill, B. (2019). *Futhark: Mysterious Ancient Runic Alphabet of Northern Europe.* Ancient Origins Reconstructing the Story of Humanity's Past. https://www.ancient-origins.net/artifacts-ancient-writings/futhark-mysterious-ancient-runic-alphabet-northern-europe-003250

Hubbard, E., Tuit, L., & Lewis, D. (2022). *Introduction to Runes*. Witchschool.com. https://witchschool.com/lesson_detail/539?page=1

Khan, M. (2019a). *Calc the Cup: Northumbrian Runes*. Heathen at Heart. https://www.patheos.com/blogs/heathenatheart/2019/06/calc-the-cup/

Khan, M. (2019b). *Cweorth: Northumbrian Runes*. Heathen at Heart. https://www.patheos.com/blogs/heathenatheart/2019/07/cweorth-northumbrian-runes/

Khan, M. (2019c). *Gar the Spear: Northumbrian Runes*. Heathen at Heart. https://www.patheos.com/blogs/heathenatheart/2019/07/gar-the-spear-northumbrian-runes/

Leeming, D. (2005). Poetic Edda. In The Oxford Companion to World Mythology. : Oxford University Press. Retrieved 2 Dec. 2022, from https://www.oxfordreference.com/view/10.1093/acref/9780195156690.001.0001/acref-9780195156690-e-1274.

Linton, M. (2013). *All About Runes A Book of Runes A Wikipedia Compilation*. http://www.1066.co.nz/Mosaic%20DVD/library/runes/all%20about%20runes.pdf#page=96

Linton, M. A. (2013). *All about Runes A Book of Runes*. http://www.1066.co.nz/Mosaic%20DVD/library/runes/all%20about%20runes.pdf#page=96

Mart, L. (2014). *Divination 1: Question 5 (Rune Meanings)*. Little Druid on the Prairie. https://prairiedruid.com/2014/06/06/divination-1-question-5-rune-meanings/

McCoy, D. (2012a). *Runes*. Norse Mythology for Smart People. https://norse-mythology.org/runes/

McCoy, D. (2012b). *Runic Philosophy and Magic - Norse Mythology for Smart People*. Norse Mythology for Smart People. https://norse-mythology.org/runes/runic-philosophy-and-magic/

McCoy, D. (2012c). *The Binding of Fenrir*. Norse Mythology for Smart People. https://norse-mythology.org/tales/the-binding-of-fenrir/

Modern Norse Heathen. (2017). *A Beginner's Guide to Rune Casting*. Modern Norse Heathen. https://modernnorseheathen.wordpress.com/2017/09/13/a-beginners-guide-to-rune-casting/

Newcombe, R. (2019). *Rune Guide - An Introduction to using the Runes*. Holistic Shop. https://www.holisticshop.co.uk/articles/guide-runes

Omniglot. (2019). *Anglo-Saxon runes (Futhorc)*. https://www.omniglot.com/writing/futhorc.htm

Rhys, D. (2021). *Algiz Rune – History and Meaning*. Symbol Sage. https://symbolsage.com/algiz-rune-symbol-meaning/

RODNAE Productions. (2021). Top View of Astrology Items [Online Image]. In *Pexels*.

Rune Secrets. (2020). *How to Interpret the Runes*. Rune Secrets. https://runesecrets.com/rune-lore/how-to-interpret-the-runes

Saul, F. (2017). *Elder Futhark*. Auntyflo.com. https://www.auntyflo.com/spiritual-meaning/elder-futhark

Sawyer, A. (2021). *Elder Futhark Runes — Meanings And Rune Casting Basics*. YourTango. https://www.yourtango.com/2018316703/how-to-read-cast-interpret-rune-casting-astrology-zodiac-horoscope

Starfire, L. (2018). *The Three Aettirs of the Elder Futhark Runes*. Witches of the Craft®. https://witchesofthecraft.com/2018/09/12/the-three-aettirs-of-the-elder-futhark-runes/

Symbolikon. (2023). *Thurisaz - Norse Runes symbol - Symbolikon Worldwide Symbols*. Symbolikon.com. https://symbolikon.com/downloads/thurisaz-norse-runes/#:~:text=Thurisaz%20is%20a%20protective%20rune

Taylor, K. E. (2020). *Futhorc: The Anglo-Saxon Runes & Runology*. Druidry. https://druidry.org/resources/futhorc-the-anglo-saxon-runes-runology

The English Companions. (2021). *About the Anglo-Saxon Futhorc*. https://www.tha-engliscan-gesithas.org.uk/written-and-spoken-old-english/old-english-alphabet-2/about-the-anglo-saxon-futhorc/

The Pagan Grimoire. (2022). *Your Guide to the 24 Elder Futhark Runes and Their Meanings*. The Pagan Grimoire. https://www.pagangrimoire.com/elder-futhark-rune-meanings/

The Rune Site. (2010, September 27). *Northumbrian Runes – Rune Meanings*. Www.therunesite.com. http://www.therunesite.com/northumbrian-runes-rune-meanings/

The Viking Rune. (2008). *Younger Futhark Runes: The Rune Set Used by Norse Vikings*. Vikingrune.com. https://www.vikingrune.com/2008/11/younger-futhark-runes/

Two Wander. (2020). *Rune Meanings and How to Use Rune Stones for Divination*. Two Wander. https://www.twowander.com/blog/rune-meanings-how-to-use-runestones-for-divination

Tyler, D. (2015). *Your Guide to Rune Divination*. Rune Divination. https://runedivination.com/your-guide-to-rune-divination/

Tyler, D. (2019). *Casting Runes*. Rune Divination. https://runedivination.com/casting-runes/

Tyriel. (2008a). *Algiz - Rune Meaning*. Rune Secrets. https://runesecrets.com/rune-meanings/algiz

Tyriel. (2008b). *Ansuz - Rune Meaning*. Rune Secrets. https://runesecrets.com/rune-meanings/ansuz

Tyriel. (2008c). *Berkano - Rune Meaning*. Rune Secrets. https://runesecrets.com/rune-meanings/berkano

Tyriel. (2008d). *Dagaz - Rune Meaning*. Rune Secrets. https://runesecrets.com/rune-meanings/dagaz

Tyriel. (2008e). *Ehwaz - Rune Meaning*. Rune Secrets. https://runesecrets.com/rune-meanings/ehwaz

Tyriel. (2008f). *Fehu - Rune Meaning*. Rune Secrets. https://runesecrets.com/

Tyriel. (2008g). *Gebo - Rune Meaning*. Rune Secrets. https://runesecrets.com/rune-meanings/gebo

Tyriel. (2008h). *Hagalaz - Rune Meaning*. Rune Secrets. https://runesecrets.com/rune-meanings/hagalaz

Tyriel. (2008i). *Ihwaz or Eihwaz - Rune Meaning*. Rune Secrets. https://runesecrets.com/rune-meanings/ihwaz-eihwaz

Tyriel. (2008j). *Inguz - Rune Meaning*. Rune Secrets. https://runesecrets.com/rune-meanings/inguz

Tyriel. (2008k). *Isa - Rune Meaning*. Rune Secrets. https://runesecrets.com/rune-meanings/isa

Tyriel. (2008l). *Jera - Rune Meaning*. Rune Secrets. https://runesecrets.com/rune-meanings/jera

Tyriel. (2008m). *Kenaz - Rune Meaning*. Rune Secrets. https://runesecrets.com/rune-meanings/kenaz

Tyriel. (2008n). *Laguz - Rune Meaning*. Rune Secrets. https://runesecrets.com/rune-meanings/laguz

Tyriel. (2008o). *Mannaz - Rune Meaning*. Rune Secrets. https://runesecrets.com/rune-meanings/mannaz

Tyriel. (2008p). *Nauthiz - Rune Meaning*. Rune Secrets. https://runesecrets.com/rune-meanings/nauthiz

Tyriel. (2008q). *Othala - Rune Meaning*. Rune Secrets. https://runesecrets.com/rune-meanings/othala

Tyriel. (2008r). *Perthro - Rune Meaning*. Rune Secrets. https://runesecrets.com/rune-meanings/perthro

Tyriel. (2008s). *Raidho - Rune Meaning*. Rune Secrets. https://runesecrets.com/rune-meanings/raidho

Tyriel. (2008t). *Sowilo - Rune Meaning*. Rune Secrets. https://runesecrets.com/rune-meanings/sowilo

Tyriel. (2008u). *Thurisaz - Rune Meaning*. Rune Secrets. https://runesecrets.com/rune-meanings/thurisaz

Tyriel. (2008v). *Tiwaz - Rune Meaning*. Rune Secrets. https://runesecrets.com/rune-meanings/tiwaz

Tyriel. (2008w). *Uruz - Rune Meaning*. Rune Secrets. https://runesecrets.com/rune-meanings/uruz

Tyriel. (2008x). *Wunjo - Rune Meaning*. Rune Secrets. https://runesecrets.com/rune-meanings/wunjo

van der Hoeven, J. (2020). *The Runes: Ōs*. Down the Forest Path. https://downtheforestpath.com/2020/11/26/the-runes-os/

van der Hoeven, J. (2022). *The Runes: Rād*. Down the Forest Path. https://downtheforestpath.com/tag/runes/#:~:text=The%20fifth%20rune%2C%20R%C4%81d%20or

Viking Style. (2020). *Viking Rune Meanings*. Viking Style. https://viking.style/viking-rune-meanings/

Wigington, P. (2020). *What Is Rune Casting? Origins and Techniques*. Learn Religions. https://www.learnreligions.com/rune-casting-4783609

Williamson, J. (2022). *All you need to know about the Elder Futhark, the oldest form of runic alphabets*. The Viking Herald. https://thevikingherald.com/article/all-you-need-to-know-about-the-elder-futhark-the-oldest-form-of-runic-alphabets/294

THE 4 PILLARS OF HERBALISM

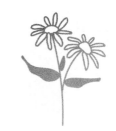 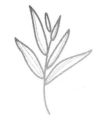  

FOUNDATION　　PROCESS　　**PROFILES**　　REMEDIES

143 Techniques & Hacks
to Improve Your Health with Medicinal Plants. Discover How to Protect Yourself and Your Family with the Power of Healing Herbs and Natural Remedies

INGRID CLARKE

Table of Contents

Introduction **101**

Pillar 1: Foundation **103**

Chapter 1: Definition **105**
    What is Herbalism? 105
    History 106
    Herbal Medicine Versus Modern Medicine 107
    Herbal Medicine in Modern Times 108

Chapter 2: Global Tradition **111**
    African Folk 111
    Arabic Unani 112
    Indian Traditional 113
    European Heritage 115
    Mesoamerican 115
    Traditional Chinese 116
    Iroquois 117

Pillar 2: Process **119**

Chapter 3: Sourcing **121**
    Foraging 121
    Growing 123
    Harvesting 125

Chapter 4: Preparation **129**
    Tools/Equipment 129
    Ingredients 131
    Methods 131

Pillar 3: Profiles **137**

Chapter 5: Herbs, Plants, Flowers, and Wood Profiles **139**
    Agrimony 139
    Angelica 140

- Ashwagandha 140
- Betony 140
- Calendula 141
- Cat's Claw 141
- Catnip 141
- Cayenne 141
- Chamomile 142
- Chaste Tree 142
- Cinnamon 142
- Cleavers 142
- Corn Silk 143
- Dandelion 143
- Echinacea 145
- Elder 145
- Elderberry 146
- Elecampane 146
- Fennel 146
- Fenugreek 147
- Ginkgo 149
- Ginseng 149
- Goldenrod 149
- Goldenseal 150
- Hawthorn 150
- Horsetail 150
- Kelp 151
- Lavender 151
- Lemon Balm 152
- Licorice 152
- Linden 152
- Marshmallow Root 153
- Meadowsweet 153
- Milk Thistle 154
- Motherwort 154
- Mullein 154
- Nettle 154
- Plantain 156
- Red Raspberry 157
- Red Clover 157
- Rose 157

    Rosemary 158
    Sage 158
    Saint John's Wort 159
    Saw Palmetto 159
    Self-Heal 160
    Solomon's Seal 160
    Thyme 160
    Tulsi 161
    Turmeric 161
    Uva Ursi 162
    Valerian 162
    Wild Lettuce 162
    Yarrow 163

Pillar 4: Remedies 165

Chapter 6: List of Remedies by Symptoms 167
    Acne 167
    ADHD 167
    Allergies 168
    Amoebiasis 168
    Anxiety 168
    Arthritis 169
    Asthma 169
    Back Pain 170
    Bloating 170
    Bronchitis/Chest Cold/Pneumonia 170
    Chickenpox 171
    Cold and Flu 171
    Constipation 172
    Cough 172
    Depression 173
    Diarrhea 173
    Dry Mouth 173
    Ear Infection/Earache 174
    Eczema/Dermatitis/Skin Inflammation 174
    Edema 175
    Endometriosis 175
    Eye Problems 176
    Fatigue and Exhaustion 176

Fever 177
Gingivitis 177
Headache and Migraine 178
Heartburn/GERD/Acid Reflux 179
Heart Palpitation 179
High Blood Pressure/Hypertension 179
Hypoglycemia 180
Hypothyroidism 180
IBS/IBD/Ulcerative Colitis 180
Indigestion/Dyspepsia 180
Insect Bites 181
Insomnia 181
Jet Lag 181
Joint Pain 182
Leaky Gut 182
Menopause/Andropause 183
Menstrual Cycle Irregularities 183
Muscle Pain 183
Nausea 184
Pain Management/Relief 184
PCOS 184
PMS 184
Postpartum 185
Rash/Skin Allergy 185
Sinusitis 185
Sore Throat 186

Conclusion **187**

Glossary **189**

References **191**

Introduction

In this book, I will share the four pillars of herbalism that can shape how you understand herbal healing. As such, plants are potent in helping our bodies return to normal function by stimulating, supporting, restraining, and retraining different parts of us. Herbalism will also help you to realize your connection with the planet and re-establish a trusting relationship with nature.

Moreover, herbalism is deeply rooted in your genes, and when used wisely, it can be an excellent asset for restoring balance to your body. During challenging times in one's health journey, herbalism can show you how to restore harmony among the different elements of your being. In fact, plant-based healing has a remarkable influence that can help to bring shifts back into alignment. With its therapeutic effects, herbalism works harmoniously with your body for the most balanced outcome.

Amid daily stresses and duties, we often forget to take time for self-care. Work and family responsibilities, anxieties, unexpected events, and inevitable life changes can leave us unhealthy, unhappy, and feeling like we cannot do anything about our compromised state. Having suffered severe burnout before, and as someone who hailed from a Scandinavian family with neo-pagan roots, I devoted myself to studying different healing methods and accumulated pearls of wisdom from metaphysical practices and occult traditions from around the world. As an empath, it is my mission to share my lifelong experiences and comprehensive knowledge from years of research with those who need healing.

This book takes a simple approach to herbalism. The first two chapters overview how people use herbs to feel better in difficult times and uncover herbal traditions worldwide. It will also share foundational concepts on natural health and how to integrate them into your life. Meanwhile, a deeper dive is taken in chapters three to five, exploring how to source, prepare, and safely handle healing herbs. Then chapter six reveals the healing properties of over 60 plants, herbs, and flowers, while the last chapter provides beginner-friendly remedies for 50+ typical health issues. You will find 143 techniques, tips, and strategies to improve your health naturally. It's peppered throughout the entire book and it's intentionally designed this way to serve as your guide along each step of the process. As a beginner, this book gives you all the information you need to start your journey with herbalism.

Since I have struggled with physical and mental pain, I always sought solutions to ease my stress and improve my well-being. Fortunately, I got to open my eyes to the countless simple yet powerful ways of herbal healing. All the research and techniques I found were outlined in this book. Through these herbal healing methods, I gained a sense of comfort and relief. Now, when I am feeling distressed, I can confidently turn to the power of medical herbs. Likewise, this newfound knowledge has helped me become more in tune with my body, enabling me to identify the root cause of my ailments. I no longer feel helpless or in the dark about my physical and mental health. Instead, I have taken control of my recovery and well-being.

The end goal of this book is to help you in your healing journey to self-care. Yet, it is not designed to replace any doctor's recommendations. Instead, it offers a different perspective on medicine and will help you integrate medicinal plants into your life when the situation deems fit. To become more capable of taking care of yourself and gaining a sense of empowerment, this book will provide you with all the guidance you need. With various paths in the plant medicine world, it will be your blueprint for self-reliance and confidence.

Overall, this book aims to make the ancient knowledge of herbalism available and understandable to anyone interested in discovering it. By simplifying and organizing the information, I have created a resource that provides an efficient path to learning about herbal medicine. With some education, you can begin to take care of yourself through the healing power of herbs, and you may find that the ailments you face become less chronic or disappear altogether. Likewise, pains that have plagued you for years will diminish, and you will become revitalized and refocused on your overall health and well-being. Hence, when you finish reading this book, you will have peace of mind that you can have a better proactive and backup plan for your health.

Attaining balance and restoring connection with nature are the guiding principles behind my techniques and strategies to unlock the power of herbalism. With many ancient remedies discussed throughout this book, you can use thousands of years of wisdom to reconnect with your body. Each chapter in this book will teach you the different theories and techniques you can use in your plant healing journey. It will allow you to learn alternative ways—through medicinal herbs—to care for yourself and your loved ones while fostering independence and self-sufficiency.

Pillar 1
Foundation

With the ever-growing interest in herbalism and alternative medicine, it is time to dig its roots. In this pillar, we uncover the definition, history, and development of herbalism and various world traditions in this field. As such, chapter one will discuss what herbalism is, while chapter two dives into African Folk, Arabic Unani, Indian traditional, European heritage, Mesoamerican, Traditional Chinese, and Iroquois systems of herbal-based medicines. By the end of this discussion, you will have enough information to help you decide if herbalism is right for you and understand your next steps.

1

Definition

The practice of herbalism has been around for millennia and thus has been well-defined alongside modern medicine. In this chapter, we will define herbalism, investigate the history of herbal practices, and draw similarities between herbal medicine and modern medicine to understand the historical significance of herbalism in medicinal culture.

What is Herbalism?

Herbalism can be defined as *"a traditional medicinal or folk medicine practice based on the use of plants" (Wiki Contributors, 2021)*. These medicines make use of therapeutic remedies and allopathic medicines for the treatment of illnesses. Herbalism or botanical medicine often includes organic products like fungi and bee products. Many people from different cultures often locate these herbs in various locations for healing. Other materials, such as minerals, shells, or animal byproducts, are also used in herbalism. Likewise, organic materials are essential in herbalism to provide health benefits, aid with health concerns, and maintain overall health. Also, herbs and spices used in seasoning food have medicinal properties, as they have antimicrobial capabilities which can be harnessed to fight against any foodborne pathogens. By understanding and utilizing these organic materials, herbalism enables us to use natural remedies to look after ourselves and our animals.

Medicinal plants are often rich in secondary metabolites, such as tannins and alkaloids. These chemicals often have antiviral, antibacterial, and antifungal properties for various medicinal uses. They can be used in a variety of different ways. Aromatherapy is a form of herbalism that incorporates oils and aromatic herbs for relaxation and mild relief. Similarly, herbal practices such as Indian herbalism, Ayurveda, and Chinese herbal practices enforce good health through the balance of the mind and body. In this way, herbalism takes many forms to provide relief, including plant leaves, stems, flowers, seeds, bark, and fruits. These herbal medicines not only cure the disease but can help to prevent bodily ailments in the future. Herbalism also provides a great alternative to allopathic alternatives. Around 88% of the world's population is estimated to integrate herbal medicinal practices into their daily lives *(World Health Organization, n.d.)*. The herbs used for common illnesses will depend on those available areas.

For example, herbalism employed in wetlands may look completely different from those in drier land areas. Likewise, the most common herbs used will vary depending on the illnesses most likely to be contracted in those areas. In some cases, herbal remedies treat ailments better than allopathic care. Alternative medicines are often extracted from plants and herbs to form extracts, pills, syrups, or powders. In the modern age, they have been commercialized to the point that herbal remedies can be found at your local drugstore. On the other hand, Herbalists have diagnosed these problems by conducting interviews to identify the symptoms to be treated. After which, a herbal remedy is recommended with the required dosage. Only the recommended dosage should be taken to avoid poor side effects due to over-dosage.

Meanwhile, dried leaves and herbs are often preferred over fresh ones, as dry herbs are more nutrient-rich. This is usually done by hanging these plants in a well-ventilated, shaded, and cool area. The sun tends to dry these plants out, stripping them of oils that may remove their healing properties. Roots, on the other hand, have to be chopped and cleaned before they are dried. They are stored in glass jars and non-metallic containers in a cool, dry area until needed. Lastly, home-brewed medicinal teas are the best way to consume herbal remedies. The herbs are steeped in boiling water to brew a strong tea. Unlikely with the commercialized versions of these teas, which only have a fraction of the healing properties.

History

It has been noted that the study of herbs dates as far back as 5,000 years to the Sumerians *(Wiki Contributors, 2021)*. Sumerians employed herbalism by using medicinal plants such as laurel, caraway, and thyme. Furthermore, it was noted that throughout history, Egyptians used garlic, castor oil, coriander, and mint, amongst other herbs, for medicinal purposes. The first recorded test of Chinese herbalism can be dated to about 2700 B.C. and listed close to 365 plants and their uses *(Wiki Contributors, 2021)*. One of these plants included ma-Huang, a scrub from which the modern drug ephedrine was derived. Modern medicine still uses this drug to prevent low blood pressure during anesthesia. Greeks and Romans have also been known to make use of herbal practices. These practices were recorded by physicians such as Hippocrates and Galen and referenced later in Western medicine. Likewise, Galen compiled the first European dissertation detailing the properties and uses of medicinal plants; this aided European herbalism greatly over time.

Attitudes towards herbalism during the Middle Ages changed due to the advent of the Christian church, as they discouraged the practice of herbalism and medicinal healing. Yet, Greek and Roman practitioners preserved medical knowledge in monasteries, later becoming centers for medicine and medical expertise. Monasteries often grew herb gardens to treat mild illnesses and disorders. Then in villages, herbalism continued to grow to provide remedies for local herbalists.

In the 11th century, Arabians became more advanced in medical science than Europeans. As a result, Arabs imported herbs from foreign places, such as China and India, and acquired knowledge at medical schools using Galen's system and teachings. This influenced Western medicine greatly. At the same time, folk medicine was used widely, resulting in many herbalist publications in the 15th century due to the invention of printing. Hence, the 15th, 16th, and 17th centuries saw a spike in herbalism; herbalist texts were now available in English, Latin, and Greek.

Grete Herball, the first English herbalist text, was published anonymously in 1526. Then, John Gerard's *The Herball or General History of Plants*, published in 1597, and Nicholas Culpeper's *The English Physician Enlarged*, released in 1653, were essential works from this period. However, Gerard's book was plagiarized from a Belgian text called *Dodoens*, and he also used German botanical works as reference material for his herb illustrations. On the other hand, Culpeper's publication incorporated herbalism with astrology and folklore; it was met with ridicule by some practitioners due to its reliance on mysticism.

The Age of Exploration and the Columbian Exchange led to the widespread use of medicinal plants in Europe. During this time, *The Badianus Manuscript*, the first herbal script, was translated from Aztec into Latin during the 16th century. By the second millennium, the influence of herbalism began to dwindle. This paved the way for modern physicians who used over-the-counter prescriptions, leading to the chemical sciences' development in contemporary medicine.

Furthermore, various medicinal herbs have been discovered by ancient Indians, Chinese, and Europeans and have been used historically for healing illnesses. These practices have been carried over for generations using historical texts. In Indian tradition, herbalists have taken to wild forests to use the 1,100 medicinal plants grown there *(Watt & Hayes, 2013)*. Almost 60 of these genuses have been used in herbal practices to cure ailments and diseases where they are grown naturally without farming. Meanwhile, the demand for herbalism in China has resulted in governmental controls for the research and development of these plants. Such plants are grown in controlled areas with over 600 plant types for medicinal use alone *(Watt & Hayes, 2013)*. This system of herbal practices has been accumulated using a knowledge database, observation, clinical trials, and experiments over several years. As a result, it has led to a sustainable industry of herbalism. Acupuncturists and commercialized Eastern medicine have further popularized this.

In the culture of Chinese herbalism, natural plant remedies is the go-to for almost any medical ailment. Minor ailments like digestive problems, coughs, flu, mild headaches, and rashes are often treated using herbal remedies. This is done through a series of biochemical responses induced by plant chemicals. For example, Native Americans have often chewed the interior bark of medicinal willow trees to treat mild headaches and pain. The salicylic acid in the bark is an active ingredient to relieve headaches and can be considered a natural aspirin. White willow has been used in the same way as a mild treatment for headaches, arthritis, and pain symptoms. Yet, use herbal manuals to identify the proper dosage of these remedies and avoid overuse.

However, herbal medicine is often used without consulting qualified medical professionals in India and China. As it has few side effects when taken as part of a diet, it provides accessible and affordable health remedies in areas where allopathic medicine may be unavailable. These remedies have also played a significant role in healthcare improvements and have been combined with allopathic treatment to relieve symptoms of chronic illnesses.

Herbal Medicine Versus Modern Medicine

Throughout history, medicinal plants have been used to treat the ailments of indigenous people. By observing animals that seek out healing plants when ill, humans have been able to experiment with various plants without being poisoned. As a result, tribal communities have gained access to generations of knowledge about medicinal plants, leading to the development of herbalism and the formation of herbalists. Similarly, field biologists use this same technique when studying chimpanzees. Based on the observation, lowlands often consumed ginger plants as an antimicrobial for infection. These could then be used to incorporate herbalism into modern medicine. However, there is still a chance that a nontoxic plant to animals may be harmful or poisonous to human beings. For example, koalas can ingest eucalyptus, while most animals may not. This knowledge was also passed on to form herbalism as it is known today.

Herbal Medicine in Modern Times

Investigating the use of herbalism in the Middle Ages, a group of German researchers integrated medieval medicine and modern science into medical practice. Dr. Johannes Meyer, a medical historian, has researched how traditional herbal medicine described in medieval texts can be applied to treating diseases, such as cancer, today. This project has gained the support of pharmaceutical companies such as GlaxoSmithKline, showcasing how effective herbal medicine is in modern-day treatments *(Watt & Hayes, 2013)*.

During his research at the University of Würzburg, Dr. Meyer has taken monastic manuscripts dating back to the 8th century to investigate herbalism. He has translated and published plant remedies for various ailments over the past few years, detailing what the medications intended to treat. In this way, herbalism has been integrated into modern times. His work has not only incorporated historical text but relied on science to substantiate his findings. The physiological effects of herbal remedies were investigated using scientific knowledge. With the funding of GlaxoSmithKline, the research group is now actively looking for modern remedies that can be derived from medieval monastic wisdom. Likewise, owing to the invaluable herbalist texts, treatments for common colds have been developed and distributed commercially. This success has prompted the group's growth, with more pharmaceutical companies joining as partners, and led to a collaboration with Würzburg University Hospital.

The scope of research has grown from plants documented in monasteries in the 8th and 12th centuries to the entire history of medicinal plants in Europe being investigated for medicinal properties. Findings as a result of this expansion could accelerate modern medicine significantly and be used to aid Westernized medical treatment. Also, Dr. Meyer and his teams incorporate current medical research practices such as testing herbal ingredients in laboratories at Würzburg University Hospital or their partner pharmaceutical companies to identify healing physiological properties. As a result, scientists in this hospital's ear and nose department have used these findings to find remedies for ear cancer. Once found successful, it will then be taken for hospital clinical trials and could be developed into new drugs after fulfilling specific legislative requirements. In this way, herbal medicine has again been incorporated into modern medicinal practices.

Many modern multidisciplinary techniques were incorporated into Dr. Mayers' research into medieval herbalism. These techniques were derived from a team of medical historians, Latin and ancient Greek scholars, chemists, biologists, and pharmacists. Then, to conduct their research on medicinal practices with a multidisciplinary approach, the herbalist texts were initially written in Arabic and later translated into Latin. This information was further preserved by ancient Greek authors such as Aristotle, making it even more valuable. Since European literature on herbalism during the early Middle Ages was lacking, much of the research relied heavily on works by non-European authors. Only in the 11th century, when Arabic texts were translated into Latin, many new plants emerged in European medicine. One such example is Alpinia officinarum, which is often used to treat respiratory problems and could be used as a mild relaxant. Even though this plant is indigenous to parts of Europe, it had only been used in herbal medicine practice once Arabic texts of herbalism were translated. During this time, monastic medicine led the forefront at universities in the 13th century; this changed only when Arabic herbalist texts were translated. After this, monastic medicine became less cemented in European society, and professional physicians took the forefront of modern medicine.

The resurgence of monastic medicine in the 16th century happened when missionaries explored the Americas. They were interested in Native American herbalism and the medicinal plants of Central and South America and brought their discoveries back to Europe. In modern times, Dr. Mayers' group of researchers has collaborated with the medical industry and monasteries to incorporate unique herbal plants used in monastery gardens for tea and lotion. Dr. Mayers has further included herbal medicine using modern practices by running herbalism courses for the public at the Oberzell local monastery, where students research herbal medication. This has resulted in additional funding for the research group.

2

Global Tradition

Herbal medicine is not isolated; it often changes with time, availability, and culture. Healthcare can be considered political; when people need remedies for ailments, they often rely on social or cultural means to get them. Thus, it is no surprise that the global tradition of medicine for African, Arabic, Indian, European, Mesoamerican, traditional Chinese, and Iroquois cultures are not the same. In this chapter, we will explore them.

African Folk

African folk medicine can be dated as far back as 1619, during the slave trade in the United States *(Fletcher, 2020)*. Healthcare for enslaved people was also often limited during that time, and these limited options led to the progression of African folk medicine. Likewise, enslaved people were at the hands of harsher medical treatment by white doctors during this time, leading to self-treatment by friends and herbal doctors. Similarly, in African American folk healing, the inability of a general practitioner or medical doctor to arrive at a remedy resulted in herbal alternatives being used. In some cases, allopathic forms of care worsened the symptoms of certain illnesses, and thus, African folk medicine was used.

In African American folk tradition, illnesses are often categorized as natural or unnatural. As mentioned, natural diseases are pre-determined by nature, while artificial conditions go against its laws or the will of God. Mental health issues, stress, and anxiety can cause these ailments. These illnesses could also be connected to physical or spiritual sources, thus making it hard to pinpoint their causes. Treatment of this depends on the origin of the disease and its nature. But when new information is discovered, the treatment strategy is revised and managed by traditional healers entrusted with medical care for their community. For instance, spiritual healers can have different titles, such as *sangomas* in South African culture, *akomfo* in Ghanaian culture, or *mugwenu* in Tanzania. To be identified, they typically wear headbands, don feathers, and paint their eyes using native chalk.

Many African folk healing traditions are strongly linked to the idea that certain plants possess beneficial therapeutic properties. Belief in this notion has been fused with the practices of traditional healers, offering an opportunity to treat ailments naturally. As such, African folk herbalism comprises three levels of specialty: *divination, spirituality, and herbalism.* Thus, illnesses are treated physically and spiritually using divination, incantations, and herbalism. Traditionally, African folk herbalism has significantly relied on the influence of ancestors and the supernatural for healing and protection. This collaboration with spiritual healing has led to the recovery of the mind in African medicinal practice. Meanwhile, healers of the body have relied on plant remedies to cure ailments incorporating animal and mineral-based medicines. This way, herbal medicine has been used with supernatural forces for healing to provide a holistic approach to medicinal practice.

Traditional medicine not only eliminates disease but aims to prevent it. These practices are usually traditionally disseminated to initiates carrying classic African traditions. In colonial periods, these conventional medicines were often dosed with stigma. They were viewed as inferior to Western medicine and even outlawed in other countries. Regardless, African folk herbalism thrived. Methods of African folk methods vary greatly depending on the region. Herbs are often used wet or dry and can be prepared by—

- **Extractions.** A solvent concocts an herbal remedy in a specific weight-to-volume ratio. During this process, the solvent often evaporated.
- **Infusions.** Crude drugs or herbs are crushed for short periods. This is done by submerging the herbal mixture in cold or hot water. Honey can be added to this mixture to prevent spoilage.
- **Decoctions.** Made to extract nutrients from woody pieces by boiling them in water. This is usually done for an extended period. After which, the remaining concentrated mixture is filtered. Additional preservatives like potash should extract nutrients and preserve the mix.

Arabic Unani

Unani medicine, also known as *Unani-tibb*, is a medicinal practice based in India with the influence of Greco-Arabic medicinal teachings. These teachings have been translated from Greek texts to Arabic and included the teachings of Greek physicians, such as Hippocrates, Galen, and other Arab physicians. The main goal of Unani medicine is to achieve balance and equilibrium in the body, divided into three categories: *temperaments, organs, and four types of humor*. This form of treatment has become increasingly popular in India since the 11th century and is widely used today. Meanwhile, medicinal practices of Greek origin, such as those of Hippocrates, were introduced to India by Arabs during the Mongol invasions in Central Asia and Persia. In this time of upheaval, their scholars took refuge in India, bringing new knowledge.

The public reception of Unani medicine was widespread throughout the country between the 13th and 17th centuries when Unani medical practitioners adopted Indian herbalism. Medical practitioner, Hakim Ajmal Khan *(1868-1927)*, advocated for this practice, which led to the inception of the Ayurvedic and Unani Tibbia College in Delhi *(Poulakou-Rebelakou et al., 2015)*. The system of Unani medicine thrived after the independence of India. In 1946, the Ministry of Health approved the development of Ayurvedic and Unani medicine through research by teaching them in educational institutions *(Poulakou-Rebelakou et al., 2015)*. A couple of years after that, in 1969, a Central Council for Research in Indian Medicine and Homeopathy was established by the Indian government. This was done in various disciplines, such as naturopathy, homeopathy, yoga, Unani medicine, Ayurveda, and Siddha. These endeavors were supported by the World Health Organization (WHO) and are endorsed by WHO to this day.

In 1978, the philosophical basis and practical application of Unani medicine were studied. This government-backed research resulted in a surge of support from hospitals and research centers for herbalism. Subsequently, the Unani Tibb system was established to meet the demand for healthcare services. Today, citizens of India can take advantage of over 100 free hospitals and 900 dispensaries that provide medical care under this system, with more than 30,000 practitioners in total.

As per noted, Unani medicine consists of five basic principles, such as:

1. Elements (arkan)
2. Temperament (mizaj)
3. Humors (akhlat)
4. Spirit (ruh)
5. Nature (tabiat)

According to Unani Tibb, elements are smaller material parts, often with identical shapes, characteristics, and properties. These components take from Ionian philosophers' concepts of water, fire, air, and earth, while Indian philosophers believe in aab (water), aatish (fire), bad (air), khak (earth), and Akash (sky). Arabic philosophy maintains that water, air, and earth are the three core elements. Out of the 92 natural elements, 80 have been detected in the human body; their presence is crucial for healthy functioning; hence, their absence may lead to health issues in Arabic Unani medicine.

Moreover, in Unani medicine, the temperament or mizaj, the balance of humor, leads to health (eukrasia) and balance from disease (disbalance). It is said that humor handles temperament and character. Each person's personality is set due to their humor and prevailing elements. These senses of humor can be categorized as the following:

- Warm—Blood Prevalence—Sanguine (dam)
- Liquid—Phlegm Prevalence—Phlegmatic (balgham)
- Dry—Yellow Bile Prevalence—Bilious (safra)
- Cold—Black Bile Prevalence—Melancholy (sawda)

This theory of humor is derived from Hippocratic principles, which state that the four senses of humor *(blood, phlegm, bile, and black bile)* must be balanced in the body for health maintenance. In Arabic Unani, diseases are then classified according to their humor; this humor is thought to be the cause of disease or disorder.

Within Unani medicine, the spirit or 'ruh' concept is linked to the notion of a soul or 'nafs.' This spiritual attachment is philosophically and religiously significant and is thought to be intertwined with the physical body. It is paramount for a healthy metabolism and an extension of positive mental well-being.

Lastly, in Arabic Unani, it is said in the theory of nature or tabiat that humoral balance is achieved through self-empowerment and self-preservation. The disease is then considered disturbed equilibrium, which can only be restored with the same self-empowerment achieved in humoral balance. Medication in Arabic Unani aims to treat this with the healing power of nature.

Indian Traditional

Indian traditional medicine, or Ayurveda, is India's *"indigenous holistic healing system" (Khalsa, 2009)*. Ayurveda is a healing practice incorporating healthy meals, physical activity, psychotherapy, massages, and herbal medicine into holistic healing. A self-care technique employs preventative techniques to restore health and balance. In Ayurveda, there is a strong presence as one of the four primary forms of herbal medicine. It includes many traditional texts and therapeutic techniques from Oriental, Western, and Unani medicine, offering an efficient and inexpensive approach to healthcare. The widespread of its popularity has made South Asian herbs more widely available.

Ayurveda has been practiced for thousands of years in Indian traditional medicine. These practices have been recorded in the *Ayurvedic Pharmacopoeia Asava*, in which more than 1,200 species of plants have been recorded. This text comprises nearly 100 minerals and 100 animal products that make up herbal remedies, with the recommended dosages for each remedy detailed according to the standards of Ayurveda. Such treatments are designed with a long shelf life and can be stored for prolonged periods. By doing so, the therapeutic properties of the herbs in the mixture become more concentrated, making it possible to draw out their beneficial nutrients and chemicals. Nicknamed "The Science of Life," Ayurveda is one of the oldest forms of herbal medicine. Meanwhile, the core concept of Ayurveda is prevention rather than cure. That said, health is promoted to ward off disease and is maintained by balancing the individual with nature to promote health.

Eight branches of science categorize the practice of Indian traditional Ayurveda. It is used in unison with ten diagnostic tools based on the three senses of humor of the body, or tridosha theory, to diagnose ailments. The herbal practice also consists of various types of herbal medicine, namely fermented and unfermented infusions termed *arishtas* and *asavas*, which are valued due to their high efficiency. Arishtas and asavas can be thought of as alcoholic extraction methods. It is highly effective and is prepared with herbal juices and sugars. Arishtas are decoctions of herbs in hot water, while asavas are fermented using fresh juices. Adding *dhataki* flowers and spices also aids fermentation, leading to a slightly alcoholic, sweet, and acidic mixture.

The benefits of alcohol in the fermentation process are that it improves the quality, boosts the therapeutic and herbal properties, and aids the efficiency of the extraction of the herbal mixture, which allows the medicine to reach the target area much faster. These medicinal practices can be found in Indian traditional text, namely: Charaka Samhita, Sushruta Samhita, Astanga Hridaya, Bhaishajya Ratnavali, Sarngadhara Samhita, Khadhan-graham, Arsaschikitsha, Sagasrayogam, Chikitshasthanam, Yogaratnagaram, and Asavarishtasangragam, to name a few.

In Indian traditional medicine, the preparation of arishta and asava is known as sandhana kalpana. Infusion and decoction are usually used in the extraction of medicinal plants. During decoction, a specified volume of water is used for cooking down a herb and releasing its concentrated nutrients. The concentrated boiled mixture is then cooled down, after which the remaining herbs are strained. To extract water-soluble nutrients from plants resistant to heat, Ayurveda uses a technique in which the ratio of herbal mixture to water stays fixed during boiling. This boiled-down concentrate is called "quath" or "kawath." Boiling alone reduces the total amount of water, and the remaining liquid is extracted and further processed for use.

Meanwhile, traditional Indian infusions are made by mashing herbs and submerging them in boiling or cool water. This is done for limited periods to form diluted solutions of herbal concentrate. To concoct a traditional Indian infusion, the following equipment is needed: a large earthen pot, a medium-sized porcelain jar, a lid, a ribbon to seal the mixture, a wooden spoon for stirring, a mesh cloth to filter out the remaining herbs, a pot to capture the remaining juices. An infusion consists of four components, each with its purpose. The herbs used to create the concentrate are integral to herbal medicine mixtures. Likewise, flavoring agents used in these mixtures are for added flavor but also have healing properties that contribute to the medicinal properties of herbal medicine.

European Heritage

British herbalism has a history of monopolized medicinal practices, often under the influence of orthodox British medicine. In the 19th century, British medicinal practice was under fire due to Thomsonian medical botany, a form of extreme herbalism that relied on local plants to induce vomiting and bowel movement to "cleanse" the body. This excitement eventually died down, leading to more discrete forms of herbalism. However, a small group of herbalists persisted in their struggle for professional recognition and acclaim but suffered at the hands of orthodox medicinal practice, which aimed to monopolize early British herbal practice. Regardless, British herbalism persisted and thrived, birthing writers such as Griggs, Stuart, and Inglis, who promoted British herbalist literature. Toxic medications and patient neglect employed by orthodox British medical practitioners also resulted in the migration towards British herbalism. That said, the final straw was embedded social changes, resulting in patients seeking alternative medicine. There was a striking increase in herbalism in European nations due to industrialization. The Great Depression also influenced the number of herbalists in that area.

Herbalism was incredibly diverse in early-century Great Britain, with businesses spread all around the country. These businesses were successful due to generations of practiced herbalism among well-respected local communities. This community of respect resulted in herbalists being elected to county positions or as mayor or alderman. Yet, not everyone was swayed by the support of herbalists, making it difficult for them to gain public trust. Often, they were labeled as untrustworthy, exploitative, or ambiguous for their inflated prices and lack of scientific evidence for their methods.

In European heritage, herbalists often had a standard body of beliefs or a fixed system of principles under which they conducted alternative medicinal practices. Herbalism was thought to be an entity entirely separate from orthodox and allopathic forms of medicine. Within these practices, herbal remedies were often a mix of vegetable substances, and herbalists tried not to use inorganic materials in their remedies and relied only on natural ingredients. It is believed, in European heritage, that the best way for the human body to receive the minerals it needs is by ingesting plants and incorporating them into daily life as food and medicine. The practice of herbalism was further developed by taking traditional herbal remedies and separating the ingredients to be used individually to enhance different healing properties. As herbalists became increasingly successful in creating effective herbal remedies, plant material was increasingly emphasized in early Britain. During the 19th century, with American herbalism's influence on alternative medicinal practices, British herbalists such as J.H. Blunt laid the foundation for concentrates, alkaloids, and resinoids to become commonplace.

Mesoamerican

Mesoamerican healthcare practices' cultural diversity and richness had existed since the early pre-classical period when various indigenous peoples began inhabiting the region. During 2000 B.C., the San Lorenzo Olmecs emerged in Veracruz, Mexico. Concurrently, the Mokaya established the first socially stratified sedentary culture in the Soconusco region, spanning Mexico and Guatemala's Pacific coast.

What sets Mesoamerica apart and defines its cultural identity are the common fundamental traits that distinguish it from other parts of the Americas. For instance, it encompassed a vast area from central Mexico to northern Central America, harboring renowned civilizations like the Olmecs, Maya, and Aztecs. These civilizations collectively contributed to Mesoamerica's rich cultural tapestry. Within this context, Aztec medicine emerged as the pinnacle of a longstanding tradition that unified diverse cultural groups in the region.

In Southern North America and Central America, social inequalities have made healthcare access difficult, spurring the rise of various alternative healthcare systems. To ensure that universal healthcare can be achieved, integration has become vital in Mesoamerica. Traditional medicine has made health services more accessible, while herbalism has been recorded to preserve this unique culture. However, there is a lack of evidence for traditional medical practices, hindering the implementation of systemic changes in healthcare. Fortunately, public health advocacy has recently made these changes possible by discussing the decolonization of herbal practices in Mesoamerica.

The core concept of traditional Mesoamerican healthcare is sovereignty, and the medicine aims to provide independent healthcare practice to indigenous peoples. Since transitioning to a modern lifestyle and emerging modern lifestyle diseases, Mesoamerica has undergone a rapid health transition, leading to higher life expectancy. The great demographic expansion of Mexico in the 1940s, with the economic growth experienced along with it, led to more outstanding health implementations by the Mexican Ministry of Health *(Geck et al., 2020)*. As a result, the Mexican Ministry of Health and the Mexican Institute of Social Security developed family planning, counseling, and contraceptives free of charge. This expanded the number of rural health posts and hospitals and extended the availability of proper health care to communities that may have only relied on traditional forms of medicine. Those without access to these services relied on conventional healers with generations of medical healing.

These investments in free healthcare have only covered 40% of average healthcare costs in Guatemala. Marginalized communities have used traditional medicine in these cases, such as conventional Mayan practice, to bridge the gap. As a result, models for combining traditional medicine, such as herbalists or ajkum, midwives or ajiyom, and physicians known as ajq'omaneel—are often combined with biomedicine by collaborating with those employed in community health posts. This led to treating unconventional conditions in formal settings, including cultural syndromes. One of them being susto (fright), ojeado (evil eye), or wuqub' siwan (disease of the seven ravines). This is treated using various botanical drugs and therapeutic services to treat patients in collaboration with Maya specialists. These specialists have collaborated with traditional medicine practitioners and healthcare staff to bring these affordable solutions to people. *"In the Cuilco health district alone, located in the western highlands of Guatemala, 360 traditional medicine practitioners coordinated interventions with 78 medical health staff"* (Geck et al., 2020). With that, Mesoamerican traditions are maintained in modern medical practice. It is unconventional that in Mesoamerica, this inclusive health model has even been promoted by the ministry of health.

Traditional Chinese

Traditional Chinese medicine dates back to 2852 B.C. *(Cheng, 1984),* with more than 2,600 herbs and remedies used to treat various illnesses. This practice is based on the fundamental principles of Taoist philosophy: the law of nature, consisting of the opposing forces of Yin and Yang. According to this concept, an imbalance in these forces can result in ailments; Yin occurs when there is too much sedation in the body, and Yang appears when there is too much tonification. These forces are then balanced using herbal medicinal remedies to restore the Yin and Yang balance. In Traditional Chinese medicine, Yang represents sunlight, heat, light, life energy, hypertension, fever, being overweight, pain, coughing, strong heart pulse, inflammation, shoulder problems, and constipation. On the other hand, Yin is negative and is tied to the moon, nighttime, coldness, dark, water, female energy, dying, hypotension, hypothermia, underweight, weakness, and diarrhea. When these two harmonize with each other beautifully, Yin and Yang are balanced.

Yin and Yang are believed to constitute a person's life energy, otherwise known as 'chi.' Chi is said to flow through the body via networks of channels termed meridians. According to traditional Chinese medicine, chi originates from the vital organs before being distributed throughout the body. Amongst many other treatments, acupuncture focuses on these points to address any health conditions at the source. Aside from that, Chinese traditional medicine takes a cyclic approach to life events rather than the linear progression seen in Western philosophies. As such, when diagnosing an illness or treating ailments, TCM practitioners consider a person's entire body rather than just focusing on the affected area.

Moreover, Chinese traditional medicine has been cultivated using a system of knowledge, observation, and clinical trials to form a well-organized system of medicinal practice. Both doctors and staff in the medical industry and government institutions have collected this accumulation of knowledge. These remedies are often not based on science but have repeatedly been proven effective by science. Acupuncture is one of them, which has been scientifically shown to release endorphins and serotonin in the body.

However, unlike Western social norms, traditional Chinese medicine is respected as equal to modern allopathic remedies. Chinese medicines are then used to develop modern medicine by incorporating healing extracts into conventional mixtures. One such example is ephedrine extracted from ma-huang to be used as a remedy for asthma. Other excerpts, such as digitalis, derived from Mao ti-huang, and coumadin, extracted from leeches, have been used traditionally for over 1,800 years *(Cheng, 1984)*. Likewise, restorative materials and old formulae of plant material have been used in unison to provide Chinese medicine using more than 2,600 medicinal materials. For this reason, Chinese medicine is valued for medical and scientific research.

Iroquois

Iroquois used simple remedies for common illnesses like gastrointestinal disorders, fevers, wounds, and fractures. These illnesses were very intelligently treated. They often relied on God and spiritual powers in unison with treatment, which is why we will explore the religious beliefs of Iroquois indigenous peoples to explore Iroquois herbalism. From pantheistic beliefs, the Iroquois assumed all living beings were connected to the divine. Specifically, this included animals, plants, and trees and an overarching presence known as the Great Spirit, believed to have created everything and to be responsible for humanity's desires. Thus, Indian medicine can be branched into two distinct categories: *practical herbalism and spiritual herbalism.*

Practical medicinal practices were developed through trial and error and often consist of fsimple yet valuable restorative practices. Herbal remedies often consisted of indigenous plants and tree bark. Physical therapy was also included as part of the diagnosis; this often-included sweat baths. In the case of fevers, treatment often included rest, sweating, purgation, diuresis, and a limited diet of primarily liquids. Treatment also had infusions, such as elderberries combined with elder bark, served hot for additional sweating. When cleansing or purgation was desired, treatment often included bonesets served in a hot decoction or bush bean to be chewed. Then, phlebotomy was used in treating fevers, in which a sharp flint punctured the vein, which was compressed at a certain point. This was done to relieve mild edema or fluid retention.

Likewise, Iroquois also made use of emetics to induce vomiting. This was done to treat stomach and intestine problems and formed a part of ceremonial purification. In Iroquois practice, cleansing was done through emetics and sweat baths in combined deep spiritual meditation to communicate with the spiritual realm. Emetics usually consisted of sanguinaria canadensis or lye created from corn cob ashes. Warm water was usually ingested after emetics were taken to induce vomiting. The Iroquois also use treatments for rheumatism or neuritis, consisting of sweat baths and boiled sprouts of asparagus, wild peas, pokeberry, cowslip, or mustard. Also, they use hot poultices and moxas of cone and fir twigs to ignite over the affected area after moistening. Aside from that, moxas included a blend of aromatic leaves; the affected limb was held over embers to be covered with a robe to breed medicinal smoke. Additional treatment of mashed leaves of wintergreen and berries was also applied to these swollen joints.

The Iroquois developed a branch of medicine dedicated to obstetrics. In prolonged labor, they employed herbal remedies such as partridge berries to induce childbirth. For excessive menstrual bleeding, Amelanchier canadensis infusions were combined with burning corn husks to remedy hemorrhaging. Furthermore, white Tuscarora corn kernels were cooked between hot stones and smeared onto the umbilical cord until detached. To ensure the health of newborns, the Iroquois developed unique feeding programs consisting of a mixture of butter, dried or crushed hickory nuts, and ground bear meat infused into milk bottles. This method supplied babies with essential nutrients and promoted healthy growth to prevent potential health issues.

For wound treatment, the Iroquois used bandages made from corn leaves, mainly when there was considerable bleeding. Exposed wounds were sewn up with needles that were either made of bones or the horns of animals. Then, chewed tobacco was packed onto healing wounds to drain and close these wounds by changing the packing periodically while allowing the wound to heal. Before the wounds were sealed, they were also inserted into a thin sheet of gut or the inner bark of slippery elm.

Meanwhile, during times of war, the Iroquois tribe is known to have developed their treatment of gunshot wounds, borrowing techniques used in World War I. Their approach to gunshot wounds, for example, involved wide debridement and the removal of ball and bone fragments. They did not shy away from the gruesome aspects of medicine and became skilled in performing these procedures. The Iroquois tribe also relied on natural remedies to aid the healing process, such as using a lotion made from the juice of corn roots and stalks.

Besides that, their use of poultices on wounds, contusions, and swellings is another example of their extensive knowledge of medicine. One of their most famous poultices was made from boiled flowers of maize and was known for its healing properties. However, the Iroquois tribe's surgical treatments were limited to boils and digit amputations.

Pillar 2
Process

Working with natural ingredients and remedies requires responsible sourcing, preparation, and safety. This pillar explores the steps needed to source herbs ethically and safely, handle them responsibly during different stages of their growth, prepare them for use, and store them properly. Likewise, it includes everything from foraging wild plants to growing them in your garden to harvesting roots, seeds, and berries. Hence, in the following chapters, you will gain knowledge of all things related to harvesting herbal medicine in the most effective way possible.

3

Sourcing

Herbalism is more than using a remedy; it is often a practice of preparation which includes foraging, growing, and harvesting before a plant remedy can be made. In modern-day herbalism, plants are often sourced by buying them directly from nurseries. These various methods are employed so plants can be sourced safely and accurately before making plant remedies.

Foraging

An urban forager is generally defined as anyone who collects rocks, materials, or plants in an urban environment. It is widely believed that foraging attempts to illustrate the spiritual aspect of its practitioners. Through their search, they foster a connection with the environment, whether in nature or an urban setting. Foragers must also be mindful when collecting herbs to preserve the natural environment and protect themselves from dangers. By following these steps, those engaging in foraging can enjoy safety and help maintain the ecosystem.

Furthermore, property laws of public spaces should also be respected in modern-day foraging to be aware of the social norms we currently find ourselves in. To harvest plants responsibly, they must be harvested without killing the plants or roots in these areas. Precautions should also be taken to avoid toxic chemicals that may have met plants, such as pesticides, insecticides, and poisons sprinkled onto lawns; this applies to both ingested plants and plants used externally on the body.

Guidelines for Foraging

Being able to forage safely is integral to safe herbalism practice, especially when plants are harvested in their raw states. The following foraging guidelines can be used when harvesting plants before boiling or tincturing:

- Before harvesting herbs, it is vital to investigate the best time to gather them thoroughly. Otherwise, the herb could be harvested at an inappropriate time and go to waste.
- When foraging, handle with care and make sure not to damage the roots. Doing so would render the plant unable to grow adequately and be reused.
- Before plucking any plant from its natural home, be mindful of the consequences: its displacement could harm the balance of the forest's ecosystem. Guard the preservation of this special community of plants; each one is an integral part of nature's cycle.

- Exercise caution when foraging in nature, as wildlife can live in the same areas.
- Be mindful when picking, and practice good medicinal practice and intention.
- Express your gratitude for the harvest and the help from the resource you have received.

The following guidelines should be considered when foraging wild herbs:

- A plant's medicinal or edible parts should be investigated before use.
- Investigate the appropriate harvest times of plants.
- Observe how long it takes for each plant to grow for future purposes.
- The natural life cycle of the plant should be observed when harvesting.
- Take caution against poisonous plants that look like the plant being harvested.
- Study the history of the soil used before planting more herbs to understand the effect of old plant chemicals on new crops.

Foraging With Intention

While foraging, herbalists in natural and urban environments often walk amongst nature to connect with the plants around them. They do this to be attractive or guided toward plants they feel drawn to the most. This approach helps them find plants most suited to their lives. The setting of these walks is not restricted to nature only but can occur anywhere nature is available, including the city and city parks. Subsequently, the spiritual nature of foraging requires herbalism to connect with herbalist practice intuitively. Some helpful tips for navigating foraging with intention include:

- Never take more than you need. Responsible foraging means being aware of the long-term effects of over-harvesting on the environment and always avoiding it.
- Focus on the leaves instead of the plant body when picking plants.
- Pick plants before the fruits and seeds start to form to ensure the plant's natural life cycle is not disrupted.
- Harvest flowers, stems, and any part of the plant that will be eaten raw before noon to prevent the sun from causing them to wilt and lose their freshness.
- Preserve rare wild plants instead of picking them to assist nature conservation in the area.
- Stay well informed of endangered plant species in the area.
- When plants do not produce enough fruit to be harvested, they should remain in their natural environment to provide habitats for birds and other species.

Plant Identification

Foraging research has cultivated tools for plant identification. A set of basic questions have been developed for the classification of plants during foraging. These identifiers have been let in layperson's terms so that they can be understood by all herbalists alike. The desired plant can be identified by making use of the following questions:

- Is the foraged plant more commonly found in dry climates, wet climates, or sunny fields?
- What is the ideal environment for this plant to thrive?
- What are the temperature and rainfall conditions of the plant?

- What sort of plants share the same climate?
- What animals often feed on these types of vegetation?
- What types of insects can be found near this type of vegetation?

When considering the physical characteristics when foraging, the following questions should be asked:

- What physical traits can the plant be expected to show when harvesting? Will it be flowering, gathering berries, bearing seeds, or harboring green leaves?
- What is the type of leaf of the plant harvested? Is it toothed, lobed, divided, or oblong?
- In what ways are the leaves arranged?
- What do the flowers look like?
- What do the colors of the petals look like?
- What are the plant root structure and stem shape?
- Does the plant have thorns or hairs?
- What is the size of the plants and all their flowers?

Growing

Growing herbs in herbal practice often take more time and effort than buying them at the store. On the bright side, many medicinal herbs are easy to grow in almost any environment—indoors, inside, using a windowsill—to provide herbalists with year-round tools. When planning an herb garden, the following factors should be considered:

- **Space available for medicinal plants.** As such, medicinal trees require more space and sunlight to grow than small shrubs of herbs.
- **Exposure to sunlight.** Windows are great for plants that need minimal sunlight but can provide too little sunlight for plants that need maximum exposure.
- **Soil used.** The soil quality will affect the herb's medicinal properties. Hence, high-quality soil will lead to nutrient-rich plants.
- Other conditions, such as the climate, must be considered, as different plants thrive in different temperatures. For example, certain plants cannot be overwatered, or they will die; the converse is true for plants that have high water needs.

Herbalists often employ three standard gardening practices. These include outdoor gardens, container gardens, and growing plants under covers such as greenhouses. For outdoor gardens, consider the following:

- A range of herbs can be grown together at once if so desired.
- Look for those who can thrive regardless of external conditions. This is especially so for outdoor gardens since they are often exposed to unpredictable and harsh weather.
- Plenty of foliage should be incorporated into outdoor gardens to improve the soil's nutrients, which are exposed to harsh winds and rains.
- Plants requiring special conditions should be planted outside in containers or shady, sheltered areas.

In the case of container gardens, herbal plants such as peppermint and bay laurel are often grown in pots, hanging baskets, or window baskets for easier access during everyday herbal practice. To keep your plants healthy, make sure they are not getting overly exposed to the sun. It is also essential to loosen the soil around them regularly, as this can help prevent the roots from becoming bound in cases where they outgrow their pot. For container gardens, try to move them to sheltered areas when harsher weather is expected.

Lastly, greenhouses can create the right environment for plants that require special conditions. These may include plants that need protection from the elements or those that are delicate and exotic. Plants such as lemongrass, often used in herbal practices, are planted in greenhouses using seedlings. Likewise, such plants are usually safer for culinary use because they are kept indoors and poison-free. Other plants, such as holy basil, prefer indoor climates. The same can be said for aloe vera plants, with the added benefit of taking poisonous chemicals from the air around us.

Plant Cultivation and Growing

The following tips should be remembered when planning a garden and choosing herbs:

1. **The site:** Most medicinal plants require a sunny area with well-drained or airy soil. The site can be improved by planting hedges nearby to protect grown herbs from the wind. Delicate herbs can be planted in sheltered sunny corners. Land used previously under harsher conditions—such as construction and industrial use—should not be used for delicate plant flowers as they might have been contaminated.
2. **Temperature:** Plants are sensitive to changes in temperature. Some plants only survive under very specific temperature ranges and will not survive extreme heat or frost. Rosemary, for example, is very susceptible to changes in temperature. Likewise, plants should also be planted out of direct contact with the wind to avoid wind-chill factors; most herbs should be grown in spring. Meanwhile, a greenhouse is a way to maintain stable optimal temperature conditions for a specific plant type. This is often the only way to keep subtropical plants cool. On the other hand, certain plants will be provided with warm sunny conditions all year round using a greenhouse.
3. **Soil quality:** Soil type varies greatly depending on the constituents of soil and clay mixtures. Sandy soils, for example, drain quickly and need constant feeding to provide plant nutrients. On the other hand, clay soils often become waterlogged and need to be drained.
4. **Pruning techniques:** Certain plant parts should be removed using delicate pruning techniques to stimulate plant growth. As such, pruning removes dead wood and leaves to improve plant shape, size, and quality. Subsequently, it should be timed to the correct harvest for each plant. Deadheading, or removing dead flowers from your plants, encourages new growth. This also reduces pests and diseases by keeping the plant healthy.
5. **Watering:** After planting, it is crucial to water your plants properly. Aim for at least once a week and split it between the morning and evening. Do not over-water them; some herbs usually do best in drier conditions. Also, if you transplant a potted plant into the ground, give it some water before doing so.
6. **Plant care:** Weeding is essential to keep plants healthy and prevent them from competing for resources. Pots, beds, and containers should be regularly weeded as well. Medicinal plants should not be fertilized or mulched to preserve their strength and healing properties. However, soils

should be supplied with good-quality fertilizer for adequate plant growth. Sandy soils need higher amounts of fertilizer to ensure proper plant nutrition.
7. **Pests and disease:** Organic remedies can be a great way to treat plant pests. Soapy and garlic water, made up of garlic skins steeped in water for two days, are a few examples. Once decontamination is complete, keeping infected plants separate from healthy ones is necessary.

Propagation Methods

Propagation methods often vary from plant to plant. The process that is most suited to the plant should be chosen. Various propagation methods include the following:

1. **Seeds.** When planting seeds, you can sow them directly into healthy soil or the ground. Once they have grown into seedlings, wait until the right season before transplanting them outdoors so that they can reach their full potential. Annual and biennial plants can proliferate from seeds and will continue to grow strongly through summer once they have sprouted. The germination requirements of each plant should be investigated to assess if the plant will be available for herbalist needs.
2. **Plant cuttings.** Plants such as woody perennial herbs can be grown from plant cuttings. These cuttings are usually taken from the plant stem or roots. It is recommended that cuts are made just below the leaves and stem using a sharp, clean knife. Any remaining leaves are stripped from the stem, which should be covered in hormone-rooting powder before planting into soil. This method only works for some, and proper care should be taken to ensure it suits the chosen shrub.
3. **Root splitting:** Plant germination that grows in the ground can be done by root splitting. Autumn is usually when herbalists divide spring-flowering herbaceous plants, while those flowering in autumn typically get divided in spring. To do this, gently remove a fully grown plant from its soil and break it into sections. Then those sections can then be replanted.
4. **Layering.** A propagation method called layering is when a root or stem is encouraged to produce roots by cutting its underside, burying it in soil, and watering it. The tip must remain above the ground until the layer of roots has formed, at which point it can be taken out of the pot where it had been planted. This practice is also referred to as mold layering.

Harvesting

Homegrown plants offer herbalists a constant source of fresh material. Before gathering, the garden must be kept up with pruning and eliminating undesirable weeds. Likewise, when harvesting, the plant should be cut carefully to avoid damage and encourage quicker regrowth for perennials. Harvesting equipment usually features trays or baskets crafted from wood to collect harvests as necessary. These trays help preserve the plant during collection. If harvesting in wild settings, non-nylon rucksacks are suitable for picking foliage. In any case of uncertainty regarding the identity of plants, a field guide can prove helpful in proper identification.

After harvesting, handle them as little as possible and make small incisions to minimize damage. Wear gloves in case of an allergic reaction. Also, it is essential to harvest only those free from disease, damage, and insect infestation and refrain from mixing up any harvested plants in case of confusion. To avoid wastage, do not gather additional plant material, as these can deteriorate very quickly, thus weakening the active ingredients. Lastly, harvest the correct plant part, as not all components can be used.

Processing of Herbs

Once herbs are pulled from the ground, they typically undergo processing for various uses. Keeping their freshness and flavor intact, these plants are often preserved through either air-drying or oven-drying. Sometimes, a warm, dry place can be used to do this. Then, a plain paper should be used over printed paper when drying herbs. Yet, it should be noted that different parts of plants are stored differently. In the case of parts of the plant growing above ground, these include stems, leaves, flowers, berries, and seeds. Stems are usually cut a few inches above the ground after the plant flowers. Perennial flowers, on the other hand, are often cut higher above the ground so that growth can happen much faster. Then, large flowers and leaves should be removed and dried separately. Smaller leaves, however, should be dried on the leaf's stem.

How to Dry Herbs

1. Bunches of herbs of— eight to ten stems—are strewn together and hung in a warm, airy, dark place. The herb bunches should not be tightly packed, and air should circulate freely.
2. Once the herb leaves are brittle but not completely dry, the stems and leaves of the plant should be separated. This can be done by rubbing the bunches of dried shrubs over a piece of paper to separate the leaves, stems, seeds, and flowers from each other.
3. Dried-out separated herbs are carefully poured from the paper sheet into a dark jar for safe storage. Then the glass jar is then sealed and stored away safely.

Processing Large Flowers

Large flowers are often harvested just after blooming; this happens during spring or summer. Often, with flower harvesting, only the petals of flowers are harvested. This can be done as follows:

1. Separate the flower heads from the stems once fully bloomed and remove any dirt or insects.
2. Place the flowers on an absorbent piece of paper to dry and leave them air-dried, allowing circulation.
3. When dried, take off the petals and store them in a dark jar or brown paper bag.

In the case of small flowers, the process of drying is much different:

1. Pick smaller flowers with the stalk still attached.
2. Enclose them in a paper bag over a tray and hang them upside down to dry, especially for smaller flowers such as lavender.

Harvesting Fruit and Berries

Fall is the perfect season to pick fruit and berries for the best results. Yet, ensure they are firm and not overripe when harvesting, which will affect the drying process. These berries can also be picked individually or in bunches, then placed on absorbent paper. They are then put into a warm oven—wholly switched off—with the oven door left slightly open for about three hours until completely dried. After this, the berries are removed and left in a dry, warm site in the dark, where they are turned occasionally. Removing moldy fruit or berries from the rest of the batch is essential, so they do not become infected.

Harvesting Roots, Rhizomes, Tubers, and Bulbs

In the case of root harvestings, roots such as *Eupatorium purpureum, Phytolacca Americana,* and *Urtica dioica* are usually gathered in autumn harvest time. For instance, Phytolacca americana is harvested after the parts of the plant above the ground have died and before the soil becomes too hard or soggy. Alternatively, some roots can be harvested in the earliest spring before it becomes old or unusable due to exposure to air. One should dig deeply around the plant body to remove it carefully from the ground to harvest plant roots. When roots are hard to pull out, a tap from the bottom is often used to release them from the soil. Then, the needed section is removed while the rest of the plant remains in place.

The process of harvesting roots is as follows:

1. Rinse dirt from the roots under warm water and shake off excess soil.
2. Discard all small or damaged roots.
3. Slice the root or tuber into pieces using a sharp knife.
4. Place the pieces on absorbent paper on a tray and place them in a warm oven with the door open for three hours.
5. Allow drying thoroughly in a warm location afterward.

Harvesting Seeds

Fundamental in the plant life cycle, harvesting seeds involves gathering mature seeds from various plants, ensuring their viability for future growth and propagation. To start, identify when the plants have reached maturity and their seeds are developed. Carefully remove the seed heads or pods and place them in a dry and well-ventilated area. Allow the seeds to dry, ensuring they are moisture-free to prevent mold or rot. Once dry, gently extract the seeds from their casings or pods and store them in labeled envelopes or airtight containers. Remember to store them in a cool and dark location to maintain viability.

Buying

For those who are not growing or foraging plants, buying is always an option. Many nurseries provide the necessary tools for safe herbal practice, offering a variety of medicinal herbs to purchase. Ensure that you buy standard medicinal shrubs and plants if you intend to use them for therapeutic benefit, as opposed to genetically enhanced ones. Dried herbs can be purchased too, so herbalists do not have to prepare and dry them before use. Tips for storing and buying both dried and wet herbs are also available, such as:

- Avoid using transparent jars that let in sunlight, as this may cause unnecessary oxidation and reduce the effectiveness of dried herbs. Instead, choose clean dark glass containers with airtight seals to ensure longer storage.
- Store herbs in brown paper bags away from direct sunlight if jars are unavailable.

- Do not use metal containers, as they contaminate dry and wet herbs.
- Herbs can be kept up to 12 months before discarding; those frozen in plastic or zip-lock bags should only be kept for six months.
- Labeling the herbs with their date of harvesting is helpful so you can keep track of how long they should be kept.
- Good quality dried herbs are aromatic and brightly colored; check for signs of infestation or adulteration before purchasing them.
- Assess the age of the herbs. For instance, calendula can usually be a vivid yellow or orange, which can turn drab or pale when left on the shelf for too long.
- Observe the expiry date.
- If any infection is observed in stored herbs, remove affected areas, and discard them in a plastic bag; sterilize the container before placing the remaining herbs back into it.

4

Preparation

No herbalist practice is complete without tools. This chapter will expand on the most common tools needed for herbalism practice.

Tools/Equipment

Below you will find a list of essential tools for any aspiring herbalist.

Storage Containers

Keeping and storing herbal remedies can be made easy using containers. Mason jars, glass bottles, and tins are some of the most recommended containers to store dry herbs, herbal products, or mixtures. If you want to give away these remedies as gifts, wrappers, and decorations can make them look beautiful. For a more economical option, reuse and recycle jars previously used for spaghetti sauce or jam. Just remember to properly clean and disinfect the container before use. Yet, if you cannot find suitable containers from store-bought items, many shops offer spray bottles, tins, or cans that can be useful alternatives.

Kitchen Scales

Accurate measurements are essential when making herbal remedies, so weight-sensitive kitchen scales are necessary. These should be measured in either grams or ounces, as exact measurements must be calculated for tinctures and other ratio-dependent formulas. Investing in such scales ensures you get the right ingredients every time.

Mixing Bowls and Saucepans

For accurate measurements and mixing of herbs, a kitchenware collection is recommended. It is best to stock up on glass, stone, or enamel-coated saucepans and stainless-steel bowls and pans for stirring. A range of different bowl sizes is also helpful for various other purposes. At the same time, enamel-coated pans are preferable as they are more durable and do not stick as quickly.

Measuring Utensils

Measuring utensils like cups, spoons, and cylinders are helpful when preparing herbal remedies. These tools can help ensure the correct amounts of solvents, herbs, and waxes for a specific treatment. Fortunately, these items may already be part of your kitchen supplies and have been used for precise measurements. With this equipment, you can measure accurate portions of solvents or tinctures whenever needed.

Kitchen Utensils

To mix ingredients into a herbal remedy, it is best to keep tools such as spoons, spatulas, knives, kitchen scissors, and cutting boards on hand. This allows one to cut, whip, and mix the components of a remedy into smaller sizes. A mortar and pestle can also be kept on hand for grinding dried and fresh herbs. Another handy kitchen tool for herbal mixtures is a spice grinder which can be used for grinding down spices for herbal remedies. Other kitchen utensils such as funnels, strainers, and cheesecloths can also be used for straining and bottling herbal remedy mixes.

Foraging Bag

Put some thought into the type of bag used for collecting your herbs. A lightweight cotton or canvas bag can be perfect for gathering plants and mushrooms without risking damage to your haul. Such a foraging bag also offers valuable storage space for any harvested items.

Scissors, Shears, Knives, Hand Lens

Having the right tools when foraging herbs for herbal remedies is essential. Scissors are handy for clipping flowers, stems, and other small branches. If you need to cut bigger roots or branches, pruning shears should do the trick. For harvesting bark, a pocketknife will suffice. Before you collect any plants, a hand lens can be used to look for signs of disease, pests, or bacteria.

Notebook

Taking notes while creating herbal remedies or recipes is a great way to track adjustments. Plus, having everything written down when collecting herbs from a store or in the wild is beneficial. Memory can sometimes fail us, so having something to record important information in is essential for any herbalist. If you do not have a notebook, loose papers can be organized in a binder with all your notes and recipes.

Writing Utensils

Other writing utensils, such as pens, paper, or colored pencils, can be used when writing down recipes or information when making herbal remedies. These writing utensils can also be used to sketch, draw, or even paint plant sketches, so they can be identified when foraging or buying herbal remedies online.

Source Materials

Books are a must-have for identifying herbs and herbal remedies. As such, books can offer a wealth of knowledge when looking for herbal remedies or trying to understand the properties of plants and their healing benefits. But nowadays, computers have become a powerful source of information as well. Not only can they help with research, but they also facilitate communication with other experienced herbalists. With many online techniques and resources, computers are essential to any modern herbalist's tool kit.

Ingredients

To successfully create herbal remedies and recipes, it is essential to use the right ingredients. Below you will find the ingredients necessary for any budding herbalist's repertoire.

Herbs

No herbalist practice is complete without herbs; this is a given. Depending on the practice you choose, herbs can be sourced from your backyard, or they can even be purchased from your local shops. They can even be sourced online. An array of herbs is often needed depending on the treatment to be made or your health and wellness needs. Starter herb collection kits are also available for those who are starting. It is essential to assess the quality of herbs before purchasing, which is why store-bought or self-grown herbs are recommended.

Solvents

When crafting herbal preparations, solvents are essential to provide a stable base for the mixtures. Common solvents used in such recipes include alcohols, syrups, tinctures, and infused oils. Carrier oils are also popular, including almonds, jojoba, grapeseed, and coconut oil. Each carrier oil offers its unique benefits and can be used to enhance the effects of the herbal remedy.

In addition to other solvents, alcohols can also be utilized in herbal preparations. Selecting the appropriate type of alcohol depends mainly on its percentage; some common examples include vodka, gin, rum, brandy, and whiskey. Moreover, alcohols are the basis for herbal tinctures. Vinegar, such as apple cider or white wine vinegar, is also used as a solvent. Natural solvents also often include honey and glycerin, popular in herbal mixtures and recipes.

Wax and Butter

Salves, creams, and body butter often contain waxes and butter as principal components. Beeswax and other natural solvents such as candelilla, carnauba, and soy are usually included in the recipe. Additionally, cocoa, shea, avocado, and kokum are common types of butter used in salves. It is important to remember that waxes and butter have a limited shelf life; they expire between several months to a year. Thus, purchasing smaller quantities of waxes and butter is recommended, so they can be replaced once they expire.

Methods

Different methods of utilizing herbs have evolved, providing various options for individuals to utilize in achieving their desired outcomes from herbal remedies. Below are some strategies commonly used in the practice of herbalism.

Powdering

Powdered herbs are a convenient and easy way to incorporate herbal remedies into one's daily routine. Generally, they can be taken as capsules, sprinkled over food, mixed with water, or applied directly to the skin or wounds. Additionally, powdered herbs can be combined with other forms of medicine, such as tinctures and poultices, for more potent effects. Quality is essential when choosing powdered herbs; grades that have been more finely milled are typically considered superior. For those wishing to make their herbal capsules at home, store-bought gelatin or vegetarian capsules can be filled with powder for maximum convenience and control over ingredients used in remedies. The steps on how to make sure such capsules are outlined below.

1. Pour the powder into a saucer or capsule-making tray.
2. Slide vegetarian pill capsules towards one another on the saucer to scoop up the powder.
3. Fill each capsule until it is half full and store it later.

For herbal capsules:

- Size 00 capsules should be filled with up to 250 mg of powder.
- The recommended dosage is two or three pills a day, depending on the strength of the herbal remedy.
- Store the capsules in airtight, dark glass containers in cool, dry places.
- Discard capsules after three to four months.

Crushing

A mortar and a pestle are often used for crushing and mixing dried herbs and can be used as follows:

1. Place your herbs and spices into the mortar bowl and hold steady with one hand.
2. Using the other hand, hold the pestle and press the pestle down into the mortar to grind or blend the herbs.
3. Move the pestle back and forth in the mortar to blend the herbs.

Grinding dried and fresh herbs using a mortar and pestle is an effective way to prepare your desired ingredients. For this purpose, it is advisable to have a separate one for edible herbs so that no harmful plants or their remnants are consumed.

Infusion

Creating an herbal remedy, tea, or a soothing beverage, infusions are ideal for gently extracting the delicate parts of herbaceous plants like leaves and flowers. These can come as single herbs or blends of multiple herbs, either hot or cold, per your preference. To make them, you need to follow the instructions provided:

1. Place the herb in a strainer and submerge it into a cup of boiled water.

2. Cover the cup with a lid and let the boiling mixture infuse for 10 minutes.
3. Remove the strainer and herbs afterward, leaving a concentrated herbal mixture behind.
4. Add a teaspoon of honey or sugar, then drink as desired.

Likewise, making a pot infusion is easy and can be tailored to your liking. Simply fill the pot with herbs and cover it with boiling water. Put a lid on and let the contents infuse. Once infused, strain the herbs, add any desired sweetener, and enjoy your concoction.

Cream

Making medicinal creams or lotions is a simple and effective way to provide soothing relief for various skin ailments. Here are the general steps for making your medicinal creams or lotions:

1. **Choose your medicinal herbs.** The first step is choosing the herbs you want to use in your cream or lotion. You can choose from various herbs, such as calendula, chamomile, lavender, and plantain.
2. **Prepare your herbal infusion.** Once you have selected your herbs, you must prepare an herbal infusion by steeping the herbs in boiling water. Either you use fresh or dried herbs for this step. Then, allow the herbs to soak for about 20 to 30 minutes before straining out the plant material.
3. **Melt your base ingredients.** In a separate pot, melt the base ingredients for your cream or lotion. Typically, a mixture of oil and water is used as the base. For example, you can combine coconut oil and beeswax as the oil component and distilled water as the water component.
4. **Mix in your herbal infusion.** Once your base ingredients are melted, slowly add your herbal infusion while stirring. Continue stirring until the mixture has cooled down and thickened to a cream or lotion-like consistency.
5. **Add optional ingredients.** For additional benefits, you can also add other optional ingredients, such as essential oils, vitamin E oil, or honey.
6. **Store your cream or lotion.** Once you have finished making your cream or lotion, pour it into a sterilized jar or container and store it in a cool, dark place. It should last for several months.

Meanwhile, ointments are oil-based and form an applicable protective layer over the skin when injured, inflamed, or damaged. They can be beneficial in relieving problems like hemorrhoids and moisturizing dry lips or diaper rash. Unlike creams, ointments do not require water, making them an excellent choice for those seeking an effective solution to skin care needs.

Follow these steps to make ointments:

7. Put a glass bowl in a pan of boiling water and add organic oils or waxes to melt.
8. Chop herbs finely, then simmer for 10 to 15 minutes while stirring constantly.
9. Fasten a jelly bag onto the rim of a jug with a string and pour the mixture through it to filter out impurities.
10. Wearing rubber gloves, press the hot liquid from the herbal mixture through the jelly bag into the jug.

11. Pour the molten mixture into jars before it solidifies and cools, then lightly place their lids on without screwing them closed.
12. Once cooled, securely close each jar's lid.

After making your ointments, remember to label the jars and store them in a cool, dry place. Different consistencies are often used for various purposes. For instance, solid ointments can be used as lip balms and prepared with mineral oils. To make them follow these steps:

1. Melt 140g of coconut oil and 120g of beeswax.
2. Mix the melted coconut oil and beeswax with 100g of powdered herbs.
3. Place this mixture in a glass bowl and over a pan of boiling water.
4. Simmer together for up to 90 minutes.
5. Once cooked sufficiently, strain and pour into jars.

For less solid ointments, such as ointments for skin rashes, a similar procedure is followed:

1. Melt 60g of beeswax and 500 ml of olive oil in a glass bowl over a pan of boiling water.
2. Mix with 120g of dried or 300g of fresh herbs.
3. Once mixed, the mixture is covered and placed in a warm oven for up to three hours. After which, it is removed, strained, and poured into separate jars.
4. An alternative for beeswax and olive oil can be made by combining 500ml hot infused oil and 60g of melted beeswax.

Sap Collection

Collecting sap is best done in either spring or autumn, depending on the tree or plant. For example, silver birch trees are often tapped for their sap, and a hole of almost a quarter of its diameter must be bored into the trunk. A container should be placed below it to collect the fluid once it is produced. Plants like aloe vera can harvest their gel by slicing the leaf sideways and peeling back the edges. After gathering almost a quart of sap, seal the hole using resin or wood filler.

Latex Collection

Latex, a milky sap or juice, is collected from the stems of plants such as dandelions by cutting them open and squeezing them over a jar or container. However, it is essential to note that latex can be caustic to the skin, so gloves should be worn while collecting sap.

Cooking

Typically, plants added for zest, taste, or appearance in food have medicinal value. A good example is rosemary, often added to red meat because it aids digestion and holds medicinal properties.

Meanwhile, lemon is also used in the same way as an accompaniment to fish due to its strong antiseptic properties, which can help treat colds and stomach-related issues. It may even be used as a treatment for food poisoning. In China, food beneficial for your health is called "medicine." Medicinal herbs can also be incorporated into cooking in various ways, such as:

- Hot spices, like turmeric, chili powder, cardamom, and ginger, are often used in meals for protection from stomach diseases and infections.
- Medicinal herbs are great additions to smoothies and can be combined with ginseng to provide extra vitality when dealing with mental or physical stress.
- Adding medicinal herbs and tinctures to salads can enhance and bring more flavor.

Concoction

Concoctions or decoctions are usually prepared using roots, barks, and berries. At times they may have leaves, flowers, and other delicate parts of the flowers included. They can be prepared as follows:

1. Place the herbs into a saucepan on the stove.
2. Cover with cold water and bring to a boil.
3. Simmer for 30 minutes until a third of the liquid has been boiled.
4. Strain through a sieve and into a jug.
5. Pour the required amount into a cup and drink as desired.
6. Store the rest of the mixture in a cold, dry jar and use it before expiration.

Boiling and Inhaling its Smoke

Inhalation of steam, using herbs and boiling water, is an effective remedy for throat and respiratory tract ailments such as congestion, asthma, sinusitis, and hay fever. The process can help to clear airways and respiratory tracts with antiseptic herbal remedies. To create a steam inhalation using herbal remedies, do the following:

1. Fill a large bowl with boiling water.
2. Add 5 to 10 drops of herbal essential oils.
3. An infusion of 25g of herbs can also be added to one liter of water.
4. This mixture should be allowed to steep for 30 minutes.
5. Cover your head with a soft towel and close your eyes to inhale the steam.
6. Inhale steam for up to 11 minutes until the herbal remedy cools.
7. One should stay in a warm room for 30 to 45 minutes after steaming to clear up mucus completely.

Risks

Just like everything, herbal and medicinal practices must be practiced in moderation. Many plants are poisonous, so ensure you are fully aware of all the herbal remedy ingredients before ingesting them. For children, a pediatrician should be consulted before a herbal remedy is diagnosed. Also, stick to the recommended dosage to prevent overdosing. As such, herbal products should be consumed in small amounts to avoid severe side effects. Products that have worked in small doses could often have negative side effects or allergic reactions in larger doses. Hence, monitor your body's reaction for any severe side effects. In the case of rash, dizziness, heavy breathing, or severe allergic reactions, a doctor should be consulted; this may be an anaphylactic reaction.

Many herbs may be dangerous and cause reactions even with little exposure. If collecting plants from the wild, be aware that some may be toxic. When making your remedies, steer clear of substances such as aonite, arnica, belladonna, and yohimbine, as they can potentially be fatal. Thus, herbs should be inspected and adequately identified before adding them to herbal remedies.

Pillar 3
Profiles

In pillar 3, it covers different herbs, plants, flowers, and wood profiles, covering an array of natural remedies essential to holistic health. From Agrimony to Yarrow, this rich chapter dives into the medicinal properties of these wonders of nature. Focusing on plants like dandelion and garlic reveals their benefits to human health by potentially reducing fever, lowering blood pressure, and providing antispasmodic effects. Further exploration in the chapter unravels how other herbs, plants, and flowers are used for their healing powers.

5

Herbs, Plants, Flowers, and Wood Profiles

Agrimony

Agrimony is commonly used for:

- Sore throats
- Upset stomach
- Diarrhea
- Irritable bowel syndrome
- Diabetes
- Gallbladder disorders
- Antihistamine
- Sedative
- Fluid retention
- Cancer
- Corns and warts
- Tuberculosis

This herbal remedy contains tannins which have healing properties and can be applied directly to the skin as a drying agent for open wounds or to reduce redness, swelling, and inflammation. Agrimony should be taken in small doses, as tannins can be unsafe when taken in large amounts.

Aloe Vera

Native to Africa, Aloe vera is a potted plant with transparent gel often used to treat wounds and burns. It has been said that using it can accelerate the healing of these injuries while minimizing the threat of infection. The plant is also widely employed for:

- Laxative for constipation
- Skin treatments
- Treatment of burns
- Skin conditions
- Sunburn
- Varicose veins
- Treatment of ulcers and irritable bowel syndrome
- To boost appetite while drinking water

However, before using Aloe vera, there are certain safety measures to consider:

- Avoid applying bitter yellow aloe juice directly to the skin, which could cause irritation and reactions.
- Pregnant and nursing women should avoid consuming bitter aloe.
- People with hemorrhoids or kidney conditions should not consume Aloe vera.

Moreover, aloe vera can be prepared for treating burns and eczema by breaking open the leaf and collecting the gel. This gel should be generously applied twice a day for the best results.

Angelica

Angelica, distinguishable by its bright green leaves, greenish-whitish flowers, and ridged upright hollow stems, can be found in Europe, the Himalayas, and Siberia. Often grown near running water in cool, damp sites, it is harvested during early summer for its root, leaves, stems, and seeds. Known to contain volatile oils like beta-phellandrene, lactones, and coumarins, Angelica root has been used for medicinal purposes:

- Anti-inflammatory conditions
- Severe colic
- Relieves indigestion and gas
- Improves blood flow in various parts of the body
- Treatment of buerger's disease
- Dilates narrowed arteries
- Phlegm
- Bronchitis
- Various chest conditions

Ashwagandha

Identifiable by its evergreen shrubbery, Ashwagandha, also known as Indian ginseng or winter cherry, is found in many regions, including India, the Middle East, and Africa. Harvested for its roots and orange-red fruits, it has various medicinal uses, such as reducing fatigue, skin conditions, and inflammation and treating diabetes and epilepsy. Additionally, it is known to bring a calming effect to those with stress and anxiety; its ability to reduce cortisol and stress hormones affects this. It has even been shown to act as a natural pain reliever for joint pain and rheumatoid arthritis.

Betony

Found mainly in Europe, Western Asia, and Northern Africa, Betony has a long history as a medicinal herb. Dried for use in medicines by various cultures, Betony has been known to treat asthma, heartburn, bladder stones, kidney stones, and diarrhea. Likewise, it is also helpful for those suffering from high blood pressure problems; it reduces hypertension and relieves headaches and anxiety.

Calendula

With its identifiable bright orange petals, calendula has long been used as a home remedy for inflamed skin. It can stop infection while speeding up the healing process and being employed to cleanse and detoxify the body. For chronic conditions, calendula infusions are an option many have tried with success due to their essential components, triterpenes, resins, bitter glycosides, volatile oil, sterols, flavonoids, mucilage, and carotenes, which possess powerful healing properties. Their key actions include:

- Anti-inflammatory properties
- Muscles spasm relief
- Astringent
- Hemorrhaging cures
- Healing wounds
- Detoxifying properties
- Mild estrogenic

Calendula is regularly used to make infusions, tinctures, creams, and ointments, all of which may offer their benefits in terms of treatment. These preparations can help ease inflammation and combat infection, relieving the user.

Cat's Claw

Cat's claw, identified by its woody vines and hook-like thorns, has been used in parts of the Amazon and South and Central America. The barks and roots of this medicinal plant have often been harvested and used to strengthen the immune system, relax, smooth tense muscles, dilate constricted blood vessels, and act as a natural diuretic. Moreover, it has also been known to be rich in antioxidants to combat free radicals that damage cells and cause cancer and heart disease.

Catnip

Catnip, which its dark green, oval-toothed leaves can identify, has often been used in parts of Central Europe, the Northern United States, and Canada for medicinal use. Its dried leaves and white flowering tops are harvested to treat stomach cramps and indigestion, induce appetite, regulate menstrual cycles, and treat diarrhea, colic, common colds, and cancer. The herb can also be made into a tea to treat anxiety, nervous conditions, and hives. Likewise, dried catnip leaves have been smoked and inhaled to treat respiratory infections. Plus, it can be used to make a poultice, which is applied externally to reduce swelling.

Cayenne

Cayenne's hot, burning taste makes it an ideal addition to many dishes. Its medicinal properties are beneficial for circulation, digestion, and removal of toxins from the body. It can also help with arthritis, chilblains, colic, and diarrhea. The key ingredients include capsaicin, carotenoids, flavonoids, volatile oils, and steroidal saponins, which improve rheumatic and arthritic conditions. Additionally, the cayenne powder can be used in cooking with infused oils, tinctures, tablets, and ointments to relieve gas and colic.

Chamomile

Rich in terpenoids and flavonoids, chamomile flowers offer medicinal benefits that can help with various ailments. As such, drinking chamomile tea treats hay fever, muscle spasms, ulcers, insomnia and restless sleep, hemorrhoids, irregular menstruations, arthritis, and gastrointestinal disorders. Furthermore, it helps with wounds and may even have some anti-inflammatory benefits.

Chaste Tree

Known as a chaste berry, the chaste tree is widely used to combat hormone imbalances. The benefits of this herb are plentiful and include aiding with PMS symptoms such as low mood, breast pain, and bloating. As a precaution, chaste trees should not be taken when breastfeeding, taking birth control, planning for pregnancy, or having conditions sensitive to hormones, such as breast and prostate cancer. A doctor should also be consulted for any signs of a bad reaction, like throwing up, headaches, diarrhea, and changes in menstrual cycles.

Cinnamon

Since 500 B.C., cinnamon has been utilized in India, Europe, and Egypt for its healing abilities. Its uses range from treating ailments, such as:

- Colds and flu
- Digestive problems
- Antiviral remedies
- Boost blood circulation
- Nausea
- Diarrhea
- Regulates menstrual cycle

The parts often include the inner bark and twigs used to make infusions, tinctures, essential oils, and powders.

Cleavers

Cleavers, identified by their greenish-white flowers and tiny bristles that stick to clothing, have often been in parts of Europe, North America, Asia, Greenland, and Australia. Its fruits and seeds are often dried and roasted to a brew-like coffee to treat:

- Eczema
- Psoriasis
- Cancer
- Ulcers
- Burns
- Acne

- Swelling
- Swollen glands
- Urinary tract infections

They are prepared as juice, herbal tincture, and tea and are consumed according to the recommended dosage.

Corn Silk

Cornsilk or Barbe de Maïs have not only been a staple food item in South America for the last 4,000 years. They have also been used medicinally to:

- Treat urinary tract conditions
- Increase milk production
- Stop uterine hemorrhaging
- Induce childbirth
- Diuretic
- Stimulate bile secretion
- Lower blood pressure
- Reduce blood clotting
- Treat bruises
- Sores
- Boils
- Treat itching skin
- Useful diuretic for those who have trouble urinating
- Treat frequent irritation caused by the inflammation of the bladder and urethral walls
- Help prostate disorders
- Counteract kidney stone formation
- Treat chronic cystitis
- Treats fluid retention and jaundice

The critical compounds of corn and corn silk include flavonoids, alkaloids, allantoin, saponins, mucilage, vitamins C and K, and potassium, which allow medicinal healing through corn silk.

Dandelion

Also known as lion's tooth, fairy clock, or moon watcher, dandelion is an herbal remedy widely used for its healing properties. A sunflower family member, it can be found in woods, fields, urban spaces, and even lawns between concrete slabs. Blooming throughout summer and winter, dandelion's un-branched and hollow stems are easily identified by one branch per flower with year-round leaves.

They are often confused for the following:

- Wild lettuce has smaller flowers with taller plants and jagged-toothed leaves that differ from those of dandelions.
- Sow thistle bears a close resemblance to dandelion and shares its properties.
- Cat's ear or false dandelion is often confused for true dandelion but can be identified by its hairy leaves with contour wavy or jagged edges and small, tinted yellow seed ball.

Subsequently, dandelions can be identified by their:

- Sharp-toothed or jaggedly shaped leaves, with some described as spear-shaped in certain areas.
- Circular leaf arrangement, forming a basal rosette.
- Lengths up to 12 inches can also be as small as three inches long.
- Deep green and lobed, with toothed edges and no noticeable veins.
- Lack of hair on the bottom of their leaves.

Moreover, they can be identified by their stems, which have the following characteristics:

- A purple tone.
- Milky sap inside when broken open.
- Hollow interiors.

Likewise, the following features can identify dandelion flowers:

- Bright yellow flowers of approximately one to two inches in width.
- Flat and broad petals.
- Many florets.
- Curved shapes start from the underside of the flower.
- Transformation into puffballs upon flowering.

Lastly, dandelion roots are typically described as having the following:

- Fleshiness.
- Branchy tangles around the root.
- Dark brown or white coloring.

Dandelions are often favored in herbalism due to their ability to regenerate quickly. They are edible and can be used in roasted vegetable dishes, in tea, or fried in oil and butter, they can be added to a salad or dried and added to a smoothie, or they can be pickled in wines and vinegar. The stems of these flowers are often used in stir-fry, soups, salads, and smoothies, making them versatile for various uses.

Medicinal applications of dandelions include:

- Brewing herbal teas from boiled roots and leaves.
- Creating decoctions of boiled roots.
- Preparing tinctures made of boiled roots.
- Making poultices with leaves.

- Creating a concentrate to make syrup.
- Using the sap as a topical treatment for wounds.

Echinacea

Echinacea often increases the body's resistance to bacterial and viral infections. It does this by stimulating the body's immune system to act as an antibiotic, which relieves allergies and clears skin infections. Echinacea contains healing constituents, such as:

- Alkamides
- Caffeic acid esters
- Polysaccharides
- Humulene
- Echinolene
- Betaine

These healing constituents stimulate the immune system, act as an antibiotic, detoxify by sweating, heal wounds, and act as an antiallergenic.

Elder

The elder tree, recognizable from its cream-colored blossoms and blue-black berries, is often used as a remedy for various ailments, such as:

- Colds and flu
- Chesty conditions
- Mild diuretic
- Anti-inflammatory
- Fever
- Mucous linings in the nose and throat
- Allergies
- Ear infections
- Yeast infections
- Arthritis
- Rheumatism
- Erysipelas and other skin infections
- Mild laxative
- Diarrhea

As such, leaves and berries possess cyanogenic glycosides, flavonoids, anthocyanins, and vitamins A and C, which can be helpful for healing in multiple areas. This natural remedy has a variety of applications, from soothing irritation to boosting the immune system.

Elderberry

Elderberries contain antioxidants and vitamins that boost and heal the immune system. The berries and flowers are usually harvested and used as a treatment for:

- Inflammation
- Stress
- Colds and flu
- Constipation
- Joint and muscle pain
- Chest and respiratory tract infections
- Headaches and fevers
- Kidney problems
- Epilepsy
- Skin conditions
- Symptoms of HIV and AIDS

Plus, it is packed with vitamins C, B, B6, and E and antioxidants, which can help reduce inflammation. However, due to its diuretic nature, caution should be taken when using elderberry medicinally while pregnant or breastfeeding.

Elecampane

Identified by its golden yellow flowers and large pointy leaves, elecampane is a tonic herb used to treat respiratory issues. It contains essential compounds such as inulin, alantol, triterpene saponin, sterols, and polyacetylenes that benefit healing. Likewise, these elements work together to treat:

- Chronic bronchitis
- Coughing
- Worms
- Antiseptic for wounds
- Mucous and bronchial linings
- Immunity problems
- Chest infections
- Chronic chest issues
- Digestive problems
- Flu
- Tonsillitis

Fennel

Native to the Mediterranean, Fennel is identified by its yellow flowers, and its seeds are widely used as a cooking spice. Often mistaken for anise-flavored spices due to their similar look and taste, fennel also offers numerous healing benefits suitable for:

- Heartburn
- Intestinal gas
- Bloating
- Increase appetite
- Colic in infants
- Respiratory tract infections
- Coughs and bronchitis
- Cholera
- Backaches

Commonly, fennel powder is also used as a poultice to help treat snakebites. Additionally, it has been known to increase milk production in mothers, regulate menstrual cycles, ease labor and delivery, and even serve as an aphrodisiac.

Fenugreek

Fenugreek, which its clove-like appearance can identify, is native to the Mediterranean, Southern European, and Western Asian regions of the world. Its seeds have been commonly used in cooking but have also been used medicinally and can be identified by the smell and taste of maple syrup. For this reason, fenugreek is favored in spice blends, flavoring agents, beverages, and tobacco. Also, it has been used medicinally to:

- Slow down the absorption of sugar to stimulate the production of insulin.
- Lower blood sugar for people with diabetes.
- Improves testosterone and estrogen levels.
- Ease menstrual cramps.
- Lowers cholesterol levels.
- Manage obesity.

Feverfew

Feverfew is a favored medicinal herb for women; it has commonly been used for:

- Migraines and headaches
- Arthritis
- Rheumatism
- Analgesic
- Menstrual flow

It comprises volatile oils, sesquiterpene lactones, and camphor, which have healing and medicinal properties.

Garlic

Garlic, which is often identified by its strong odor and taste and is famous for home use, can be used to treat an array of health problems, including:

- Nose, throat, and chest infections
- Cholesterol
- Circulatory disorders
- High blood pressure
- Blood sugar
- Diabetes
- Blood clots
- Worms

Aside from that, garlic is high in vitamins A, B, C, and E, selenium, scordinins, allin, alliinase, and allicin.

Ginger

Ginger, revered in Asia for its uses and properties, can be identified by its stalks of white and yellow flowers and lance-shaped leaves. They have even been referenced in the Garden of Eden and have been recommended for relief for:

- Motion sickness and postoperative nausea
- Morning sickness
- Chilblains and circulation to the hands and feet
- Inflammation
- Antiseptic
- Digestive complaints such as indigestion
- Colic
- Gastrointestinal infections
- Food poisoning
- High blood pressure
- Breaks fevers
- Coughs, colds, and flu
- Respiratory problems
- Headaches
- Aching muscles
- Internal colds resulting in cold hands, weak pulse, and pale complexion
- Peptic ulcers

Zingiberene, gingerol, and shogaols are vital components that act in harmony to give the body a healing effect. Their combined power allows them to provide many health benefits effectively.

Ginkgo

Ginkgo is a deciduous tree that has often been used medicinally in China. It has been used to treat:

- Poor circulation in the brain
- Asthma
- Allergies
- Inflammation

Composed of flavonoids, ginkgolides, and bilobalide, Ginkgo can help soothe wheezing and coughing. It also has cognitive benefits, such as aiding memory and protecting against dementia. Additionally, it is often used to treat autoimmune problems and multiple sclerosis as well as for post-organ transplant recovery.

Ginseng

For almost 7000 years, Ginseng has been revered in Chinese medicine for its therapeutic effects. Easily identifiable by its round-toothed leaves and small yellowish-green flowers, it has been used to treat various ailments, including but not limited to:

- Fatigue
- Stress and emotional stress
- Colds
- Extremes of hunger and temperature
- Insomnia
- Immune deficiency and infection
- Liver problems
- Illness and old age
- Male aphrodisiac

Ginseng's constituents, including triterpenoid saponins, acetylenic compounds, panaxans, and sesquiterpenes, create a potent tonic beneficial health.

Goldenrod

Often seen in the wild, this bright yellow flower is commonly used in herbal supplements and teas to treat various ailments, such as:

- Urinary health
- Inflammation
- Yeast infections
- C and inflammation
- Free radicals
- Heart disease

This plant, native to many parts of the world, including Europe, Asia, and North and South America, is widely known for its healing properties. Beneficial elements such as saponins, flavonoids, and antioxidants like quercetin and kaempferol are among their active components.

Goldenseal

Widely used in traditional North American medicine, goldenseal has been used to heal wounds and ulcers, soothe inflamed eyes, repel insects, and treat stomach and liver ailments. It is still employed as an aid for various conditions in modern times, including:

- Astringent
- Antibacterial remedies
- Bodily mucous
- Tonics
- Constipation
- Internal bleeding
- Diuretic

The essential elements of this plant, including alkaloids, resin, and volatile oils, make it a valuable remedy for various body parts. These include the eyes, ears, nose, and throat, as well as the stomach, intestines, and vaginal mucus. Its uses are not restricted to external applications and can also be used as a mouthwash for gum infections or douche for yeast infections.

Hawthorn

In the Middle Ages, Hawthorn was often used for heart and circulatory disorders such as angina. Its healing properties include:

- Increasing blood flow to the heart and muscles
- Regulating normal heartbeat
- Dilating blood vessels
- Mild relaxant
- Antioxidant effects
- Relieve chest pains
- Acts against heart failure

Yet, precaution should be taken not to exceed the daily limit for each dosage.

Horsetail

Found in parts of Europe and Central America, horsetail, with its green and densely branched stems, has been used medicinally to treat wounds, enhance skin and hair, and boost bone health. It is also a natural diuretic that can help heal wounds as an ointment for skin regeneration. Rich in antioxidants and silica, it protects against free radicals, which can cause cell damage. This plant is very beneficial because its silica keeps skin, nails, hair, and bones healthy. Additionally, horsetail aids bone healing by metabolizing collagen to absorb calcium and increase bone density.

Kelp

Seaweed, known as kelp, is a green alga high in iodine. This nutrient is essential for proper thyroid functioning and has been used to treat various conditions, like:

- Hypothyroidism (decreased thyroid function)
- Hyperthyroidism (increased thyroid function)

Not only is kelp known for its iodine content. In fact, it has also been used to improve sensory receptors and promote healthy nails, blood vessels, digestion, and even constipation. Further, it has been applied in curing cases of various ailments, including:

- Hair loss
- Diabetes
- Weight fluctuation
- Gastrointestinal ulcers
- Breast cancer

However, caution should be taken when consuming, as too much kelp could lead to additional thyroid issues.

Lavender

Lavender can often be considered a relaxant that its purple flowers and clustering shrubbery can identify. Its key components, such as flavonoids, tannins, and coumarins can be used to treat:

- Muscle spasms
- Depression
- Insomnia
- Irritability
- Headaches and migraines
- Depression
- Indigestion
- Colic
- Gas and bloating
- Asthma
- Burns
- Wounds
- Sores

Massaging lavender oil into the temples and scalp can help to alleviate headaches. Likewise, it can be used on tense muscles to relieve tension and pain.

Lemon Balm

Lemon balm, which its white flowers and veiny leaves can identify, is a well-known treatment for the brain and memory. It can be used as a tonic for depression and the treatment of cold sores. Its key constituents of flavonoids, triterpenes, polyphenols, and tannins work in unison to treat:

- Overactive nervous system
- Antispasmodic
- Antiviral
- Wounds
- Toothaches
- Anxiety
- Depression
- Restlessness
- Digestive problems, including indigestion, nausea, and bloating
- Insect bites
- Fevers

Licorice

Licorice is a woody stemmed medicinal plant made up of glycyrrhizic acid that has been valued for its powerful anti-inflammatory properties. It can be used to treat:

- Arthritis
- Canker sores
- Constipation
- Adrenal gland disorders
- Asthma
- Digestive problems
- Gastritis
- Inflamed eyes

The key constituents of licorice include flavonoids, sterols, asparagine, coumarins, and polysaccharides.

Linden

Lindren, which is harvested for its dried flower, leaves, and wood, is commonly used in the treatment of:

- Colds
- Stuffy nose
- Sore throats
- Breathing problems such as bronchitis
- Headaches
- Fever
- Phlegm

- High blood pressure and rapid heartbeat
- Hemorrhage
- Nervous tension
- Insomnia
- Bladder control
- Muscle spasms

Meanwhile, the bark of linden trees is used for liver and gallbladder disease and swelling.

Marshmallow Root

Marshmallow root is usually harvested for its flowers, roots, and leaves for medicinal purposes. The mucilage is high in antioxidants which are good for the digestive tract. It can also treat skin irritation and digestive disorders, such as ulcers. Aside from that, it can be a remedy for:

- Cough syrups for severe dry coughs
- Respiratory tract infections
- Chronic dry mouth gum disease and dental infections
- Antihistamines
- Blood pressure
- Neurological problems and autoimmune disease
- Gastric ulcers
- Skin irritation and skin inflammation
- Eczema and skin damage from sun exposure
- Wounds

Usually, these roots are brewed as tea but can be ingested as cough syrup and root capsules, among other remedies.

Meadowsweet

Meadowsweet has been used since medieval times for gastric problems and inflammatory conditions such as arthritis. It contains salicylic acid, flavonol glycosides, phenolic glycosides, and tannins to act as the following:

- Diuretic
- Anti-inflammatory
- Ease stomach pain
- Antirheumatic
- Astringent

Salicylates can be thought of as aspirins that reduce inflammation and relieve pain. This unique cocktail of salicylates, tannins, and other properties protects the stomach's inner lining. It is also a remedy for indigestion reducing acidity in the stomach, which in turn levels acidity in the whole body.

Milk Thistle

In Europe, Milk thistle is known to be effective in treating depression. Apart from this, it has also been used to help with liver ailments, such as those caused by alcohol or food poisoning, due to its essential constituents, flavonolignans, and polyacetylenes, which protect the liver against damage and other toxic elements. Moreover, Milk thistle has even been used to treat liver damage caused by ingesting carbon tetrachloride or death cap mushrooms within 48 hours of ingestion. These treatments usually come in decoctions, capsules, tinctures, or infusions.

Motherwort

Motherwort has long been used as a medicinal tonic to address a variety of ailments, including heart failure and irregular heartbeat. Besides that, it is also beneficial in treating anxiety. Moreover, it can be used to address other health issues, such as:

- Irregular menstruation
- Flatulence
- Hyperthyroidism
- Itchy skin and shingles
- Poor eyesight

Mullein

The flowers of mullein, which are harvested in the mountainous areas of Pakistan and Turkey, contain chemicals for the treatment of:

- Infections
- Asthma
- Bronchitis
- Pneumonia
- Colds
- Coughs
- Tonsillitis
- Earaches
- Gastrointestinal bleeding
- Bruises
- Frostbite

Nettle

Nettle, which can be identified by its lance-shaped leaves and green flowers with yellow stems, has been commonly used in herbal medicine to treat:

- Septic wounds
- Nosebleeds

- Irregular menstrual cycles
- Fever
- Arthritis
- Anemia
- Skin conditions
- Prostate problems
- Hemorrhage
- Prostate enlargement
- Hay fever

Volatile oils such as bornyl acetate, beta-caryophyllene, iridoids, and alkaloids in nettle provide therapeutic properties to act as a mild sedative and relaxant, amongst other healing properties.

Olive Leaf

Harvested from an olive tree's leaves, olive leaf is used medicinally due to its antioxidant and anti-inflammatory properties. At the same time, its active ingredient, phenolic compounds, is known for its antiviral and antibacterial effects. Bearing various therapeutic properties, it has been used to treat various ailments, like:

- Digestive ailments
- Nervous system problem
- Microbial growth
- Inflammation
- Pain
- Oxidation and cell damage

Olive oil extract has also been used to help with weight loss, heart health, and the breakout of herpes. The dosage can be split up into smaller doses per day. It can reduce the risk of cardiovascular disease, lower blood pressure, treat type 2 diabetes, encourage weight loss, eradicate free radicals in the body, boost immunity from sickness, fight herpes, reduce inflammation, and prevent cancer.

Oregano

With olive green leaves and purple flowers, Oregano has been used medicinally to treat coughs and fight against certain bacteria and viruses. Oregano has been used to speed up the healing of open wounds and clear up parasite infections. Herbal medicine has been used for centuries to treat:

- Skin sores
- Sore muscles
- Asthma problems
- Cramps
- Diarrhea
- Colds and flu
- Indigestion

The main components of oregano, namely carvacrol and thyme, have antimicrobial properties that work together to fight disease.

Pau D'arco

Pau d'arco, made from the inner bark of tabebuia trees, is native to Central and South America. It has been commonly used to reduce body inflammation and aid weight loss. Its pink and purple flowers can identify it as dense wood used by native peoples to construct hunting bows. It has antibacterial and antifungal properties and can be used to treat diseases such as cancer, obesity, and heart disease. The anti-inflammatory properties have also been used to treat osteoarthritis, swelling, pain, and joint stiffness. They are available in capsule, liquid, and powder form, and traditionally the bark is simmered in boiling water before it is taken as a strong tonic.

Peppermint

Egyptians have used peppermint since 1000 B.C. for its healing properties. Greeks and Romans also favored peppermint herbs for their medicinal properties. The herb has been used to treat:

- gas and flatulence
- bloating
- colic
- secretion of bile
- muscle spasms
- antiseptic
- skin ailments
- irritable bowel syndrome
- diarrhea
- spastic colon
- headaches and migraines
- respiratory infections

Pine

The spikes, barks, and needles of pine trees are harvested to make medicine. Pine is most used to treat respiratory tract infections, swelling, and inflammation. It has also been used to treat a stuffy nose, common cold, coughs, and bronchitis. Pine has also been used in infection and blood pressure remedies and can be applied externally to treat muscle and nerve pain. It is also mildly effective in killing fungus and bacteria.

Plantain

Great plantain, which its broad leaves can identify, is native to Europe and Asia and used medicinally worldwide. The chemicals in plantain have been used to treat:

- pain and swelling
- mucous
- blocked airways
- kill bacteria and fungi
- coughs
- mouth sores
- obesity
- irregular menstruation

Red Raspberry

The sweet fruit of raspberry has been widely used for its antioxidant effects, which help blood flow in blood vessels. Raspberry has also been used to treat diarrhea and diabetes. It is commonly ingested as a fruit. Care should be taken when ingesting raspberry medicinally in pregnant women.

Red Clover

The wildflowers of red clover have been used traditionally to treat symptoms of asthma, coughs, arthritis, and cancer. It can be identified by its dark pink flowers that are popular for use as a popular garnish. It has also been used in South America as fodder to improve soil quality. It is a traditional medicine for the treatment of:

- osteoporosis
- heart disease
- arthritis
- skin disorders
- menstrual cramps and symptoms
- menopausal symptoms

Rose

Rose, or Indian cabbage rose, is a woody and perennial plant with oval leaves. Its fruit is fleshy and can be eaten. When this fruit ripens, it is called rose hip and exists in various hybrid varieties worldwide. It can be used as a blood purifier and has anti-inflammatory and aphrodisiac properties. It has also been used for the healing of ulcers and diarrhea. Its practical uses include:

- treatment of blood pressure
- heart disease
- healing of wounds
- regulates excessive sweating
- antiseptic for eye infections
- gastritis
- constipation

- relieves colic
- gargle for sore throats
- prevents scurvy
- insomnia
- burning sensation in the body

The fresh and dried petals of the rose are used to make tinctures, teas, powders, and herbal concoctions to be used medicinally.

Rosemary

Rosemary, identified by its evergreen shrub and pine-like leaves, is often used medicinally in parts of Europe. Rosemary has been used medicinally to treat:

- strengthening of memory and concentration
- improve blood circulation to the head and scalp
- energy and fatigue
- anti-inflammatory
- mild analgesic when applied to the skin
- strengthens blood capillaries
- headaches and migraines
- epilepsy and vertigo
- fainting and weakness due to poor circulation
- supports healthy adrenal gland function and can aid in improving circulation and digestion
- treats stress
- treatment for mild to moderate depression
- aching ears
- rheumatic muscles

The plants' volatile oils, flavonoids, tannins, rosmarinic acid, diterpenes, and rosmaricine act medicinally to heal these ailments.

Sage

Sage, or salvia, which is its botanical name, is a common herbal remedy for:

- gargle for sore throats
- poor digestion
- irregular menstruation
- strong antiseptic
- relieves flatulence
- regulates estrogen by reducing breast milk production
- strong anti-inflammatory

- relieves muscle spasms
- strong antimicrobial
- antiseptic
- strong nerve tonic
- treats mild diarrhea
- hot flashes and hormonal changes due to menopause
- asthma

Sage constituents, such as volatile oils, diterpenes, flavonoids, phenolic acids, and tannins, are used in unison to heal the body.

Saint John's Wort

Since the 19th century, Saint John's wort has been used to address nervous system disorders. Known for its bright yellow flower clusters, the plant comprises compounds such as hypericin, hyperforin, flavonoids, and xanthone, which serve as:

- Antidepressant
- Antispasmodic
- Astringent
- Sedative
- Pain reliever
- Antiviral
- Bile stimulant

Saint John's wort can be prepared as a tonic to treat anxiety, tension, insomnia, and depression. Likewise, it treats symptoms of menopause to regulate hormonal changes and energy slumps. Furthermore, Saint John's wort tonic can be used for treatment in the liver and gallbladder. The infused oil can also be applied externally to treat wounds, burns, muscle cramps, nerve pain, and other external wounds.

Saw Palmetto

Characterized by its yellow-green leaves and ivory flowers, saw palmetto has been used as a medicinal tonic since the 19th century. It can be employed to treat numerous ailments, including:

- Debility
- Urinary tract problems
- Enlarged prostate glands and prostate infections
- Weight gain
- Fatigue
- Estrogenic action in women
- Aphrodisiac
- Problems in reproductive organs
- Weak bladder
- Cystitis

The key components of saw palmetto, such as fatty acids, plant sterols, polysaccharides, and tannins, work in unison to provide potential healing benefits.

Self-Heal

Self-heal, a native European plant, is renowned for its healing properties. With pointed oval leaves and clusters of purple and pink flowers, it can be easily spotted in the wild. Traditionally used to treat:

- Liver problems
- Throat problems
- External wounds
- Internal bleeding
- High blood pressure
- Urinary tract infections
- Digestive problems
- Staunches bleeding and accelerates the rate of repair
- Obstructions in the liver and gallbladder
- Jaundice
- Sore throat
- Leucorrhea
- Hemorrhoids
- Fevers
- Headaches
- Dizziness
- Vertigo
- Sore and inflamed eyes
- Infected and enlarged glands, such as lymph nodes

The key constituents include pentacyclic triterpenes, tannins, caffeic acid, and vitamins B1, C, and K, which work to provide healing.

Solomon's Seal

An ancient medicinal herb, Solomon's seal is well-known for its ability to **decrease inflammation, treat various lung diseases, and speed up the healing of wounds**. Applied externally as an ointment, it can reduce redness and swelling on the skin and treat conditions such as boils, bruises, and ulcers. Studies also show that Solomon's seal has properties that can help lower blood sugar levels.

Thyme

Thyme, which can be identified by its shrub-like appearance, woody stems, small leaves, and pink flowers, has been used to treat:

- Weakened lungs
- Coughs and respiratory remedies

- Fungal infections
- Chest infections and bronchitis
- Throat infections
- Asthma
- Hay fever
- Worms in children
- Bites and stings when used externally
- Sciatica
- Rheumatic aches and pains
- Ringworms
- Athletes foot
- Thrush
- Fungal infections
- Scabies and lice

Key ingredients such as thymol, methyl chavicol, cineole, borneol, flavonoids, and tannins work together to benefit both internal and external healing.

Tulsi

Tulsi, also known as holy basil, has long been used in Indian households to treat various ailments. This bushy herb is typically found in semi-tropical climates and is a common ingredient in Ayurvedic medicines. It can help cure illnesses such as the common cold, heart disease, headaches, stomach disorders, and kidney stones. Additionally, tulsi repels mosquitoes, flies, and other insects. Even malaria fever can be treated with it. Other associated uses are:

- Alleviates nausea
- Lowers cholesterol and blood pressure
- Relieves pain
- Protects the liver
- Reduces stress
- Prevents cancer
- Expels mucus

Turmeric

Known for its vibrant yellow hue and iconic spicy flavor, turmeric is a popular ingredient in Indian cuisine. It has long been used medicinally to help with liver and digestive issues and can be employed to treat:

- Blood-clotting
- Inflammatory conditions
- High cholesterol
- Digestive tract issues

With natural antioxidant properties and powerful antibacterial capabilities, turmeric contains components such as volatile oils, zingiberene, and turmerone which are beneficial for healing arthritic and skin conditions. Curcumin, an even stronger antioxidant than Vitamin E, is especially effective when applied topically.

Uva Ursi

Often referred to as bearberry, uva ursi is a perennial shrub with striking glossy green leaves, bell-shaped pink flowers, and small red berries. Originally native to Europe, its spread across the Northern Hemisphere extends even into the Arctic. The plant thrives in damp conditions such as undergrowth and grasslands, with the harvesting of leaves and berries typically done in autumn. The constituents of hydroquinone, tannins, phenolic glycosides, and flavonoids found in them provide the healing properties so often used to treat:

- Urinary tract infections
- Chronic cystitis
- Urethritis
- Bacteria

Native Americans have also used uva ursi recreationally as tobacco. However, caution should be practiced if there is a simultaneous infection in the kidneys or for those with kidney disease.

Valerian

Since Roman times, Valerian has been used medicinally and can be identified by its divided leaves and pink flowers. Also, it has been used medicinally to treat:

- Nervous tension
- Anxiety and overexcitement
- High blood pressure
- Poor sleep quality
- Depression
- Tremors, panic, palpitations, and sweating
- Neck tension
- Colic
- Bowel syndrome
- Muscle spasm
- Menstrual pains

This way, the volatile oils, iridoids, and alkaloids have worked together to treat these ailments.

Wild Lettuce

Wild lettuce is used medicinally to treat:
- coughs
- asthma

- urinary tract infections
- insomnia
- restlessness and anxiety
- menstrual cramps
- joint pains
- poor circulation
- relieves pain

Yarrow

A traditional European plant, Yarrow has long been used to treat wartime injuries. Apart from its use in treating colds, flu, and allergies such as hay fever, it also helps with menstrual complications and issues related to circulation. Yarrow can be used to treat:

- Urinary tract problems such as bladder infections
- Internal bleeding
- Inflammation
- Poor menstrual cycles

Moreover, yarrow has key properties, including flavonoids, alkaloids, polyacetylenes, triterpenes, salicylic acid, tannins, and coumarins. These contribute to medicinal properties, including lowering blood pressure, reducing fever, acting as a bitter tonic, and acting as an antispasmodic.

Pillar 4
Remedies

In Chapter 6 of Pillar 4, we will explore many remedies that can be used to treat everything from acne and ADHD to menopausal symptoms and sore throat. From natural herbs and plants to homeopathic treatments and ayurvedic medicines, there are numerous ways to treat common ailments in the comfort of your own home. These remedies offer a practical, economical alternative or complement to modern medicine. Lastly, as we go through this pillar, we will go over the pros and cons of each method so you can decide what is best for you.

6

List of Remedies by Symptoms

Herbalism, a centuries-old practice, has been used to help people achieve holistic wellness. From treating common symptoms and diagnoses to providing a rewarding experience, those seeking healing must be aware of this ancient art's possibilities. Many go through life without knowing what herbalism can do for them.

Acne

For pimples, there is likely an herbalist solution, such as:

- **Neem oil.** An antiseptic herb that can help cleanse the skin and eliminate some bacteria that lead to acne.
- **Tea tree oil.** Inflammation is another issue that may be causing your acne. Applying some tea tree oil is a great way to reduce inflammation that can lead to additional skin redness.
- **Witch hazel.** The other big part of acne is excess oil. When this extra oil gets trapped in the pores, it leads to pimples. Witch hazel dries out the skin, allowing it to clear up and prevent the development of additional oil.

Boil the herbs with water, allow them to cool, and use it as a face wash. This process is the perfect way to take advantage of their properties for soothing acne. Likewise, it is a simple method needed to transfer the healing benefits onto your skin.

ADHD

Those with ADHD also tend to have high anxiety and difficulty calming themselves. While herbs cannot wholly cure ADHD, they can help you mitigate some symptoms and reduce some of the stress they can cause. These are the best herbs to use for ADHD:

- **Oats.** Considered a "nervine" herb, it is excellent for targeting your nervous system, which can be overstimulated if you have ADHD. Oat-top tea is thus a great calming agent for any ADHD-related stress.
- **Lion's mane.** Help target the effects of some persistent stress hormones that can make your life difficult with ADHD.
- **Velvet bean.** With many properties that can help you with some of your ADHD symptoms.

To use these herbs for treating ADHD, aromatherapy can be a useful approach. The calming properties of aromas can be paired with herbs to enhance their relaxing effects, making them more effective in managing ADHD symptoms.

Allergies

Many people suffer from seasonal and food allergies, among many others. These symptoms can be wide-ranging and are often very debilitating. Some popular herbal remedies for allergies include:

- **Butterbur.** An antihistamine for treating allergies.
- **Stinging nettle.** Though painful to touch, this herb contains organic compounds that act as an antihistamine.
- **Curcumin.** Have a property found in turmeric that can be taken as a supplement to ease congestion.
- **Garlic.** A classic kitchen staple that contains quercetin, an antioxidant that treats allergies.
- **Honey.** For those with pollen allergies, honey can be a godsend. It contains pollen which, when consumed, can help immunize you to their irritations, like a natural vaccine. The more locally you buy your honey, the better it will contain local pollen.

Various herbs can be eaten, drank in teas, or added to dishes like smoothies. Introducing them into your diet can be very effective for treating allergies.

Amoebiasis

Amoebiasis is an infection of the intestines caused by a parasite. Symptoms of intestinal parasites include fatigue and weakness, bloating and gas, diarrhea, nausea or vomiting, weight loss, and stomach tenderness. Herbal remedies are commonly used for a parasite cleanse. These remedies often include:

- Papaya seeds
- Pumpkin seeds
- Berberine extracts
- Wormwood extracts
- Garlic
- Yogurt with probiotics
- Carrots or sweet potatoes due to their beta-carotenes

These foods are often rich in vitamin A, selenium, and zinc, natural defenses against parasitic infections. Pumpkin seeds are also high in amino fatty acids, which act against parasitic infestation.

Anxiety

There are several herbal remedies for anxiety:

- **Kava.** Precaution should be taken when taking kava excessively, which may lead to liver damage.
- **Passionflower.** Caution should be taken as it may lead to drowsiness, dizziness, and confusion.
- **Valerian.** Dosage should not be exceeded as this may lead to headaches, dizziness, and drowsiness.
- **Chamomile.** Can increase the risk of bleeding as it leads to blood thinning.
- **Lavender.** When ingested orally or as aromatherapy to reduce anxiety, constipation, and headaches. It can also increase appetite, act as a sedative, and lower blood pressure.
- **Lemon Balm.** Reduce nervousness and excitability. Yet, long-term use is not recommended, as it can lead to nausea and abdominal pain.

Since aromatherapy can be great for anxiety, consider making these into soaps, potpourris, or candles. Likewise, you can drink them as teas, combining aromatherapy properties and consumption.

Arthritis

Several herbal remedies can be used to treat arthritis. These often include:

- **Ginger.** An anti-inflammatory root with a component called leukotrienes that treats arthritis.
- **Thyme.** Another anti-inflammatory and anti-microbial herb with properties to treat arthritis.
- **Turmeric.** Has anti-inflammatory properties to treat arthritis and musculoskeletal disorders.
- **Green tea.** Has antioxidant-rich polyphenols that reduce inflammation, protect joints, and stimulate immune responses to treat arthritis.
- **Cinnamon.** One of the best anti-inflammatory spices out there. Cinnamon will greatly help your joints.

Many of these herbs are ideal for adding to your existing diet. Putting spices like turmeric and cinnamon into your foods can help sneak in some of their benefits. You could switch to green tea instead of coffee for a healthier morning routine to help your arthritis.

Asthma

A common respiratory condition, asthma affects many people globally. But did you know there are some great herbal treatments for it too? Here are some of the best ways to use herbs and plant by-products for asthma:

- **Turmeric.** An effective anti-inflammatory, turmeric helps fight asthma by calming inflamed lungs.
- **Ginseng.** Studies in rats have shown that ginseng reduces lung inflammation, and human studies are underway.
- **Honey.** A sore throat remedy and antihistamine, honey can also help clear airways and encourage coughing to relieve constricted throats. Although not an herb, honey is a plant by-product used with herbs for medicinal purposes.

These herbal remedies are best consumed orally. The good news is that honey and turmeric are easy to add to your routine. Consider having a honey turmeric tea before bed every night to help stave off your asthma symptoms.

Back Pain

As an average adult, it is common to experience some back pain. While there is no perfect solution, reducing tension is one way to ease the discomfort. Here are a few herbs that can reduce tension and relieve back pain.

- **Valerian root.** Help regulate the nervous system and ease stress-related issues.
- **Turmeric.** Used to decrease inflammation in joints, turmeric can be a great aid in relieving back pain.
- **Ginger.** An anti-inflammatory and reduce back pain when added to your diet.

For back pain, you have two options: *consuming the herbs or applying their oils topically*. Consuming the herbs can help with stress relief while using the oils directly on the skin offers more immediate results. A massage with turmeric-infused oil could be a great way to see if this approach works for you.

Bloating

Eating a heavy meal with much fat can sometimes lead to bloating. Fortunately, certain herbs can help provide relief from chronic bloating. Here are some of the best ones to use:

- **Peppermint or chamomile tea.** Generally, teas will be your best bet for bloating, but peppermint and chamomile are some of the best. These teas are easy on the stomach and promote good digestion.
- **Fennel.** An excellent anti-inflammatory herb, fennel or fennel tea can significantly reduce bloating or gas pain.
- **Turmeric.** As we have seen throughout this chapter, turmeric is one of the best herbs for any inflammatory condition. In this case, it is excellent for reducing stomach inflammation.

Reducing stomach inflammation is crucial for relieving bloating. And the best way to consume the herbs is with food or drink for faster relief.

Bronchitis/Chest Cold/Pneumonia

No one likes having a chest cold. And with the recent pandemic, everyone has them these days. There are antibiotics that you can take to fight against bacterial infections. Still, there are also a lot of herbal remedies you can take conjunctively that can help reduce some of the more extreme symptoms. Below are some ways you can greatly reduce your bronchial symptoms.

- **Ginger.** Packed with nutrients, ginger is a great way to boost your immune system and relieve bronchial symptoms. Try making ginger tea or taking chewable ginger.

- **Honey and Lemon.** These two ingredients can be soothing for bronchial infections. Add them to your ginger tea or drink them separately.
- **Pineapple.** Pineapple contains the nutrient bromelain, which can help your immune system and expel mucus from your lungs.

Ingesting all these substances is a great way to battle your lung issue, but aromatherapy can also be great. Breathing in steamed lemon or ginger can help get those substances into your lungs and thus address the issue more directly.

Burns

Having a nasty burn from the sun or taking out your cookies without an oven mitt can be unpleasant. However, you can treat them with the right herbal knowledge very easily. Some great ways to use herbs to treat skin burns include:

- **Aloe vera.** Essential for relief of any burn, particularly sunburns. Its properties provide both instant relief and an effective way to heal the skin in the long term.
- **Calendula.** This flower makes a great tea that can work wonders on burns.
- **Gotu kola**. Best when turned into a cream with just 1% of the herb. Also, it is an excellent way to soothe burns quickly

These simple remedies can help you to get instant relief from your burns, as well as provide an aid to healing the skin after the burn is done.

Chickenpox

Though not as common of an illness anymore, chicken pox can be very painful and unpleasant. If you are suffering, waiting for the medicine to take effect can be a drag. In the meantime, you can use some of these herbal remedies to help you get some relief from the symptoms.

- **Chamomile.** As a soothing herb, chamomile can be ideal for treating chickenpox's painful and itchy skin rashes. A compress or a bath will work wonders for the skin and give you that much-needed relief.
- **Oats.** Another classic remedy for chicken pox. Bathing in or using an oatmeal-based soap or cream is a surefire way to relieve some of the itching and burning.

To soothe the terrible skin irritation of chickenpox, topical treatments are considered the most effective way. These treatments provide direct relief and comfort to your skin.

Cold and Flu

Few medical treatments are available to combat the common cold, but there are plenty of ways to relieve and manage your symptoms. Here we look at some of the most successful options for dealing with cold and flu symptoms.

- **Lemon balm.** An herb that can be used in many forms, such as steams and teas, and is easy to grow.
- **Echinacea.** Great for relieving cold and flu symptoms as tea or cough drops.
- **Rosemary.** Using rosemary oil on the neck, drinking rosemary tea, or taking a bath with the aroma are all effective ways of relieving cold and flu symptoms.

Finding things you can drink or breathe in that contain these herbs is one of the best ways to manage symptoms and ensure you will recover quickly from your condition.

Constipation

Constipation is a common digestive issue, and it is hard to maintain the recommended two to three bowel movements a day. Eating fiber and exercising are basic solutions, but you can also try herbal remedies to help with this issue. As such, below are the top herbal remedies for constipation that you can use to find relief.

- **Psyllium.** One type of plant you can use is natural laxatives, which can help you with short-term constipation. Psyllium is one of the best ones to use. However, use in moderation, as excess laxative use can cause long-term dangerous weight loss and issues like nausea, vomiting, and diarrhea.
- **Slippery elm.** Another herbal method, but not a laxative one. Instead, slippery elm stimulates gastrointestinal nerves, helping you pass better bowel movements.
- **Rhubarb.** Good secondary laxative option. The best thing about rhubarb is that it is delicious, so you can have it in a pie or tea. Again, short-term use only.

As we have said throughout this section, it is imperative that you use any constipation relief methods responsibly. Otherwise, you could quickly end up harming your digestive system. Use these methods only in emergencies, as needed, and not regularly.

Cough

Coughing is a common symptom of most colds but can be unpleasant. But there are a lot of herbal remedies you can enact to cure your cough. Here are some of the best ones.

- **Honey.** Besides its antihistamine properties, honey can help soothe your throat. It is also antibacterial, meaning you can nip a would-be cold in the bud with some quality honey.
- **Ginger.** Another frequently occurring plant in this list, ginger, has much to offer. It can have excellent effects on colds, including relaxing your muscles to your airways and helping you breathe better.
- **Elderberry.** If you want something soothing and immunity-boosting at the same time, look no further than elderberry. You can consume it as tea or even in capsules.

To soothe a cough, you want something that is both soothing and can help you get over the illness that is causing the cough in the first place. All three of these remedies will help you do just that.

Depression

With mental health issues increasing and more awareness around them, many people seek more holistic and varied methods to cure their depression. The good news is that there are a lot of herbal treatments that you can use to help your depression. Here are some key ones that you can try:

- **St. John's wort.** Although not the most appealing name, this is one of the most long-used methods for treating depression herbally. It can help calm your stress and give you a more long-term mood boost.
- **Ginseng.** One of the worst symptoms of depression is the cloudiness you often feel. Ginseng is a highly effective treatment because it boosts energy and mental clarity.
- **Lavender.** Another great mood-boosting herb. Lavender is both pleasant to smell and can have positive neurological effects. It can also improve sleep, which is particularly important for those with depression, as insomnia can be a major symptom of depression.

These three herbs are excellent for helping with some surface-level aspects of depression. They are best consumed with aromatherapy as candles, essential oils, or even soaps.

Diarrhea

Like with constipation, many people also struggle with diarrhea. This can be caused by many factors, including food sensitivities and gut health, so you should get these things checked out first. However, there are also some essential herbal methods you can use to try to aid in your diarrhea recovery. Here are some good ones to try.

- **Blackberry leaves.** A slightly more unusual herb, blackberry leaves can be highly effective for diarrhea.
- **Peppermint.** To help your digestive system, add some peppermint. Do it either in the form of tea or essential oils. These will both be highly effective in mitigating some of your diarrhea symptoms.
- **Ginger.** As always, ginger is a highly effective remedy. Ginger teas or adding ginger to your cooking can be a great way to help this illness.

The digestive tract is likely the best way to help with diarrhea problems since it is the digestive tract that has issues. Incorporating these things into your diet can help you quite a bit.

Dry Mouth

A dry mouth may seem minor, but it can affect your life. Fortunately, there are natural remedies specifically designed to help with this discomfort. The most effective ones are moisturizing agents, which stimulate saliva production in your mouth and bring relief. Here are a few of the best herbal solutions for this problem.

- **Aloe vera.** Refresh and hydrate your mouth by drinking this versatile plant in juice form.

- **Marshmallow root.** Highly moisturizing, this root helps replace lost saliva.
- **Black pepper.** Used as a natural remedy to stimulate salivary glands, which may indirectly help alleviate dry mouth symptoms.

As with all the other oral issues discussed in this book, these remedies are best taken through the mouth, meaning that you can eat most of them to help you get over your dry mouth.

Ear Infection/Earache

Those who have had the misfortune of an earache know just how agonizing they can be. Fortunately, there are several herbal remedies you can try to help with an ear infection, such as:

- **Ginger.** An old standby, this plant is known for its anti-inflammatory properties and can provide relief when used externally around the affected area.
- **Garlic.** This vegetable will help with inflammation and has antibacterial qualities that can fight against infection. Use it as an infused oil directly into the ear canal.
- **Olive oil.** This oil can help loosen buildup and blockages in the ear, helping to reduce pain caused by clogged ears.

Although all these herbal methods are meant to be put into the ear, be careful about what parts of the ear they are encountering, especially ginger, as you can potentially harm your eardrums this way.

Eczema/Dermatitis/Skin Inflammation

Like with acne, many types of skin irritations can cause many problems. If you have skin dryness or general irritation issues, you have probably tried everything to cure yourself. Cures are tricky because the skin can be sensitive, even to creams designed to help them. There are a lot of herbal remedies, which we will talk about, but you should also know that your skin can have adverse reactions to these too. Just because they are natural does not mean they will necessarily work for your skin type, so always make sure to do a patch test beforehand, especially if you are going to be using any of these treatments on your face, to ensure that you are not going to have an allergic reaction.

That being said, here are some excellent herbal remedies for your skin irritation.

- **Oatmeal.** Highly nourishing and moisturizing, using oat soaps, creams, or baths is a great way to benefit from this plant's properties.
- **Witch Hazel.** Good for general itchiness and inflammation, this treatment is not recommended for eczema specifically.
- **Honey.** Known as an effective treatment against eczema, you can try rubbing it directly into your skin, diluted if necessary, to help reduce rashes.
- **Coconut oil.** As a great moisturizer and healer, rubbing some of this oil into your skin will provide soothing relief. Feel free to add essential oils to create a fun DIY moisturizer.

Applying any of these to the skin can be excellent. However, there are also other ways of ingesting. Honey can promote moisture throughout the body, so even incorporating it into your diet can be ideal for your skin.

Edema

One of the lesser-known conditions on this list, edema, still affects many people yearly. It is characterized by swelling and often caused by buildup of fluids in the body. For this reason, many herbalists recommend diuretics to help drain some of those fluids that could be causing your edema. Here are some of the best diuretics to use for your edema:

- **Green tea.** A healthy tea packed with antioxidants and a stimulating diuretic, green tea is essential for any edema treatment practice. Drink or bathe in it to absorb fumes, which should help drain some of that liquid almost immediately.
- **Olive leaf.** An anti-inflammatory herb, olive leaf can also have good diuretic properties. Buy these in capsule form to make consumption easier if that suits you better.
- **Pineapple juice.** Another great anti-inflammatory substance, pineapple, is an excellent choice for curing your edema. Either buy it pre-made or blend your own from a fresh pineapple.

Since the fluid-draining nature of these diuretics primarily works through the digestive system, they are best consumed orally. However, if another method works best for you, then you should try that one instead.

Endometriosis

A painful uterine dysfunction disorder, endometriosis affects many people around the world. Although surgery tends to be the most common cure for the condition, there are also a lot of painful symptoms, such as pelvic and back pain, nausea, and menstruation issues, that can be treated with herbal remedies. Here are some of the best herbal remedies to treat your endometriosis.

- **Curcumin.** Found in turmeric, this amazing chemical has excellent anti-inflammatory properties. It is a superb symptom reliever and one of the best ingredients to incorporate into your diet if you struggle with endometriosis.
- **Pine bark.** Discoveries suggest that this ingredient might have pain-killing properties, which can be a lifesaver for the chronic pain often endured by people with endometriosis. Incorporating the extract into your diet can help relieve some of the chronic pain you are experiencing with endometriosis.
- **Peppermint.** Antioxidants are always a great thing to eat if you are experiencing a chronic pain illness like endometriosis. Incorporating some into your diet will do wonders for your pain.

To help these substances enter your bloodstream as quickly as possible, they are best incorporated into a diet. However, sometimes incense or other scent-based remedies can help as well.

Eye Problems

Many people have trouble with their eyes. The eye can be delicate, from vision problems to allergies to infections. Yet, there are quite a few herbal remedies you can do for your eyes to help you get relief from any of these symptoms. Here are some of the best ones.

- **Fennel.** For cataracts or consistent eye infections, fennel is an excellent herb. It has also been shown to prevent macular degeneration, which can lead to vision loss. With all these healing properties, you should consider incorporating them into your life.
- **Passionflower.** Another excellent eye-healing herb, this one is best used to relieve eyestrain. With excess reliance on screens, eye strain is more of a problem than ever. Using some passionflower can help reduce some of those more debilitating symptoms.
- **Bilwa.** Being prone to eye infections, bilwa is one of the best herbs. It is beneficial for curing diseases like sty and conjunctivitis. Its rich nutrient content, including iron, calcium, and proteins, can particularly help with infection relief.

Infections can be a drag, but using some of these methods could quickly relieve some of the worst symptoms. Either apply these to the eye with extreme care or consume them orally to get the substances into your body.

Fatigue and Exhaustion

Many people deal with chronic fatigue. In our fast-paced world, it is no wonder this is a common problem. However, you do not have to worry about it because there are a lot of great herb supplements you can introduce into your life that can help you manage some of this chronic fatigue you might be experiencing. Here are some excellent herbs you can use to help ameliorate chronic fatigue.

- **Ginseng.** As an excellent immunity-boosting and energy-boosting herb, ginseng is perfect for relieving chronic fatigue and restoring alertness and energy to your life. Incorporating it into your diet through teas or even into your skincare through soaps can help bring you the benefits of ginseng.
- **Echinacea.** Another immunity-boosting herb is echinacea. Immunity boosting is particularly important for people with chronic fatigue because the immune system takes up much energy. As you always fight potential illnesses, giving your immune system extra strength can significantly help you conserve that energy for other things. Taking these two immunity-boosting supplements will thus do wonders for your energy levels.
- **Sage.** Another excellent supplement for boosting your energy levels. It has also improved others, like mood, cognitive function, and memory. These things are related, so improving them can significantly enhance your energy levels.

Energy is necessary, so keeping these essential herbs around can improve your life. Many of them can either be consumed orally or used with aromatherapy.

Fever

Fevers can come along with many kinds of illnesses. In theory, a fever is part of your body's natural immune response, trying to boil the germs alive and stop them from spreading. However, it can also be dangerous and unpleasant. To help mitigate some of the dangers and discomfort of a fever, here are some excellent herbal remedies you can try.

- **Coriander seeds.** Some of the best immunity-boosting seeds on the market are excellent for helping you fight that virus without overheating your body. If you take some of these with your fever, it will help bring it down due to the immune response being redirected.
- **Garlic.** A known antibacterial substance, garlic is excellent for boosting your immune response and killing a fever. Taking it in tea or soup is a great way to help your fever while enjoying a delicious treat.
- **Moringa.** This excellent tree is packed with many nutrients and antibacterial qualities. If you introduce this into your diet, you could do a lot for your fever. Try some in tea to bring down some of the inflammation you are experiencing.

These are all great herbs to use for your debilitating fever. If you take them orally, then you should have an excellent remedy. However, you can also take them in several other ways.

Fungal Infection

Fungal infections can happen in any number of parts of the body. They can be particularly unpleasant and painful, so many seek herbal treatments. Fortunately, many such treatments can do a lot for your fungal infection, including relieving you of some of the more painful symptoms. Here are the best ones to try.

- **Turmeric.** Has antimicrobial qualities that can help fight some more debilitating fungal infections. Either apply turmeric paste, made from turmeric and water, over the infected area if it is external or drink it to get the internal benefits.
- **Oregano or oregano oil.** As an active antifungal herb, oregano is excellent for helping you deal with some of the nastier aspects of infection. Again, like turmeric, it can be applied directly to the infected area or consumed to help with internal infections.
- **Neem leaves.** Infuse some neem in water and wash the infected area to help kill dangerous microorganisms that infect your body.

As fungal infections can come in many forms, many of these remedies can be used as topical and internal treatments. Tailor the application method to the nature of your condition and find the best one for you.

Gingivitis

Oral diseases are more dangerous than people think. Not taking care of your oral health can lead to a lot more debilitating health issues down the road. As such, having a healthy body starts with having a healthy mouth. That said, herbal remedies are a great way to better care for oral health.

Some essential herbal supplements to introduce into your life to prevent and even cure illnesses like gingivitis, include:

- **Lemongrass.** An excellent plaque reducer, lemongrass has been shown to reduce gingivitis, sometimes even better than traditional commercial mouthwashes. Make your mouthwash using lemongrass essential oil or incorporate lemongrass into your diet.
- **Aloe vera.** Another tremendous natural method for reducing gingivitis is aloe vera. For instance, use pure aloe vera juice as an effective mouthwash every morning to cure some of the worst symptoms of gingivitis.
- **Guava leaves.** Finally, guava leaves can also be used as a mouthwash for gingivitis. It can be great for targeting plaque and can also be a great anti-inflammatory substance.

Mouth washing is one of the best ways to treat gingivitis because it helps to target the infected area and allows all the healing properties to seep in all the way. However, incorporating these things into your diet, in general, can also be beneficial.

Hangover

Likely, everyone had one of those nights, having drunk too much, skipped out on water or sleep, and then suffered the consequences the next day. But did you know there are remedies backed by herbalism that may help ease your hangover? These tried-and-true solutions have been around for a while and could make a difference if you find yourself in a similar situation.

Below are some of the best herbal cures for your post-party misfortunes.

- **Milk thistle.** When it comes to hangovers, the liver is the most important thing. That is your detoxifying organ; you must treat it as well as possible. Milk thistle is one of the best things to eat for your liver, helping to cleanse it and boost its detoxifying properties.
- **Ginseng.** As with many other conditions discussed in this chapter, ginseng is a foundational herbal remedy. For hangovers, it has the advantage of being a great metabolizer. It can help you to process some of the alcohol in your system, which can speed up your hangover recovery.
- **Dandelion root.** One of the best-kept secrets of the herbalist world is that this "weed" is a beneficial plant with many helpful properties. A certain type of coffee-like drink can be made from the roots, which can be particularly helpful for hangovers. It can work as a diuretic, which will also help speed up the metabolizing process and help get any excess alcohol out of your system.

Many of these substances are ideal for helping your body's natural detoxification process and helping to aid it in ridding your body of alcohol. As a result, taking these orally to transmit them into your digestive system is ideal.

Headache and Migraine

Almost everyone has suffered from headaches or migraines at some point. They can be debilitating and even cause you to miss school or work. Painkillers can help, but often they do not deal with the other things that accompany migraines, such as light sensitivity and nausea. These herbal remedies can help address your headaches or migraines more holistically.

Here are some of the best ones to use.

- Peppermint
- Ginger
- Valerian
- Coriander

Heartburn/GERD/Acid Reflux

Ever been left feeling uncomfortable after a meal, whether with heartburn or acid reflux? Some people suffer from much worse, chronic GERD. Eating can be difficult; you may even avoid certain foods to prevent these symptoms. The good news is that there are ways to alleviate excess acid and make your digestive process more bearable.

To help you out, consider the following herb.

- Fennel
- Catnip
- Papaya tea
- Marshmallow root

Heart Palpitation

Heart palpitations can be scary if you have generalized anxiety or a heat problem. There are some medications you can take for more severe heart conditions, but if you are looking for something to relieve symptoms, there are also many herbal remedies for your heart problems, such as:

- Passionflower
- Reishi
- Lemon balm
- Motherwort

High Blood Pressure/Hypertension

High blood pressure can be dangerous, but it often has simple causes. Anxiety or prolonged exposure to stressful situations can contribute to high blood pressure. Thus, herbal remedies that promote soothing and stress relief can do wonders for your blood pressure and the following symptoms. Some of the most common herbs people use to help bring down some of that blood-pressure-raising stress include:

- Parsley
- Basil

- Cinnamon
- Ginger

Hypoglycemia

Are you experiencing extreme hunger and irritability even after eating? Possibly, you could be suffering from hypoglycemia. While there are medications you can take, there are also plenty of herbal remedies to help manage your symptoms, like:

- Aloe vera
- Ginseng
- Bitter melon
- Cinnamon

Hypothyroidism

People with hormone imbalances tend to be able to trace that to their thyroid. The thyroid is an essential aspect of the endocrine system which flows through the whole body. As a result, an unbalanced thyroid can have devastating consequences on many aspects of your health. Again, you can take thyroid medication, but many herbal supplements help your thyroid in tandem with these medications. Here are some essential herbs that can greatly affect your thyroid regulation.

- Black cumin
- Licorice
- Gotu kola

IBS/IBD/Ulcerative Colitis

Problems with bowel movements, especially if they are inconsistent (i.e., oscillating between constipation and diarrhea), are debilitating. As such, it can affect your work situation, diet, and social life. People with extreme IBS sometimes cannot even go out for long stretches due to their body's excessive demands. Thus, you likely want some relief if you suffer from these things.

Fortunately, many herbal remedies help your IBS or ulcerative colitis, such as:

- Ginger
- Peppermint
- Aloe vera

Indigestion/Dyspepsia

Struggling with indigestion is no walk in the park. It can be hard on your eating habits and your entire digestive system. If you are suffering from this, you have probably tried many things to help you get relief. But if you investigate some of the herbal remedies, you will see a lot to be found there. Here, we will tell you some of the best herbal remedies for your digestive issues.

- Fennel
- Ginger
- Peppermint

Insect Bites

An insect bite can damper an otherwise fun experience, such as camping or hiking with friends. Fortunately, several herbal remedies can be used to soothe the discomfort or itchiness from these bites. Here are some of the best:

- **Green tea.** An itch-reducer with anti-inflammatory properties, making it an ideal choice to fight bug bites.
- **Basil.** Another itch-reducing herb, basil, is excellent for bites. Just create a paste from ground-up leaves.
- **Aloe vera.** One of the best plants for skin irritation, aloe vera works excellent for bug bites. Rub the paste on the infected area for immediate relief.

Curing insect bites with herbal remedies is excellent because they offer immediate relief. If you choose this solution, you will feel much better within minutes.

Insomnia

Many people have insomnia. Yet, sleeping pills have been heavily criticized for being highly addictive, causing people to develop a dependence and not be able to sleep without them in the future. Yet, plenty of herbal remedies can do a lot for your insomnia and help you get to sleep more easily, including:

- Lavender
- Chamomile
- Valerian

Jet Lag

Traveling is tiring enough, but add time differences into the mix, and you have a recipe for exhaustion. When you enter a different time zone, you disrupt what is known as your circadian rhythm, an internal clock that can help you determine what time it is without looking at your watch. Disrupting these rhythms can harm your sleep schedule, eating schedule, and energy levels. Thus, many people find traveling and jet lag to be unbearable.

And as we said above, sleeping pills can be dangerous, especially alongside stimulants like caffeine. Fortunately, many tried-and-true herbal remedies can help you re-regulate your circadian rhythms and regain control over your sleep schedule, like:

- Lavender essential oil
- Hops
- Red clover

Joint Pain

Joint pain can be annoying because of a severe condition, past injury, or creaky joints in the morning. As such, it can hurt your ability to play sports, lift heavy things, and even do simple things like walking around. If you are dealing with it, you probably face severe limitations. Likewise, you may even be a chronic painkiller-taker, which can be dangerous to your system over time. Thus, if you are experiencing a chronic issue, trying herbal remedies and avoiding some of the dangers of prolonged painkiller use might be helpful.

Such herbal to soothe your joint pain include:

- Aloe vera
- Cat's claw
- Ginger
- Green tea

Leaky Gut

Recently, health scientists have been looking into gut health's importance. The gut microbes are essential to your overall health and can make or break a diet plan. A specific condition within gut health is called a "leaky gut." This condition means that the barrier between your gut and your bloodstream is compromised, allowing anything from your intestines to reach your bloodstream. Since many toxins pass through the gut—part of its job is separating waste and toxins from beneficial nutrients—this can be especially dangerous for your health. Research still needs to be done about the lasting implications of a leaky gut and how it can impact your health, but suffice it to say, it matters. Since the research around leaky guts is still new, there are not a lot of established medical treatments. However, you can use many herbal therapies to help your leaky gut and maybe prevent your body from absorbing some of those toxins.

Here are some excellent types of herbs to use to improve your leaky gut.

- **Slippery elm.** This herb contains mucilage, a gel-like substance that can help soothe and protect the lining of the digestive tract.
- **Marshmallow root.** Like slippery elm, marshmallow root contains mucilage and can help soothe and protect the digestive tract.
- **Licorice root.** This herb has anti-inflammatory properties and may help reduce inflammation in the gut.
- **Turmeric.** Turmeric contains curcumin, a compound with potent anti-inflammatory effects that may help reduce inflammation in the digestive system.
- **Ginger.** For centuries, ginger has been used to help treat digestive issues and may help reduce inflammation in the gut.

Menopause/Andropause

When people of all genders reach middle age, their bodies undergo a powerful hormonal shift. This shift is akin to puberty and is essentially the body's reproductive organs starting to shut down. For women, this is known as menopause; for men, it is known as andropause. How the body processes these changes differs between men and women, but both undergo significant hormonal shifts throughout their lives. These hormonal shifts can be confusing. Plus, there can be a huge variation in symptoms, ranging from benign to debilitating. For many of these symptoms, there are lots of herbal remedies that you can try to help give you relief from these symptoms. Here are some of the best herbs for menopause or andropause symptoms.

- Evening primrose
- Ginseng
- Hops
- Saint john's wort

Menstrual Cycle Irregularities

For those who menstruate, that time can be tough. Some people have very easy cycles with little to no pain, but others can have debilitating symptoms that can cause them to go through extreme pain and possibly even take time off school or work. But it does not have to be that way. According to recent research, there are many links between poor overall health and painful periods. Thus, if you experience them, there might be some things you can do for the overall health that will help relieve you of these more debilitating symptoms. Consequently, there are a lot of specific herbal remedies that you can use to help improve some of your period pains. Here, we will show you some of the best ones to try.

- White peony
- Dong quai
- Vitex (or Chaste tree)
- Yarrow

Muscle Pain

Tension and strain can be an actual trial for your muscles. It can be painful for you with a lot of muscle tension. It can cause mobility issues, difficulty lifting things, and even general unpleasantness. There are muscle relaxants that you can take, but being on those 24/7 can also cause a host of problems. Instead, there are a lot of herbal remedies that you can use to help you get relief from your muscle pain. They can be easier on the digestive system and more effective than conventional drugs. Here, we will show you some of the most effective herbal remedies for muscle pain.

- Ginger
- Turmeric
- Devil's claw
- Arnica

Nausea

Having stomach issues is a complicated ailment to deal with. It is one of the more unpleasant sicknesses to have daily. It can prevent you from eating certain foods and might even stop you from eating socially. For this reason, you probably want to have some relief from your nausea, especially if it is chronic.

Herbal remedies pose a great solution since they are minimally invasive and are not hard on the body, such as:

- Ginger
- Grapeseed oil
- Chamomile
- Peppermint

Pain Management/Relief

People who deal with chronic pain, or even incidental pain, have many options available to them. Commercial painkillers are easy to come by but come with their issues. They can be expensive and, if overused, can cause health problems. More powerful or prescription painkillers can even be highly addictive and lead to substance abuse issues down the road. Thus, you should ensure that you try a wider variety of options for pain relief. Herbal remedies are great because they are not addictive and are usually less costly than over-the-counter medications. Here are some of the most effective herbal remedies for pain relief.

- Lavender essential oil
- Cloves
- Rosemary
- Eucalyptus

PCOS

A somewhat lesser-known but widespread illness, polycystic ovary syndrome (PCOS), affects the reproductive organs of women of childbearing age. This syndrome is hormonally based and can be painful for those it affects. It can also cause many other issues, from painful periods to acne to hair loss. Many people also go undiagnosed with PCOS for long periods, meaning they suffer from their symptoms in silence. Fortunately, there are plenty of herbal remedies that you can try to alleviate some of the more difficult PCOS symptoms you might be experiencing, like:

- Green tea
- Turmeric
- Cinnamon

PMS

Having difficult periods can be painful, but for the average person, premenstrual syndrome itself can be challenging enough. With symptoms from fatigue to cramping to difficulty concentrating, PMS can negatively affect many people's lives. Because fatigue is so central to PMS, stimulants are usually the answer since your body is working harder in preparation for the menstrual cycle. However, as we said earlier, stimulants can be dangerous if you abuse them, so you should use them responsibly. Herbal methods, alternatively, are an excellent method to use instead.

Here, we will look at some of the best herbs to help ameliorate the worst symptoms of PMS.

- Curcumin
- Saint john's wort
- Evening primrose

Postpartum

Having a baby is one of the most challenging and stressful things a person can go through. Then, you need to launch straight into a new lifestyle where you are entirely responsible for a vulnerable life. If that is not one of the most anxiety-inducing experiences in the world, then nothing is. As a result, many new mothers go through postpartum mental health issues, including depression, anxiety, and even worse. These can feel difficult since you have so much to do, and having a baby can be isolating. Thus, many new mothers seek relief from some of these debilitating feelings. While talking to a counselor or maybe even going on antidepressants can help, many herbal methods can help relieve some of your postpartum symptoms.

- Rosemary
- Sage
- Thyme
- Lavender

Rash/Skin Allergy

Dealing with itchy or irritated skin is very unpleasant, especially if it comes from an allergy. Many people struggle greatly with rashes and find them difficult to eliminate. Of course, there are also many topical creams that you can use and even antihistamines you can take to help give yourself relief from these issues. However, there are also a lot of purely herbal remedies that you can also use to help improve some of your skin issues. Here, we will give you some great herbal remedies for skin irritation.

- Coriander
- Basil
- Chamomile
- Marigold

Sinusitis

If you have any seasonal allergies or are prone to colds and flu, then you have probably experienced issues with your sinuses. Sinusitis is a serious condition and can affect your breathing. In extreme cases, sinus blockage pressure can cause headaches and oxygen deprivation. Thus, you should get some treatment to avoid these negative symptoms. Luckily, herbs offer a lot of great solutions to the issue of sinus blockage. This section will give you some excellent remedies for dealing with sinus issues.

- Yarrow
- Ginger
- Turmeric

Sore Throat

Several over-the-counter remedies exist for sore throats. In the same breath, the same can be said for herbal remedies. Some of these herbal remedies include:

- **Eucalyptus oil.** Up to 12 drops of eucalyptus are boiled with 150ml of boiling water and inhaled to reduce coughs.
- **Sage.** Liquid sage is ingested to relieve coughs and asthma.
- **Licorice root.** Licorice can be made into gargles or lozenges to remedy a sore throat. They can also be used to relieve soreness in the throat after injury.

Conclusion

Herbalism is an incredibly fascinating field of study, with plenty of opportunities to explore. Whether you aim to take a more holistic approach and use herbal remedies as your primary healing form or add extra help to an existing medical plan, you can find something useful here. No matter where you decide to go with it, there are always interesting aspects that could make a positive difference in your life. In this book, we have given you a comprehensive overview of the practice of herbalism and shown you how you could make it fit within your lifestyle. Now you should thoroughly understand what herbalism involves and how it can benefit you.

Before delving into later aspects of herbalism, Chapter 1 helped define the field and clarify what it entails. As such, this chapter discussed what herbalism means and sorted out some confusing distinctions. Likewise, terms like "herbalism" vs. "herbal remedies" are examined, giving you a clear idea of what they both entail and setting up the groundwork for our later exploration of this discipline. With this fundamental knowledge base set, you can confidently delve into herbalism.

In Chapter 2, we moved on to the history of herbalism worldwide. We looked at seven different herbalist traditions to illustrate both the longevity and the variation within herbalism. It is a long tradition, so realizing how important it can be to human history is essential. However, it is also important to acknowledge the people who pioneered these disciplines, who went through years of discovery and trial and error to arrive at the system of herbalism they have today. Although these practices are diverse and sometimes contradictory, you can still take inspiration from lots of them. You can either commit to one of them and try to follow it as closely as possible, or you can respectfully take from each of them as it suits your needs. Whatever your choice, knowing and acknowledging where these things come from is always important.

Then, in Chapter 3, we dove into how to source your herbs. For healing purposes, it is more important to source your herbs properly than anything else. As such, the quality of your ingredients will greatly influence the quality of your product and results. Meanwhile, the difference between foraging, growing, and buying your ingredients can thus have a massive impact on the results of your herbal practice. Now you are aware of all the advantages and disadvantages of each of these methods.

After that, in Chapter 4, we dove more deeply into how you can prepare your herbs. We covered the kinds of tools you will need for your preparation process, which is essential. Missing a tool will result in you having subpar herbalist creations and, thus, subpar results. Likely, we talked about the kinds of ingredients you will need other than the herbs themselves. These can be easily overlooked, so it is vital that you pay close attention to that part. Then we talked about different methods of preparing herbs. Since the applications of these herbal methods are so diverse, it is essential to know about all the different ways you can prepare herbs for your process.

And finally, in Chapters 5 and 6, we gave you two large lists of herbs and their uses, ailments, and their herbal cures. These sections are great for cross-referencing and can do much for your reference in herbalism going forward. If you can have a comprehensive list of both the ailments and herbs, you will have a much better sense of the scope of herbalism and all the things you can do with it. After that section, you should have a strong sense of all that herbalism can do for you and a great list to reference far in the future.

Through all these chapters, we have equipped you with the most important tools you will need going forward on your herbalism journey: the four pillars of herbalism. It might not be a simple or easy discipline, but it can add much to your life. It can help you heal illnesses, practice better mental health, connect with people, and even feel better in your body.

If you enjoyed or learned something from this book, I would appreciate you leaving us a review. I read the reviews and learned a lot from them for research purposes. Take your knowledge, get out there, and improve your life with the incredible power of herbs!

Glossary

Foraging: Finding herbs in nature and harvesting them for your use.

Fumigating: Filling an area with fumes of a particular scent.

Herbalism: The medical practice of curing illnesses or promoting health primarily with herbs.

Herbal Remedies: Cures to illnesses that are made of natural plant materials.

Iroquois: An indigenous North American culture.

Mesoamerican: An ancient Central American culture.

Propagation: The act of taking part in a plant and growing it into another new one.

Solvents: Substances to mix with your herb concoctions.

Unani: A South Asian herbal healing method.

References

Agrimony: Health benefits, side effects, uses, dose & precautions. (2021, June 11). RxList. https://www.rxlist.com/agrimony/supplements.htm#:~:text=Agrimony%20is%20used%20for%20sore

Angelica: Health benefits, uses, side effects, dosage & interactions. (2021, June 11). RxList. https://www.rxlist.com/angelica/supplements.htm

Baillie, L. (2018, May 15). *5 top herbs for muscle and joint pain*. Avogel. https://www.avogel.co.uk/health/muscles-joints/5-top-herbs-for-muscle-and-joint-pain/

Banerjee, N. (2022, November 22). *18 simple home remedies for fungal infections!* PharmEasy Blog. https://pharmeasy.in/blog/try-these-simple-home-remedies-for-fungal-infections/

Betony: Overview, uses, side effects, precautions, interactions, dosing and reviews. (n.d.). WebMD. Retrieved February 7, 2023, from https://www.webmd.com/vitamins/ai/ingredientmono-587/betony#:~:text=Betony%20is%20an%20herb

Binu, S. (2022, August 4). *Viral fever: 5 incredible natural herbs to combat viral fever*. Netmeds. https://www.netmeds.com/health-library/post/viral-fever-5-incredible-natural-herbs-to-combat-viral-fever

Bowman, J. (2021, November 19). *The many benefits of lavender for mood, sleep, hair, and skin*. Healthline. https://www.healthline.com/health/what-lavender-can-do-for-you

Brown, P. S. (2012, August 16). The vicissitudes of herbalism in late nineteenth- and early twentieth-century Britain. *Medical History, 29*(1), 71–92. https://doi.org/10.1017/s0025727300043751

Burgess, L. (2019, February 27). *12 natural ways to relieve pain*. Medical News Today. https://www.medicalnewstoday.com/articles/324572#peppermint

Burke, T. (2019, November 9). *Herbs for hypothyroid*. Blossom Wellness. https://drtaraburke.com/herbs-for-hypothyroid/#:~:text=Fucus%20vesiculosus%2C%20alternatively%20known%20as

Burns | Complementary and alternative medicine. (n.d.). St. Luke's Hospital. Retrieved February 7, 2023, from https://www.stlukes-stl.com/health-content/medicine/33/000021.htm

Calendula information. (n.d.). Mount Sinai Health System. Retrieved February 7, 2023, from https://www.mountsinai.org/health-library/herb/calendula#:~:text=The%20dried%20petals%20of%20the

Canter, P. H., Thomas, H., & Ernst, E. (2005, April). Bringing medicinal plants into cultivation: opportunities and challenges for biotechnology. *Trends in Biotechnology, 23*(4), 180–185. https://doi.org/10.1016/j.tibtech.2005.02.002

Catnip uses, benefits & side effects. (n.d.). Drugs.com. Retrieved February 7, 2023, from https://www.drugs.com/npc/catnip.html

Chaste tree uses, benefits & side effects. (2022, June 16). Drugs.com. https://www.drugs.com/npc/chaste-tree.html

Chauhan, M. (2019, April 17). *Rose (rosa centifolia) - medicinal properties, benefits, dosage.* Planet Ayurveda. https://www.planetayurveda.com/library/rose-rosa-centifolia/

Chen, S. L., Yu, H., Luo, H. M., & et al. (2016, July 30). Conservation and sustainable use of medicinal plants: problems, progress, and prospects. *Chinese Medicine, 11*(37). https://doi.org/10.1186/s13020-016-0108-7

Cheng, R. (1984, January 1). Chinese herbalism. *Canadian Family Physician*, 30:119-22. https://pubmed.ncbi.nlm.nih.gov/21283498/

Cherney, K. (2022, November 15). *9 herbs to fight arthritis pain.* Healthline. https://www.healthline.com/health/osteoarthritis/herbs-arthritis-pain

Cleavers 101. (2017, April 12). Traditional Medicinals. https://www.traditionalmedicinals.com/blogs/ppj/cleavers-101

Clonger, K. (n.d.). *Herbs for ADHD.* Remedy Holistic. https://www.remedyrx.com/blogs/the-remedy-blog/herbs-for-adhd#:~:text=Other%20adaptogenic%20herbs%20that%20have

Complementary and Alternative Medicine | Chronic fatigue syndrome. (n.d.). St. Luke's Hospital. Retrieved February 7, 2023, from https://www.stlukes-stl.com/health-content/medicine/33/000035.htm

Corn silk: Health benefits, uses, side effects, dosage & interactions. (2021, June 11). RxList. https://www.rxlist.com/corn_silk/supplements.htm

Cronkleton, E. (2018, December 12). *How to use aloe vera plant: Benefits, risks, and more.* Healthline. https://www.healthline.com/health/how-to-use-aloe-vera-plant

Cronkleton, E. (2019, March 8). *10 benefits of lemon balm and how to use it.* Healthline. https://www.healthline.com/health/lemon-balm-uses

Cunha, J. P. (2021, August 16). *Ginkgo biloba: Side effects, dosages, treatment, interactions, warnings.* RxList. https://www.rxlist.com/consumer_ginkgo_biloba/drugs-condition.htm

Dandelion information. (n.d.). Mount Sinai Health System. Retrieved February 7, 2023, from https://www.mountsinai.org/health-library/herb/dandelion#:~:text=The%20leaves%20are%20used%20to

Davidson, K. (2020, August 20). *Red clover: Benefits, uses, and side effects*. Healthline. https://www.healthline.com/nutrition/red-clover

DerSarkissian, C. (2021, August 2). *Natural cough remedies*. WebMD. https://www.webmd.com/cold-and-flu/ss/slideshow-natural-cough-remedies

Echinacea information. (n.d.). Mount Sinai Health System. Retrieved February 7, 2023, from https://www.mountsinai.org/health-library/herb/echinacea#:~:text=Today%2C%20people%20use%20echinacea%20to

Egan, N. (n.d.). *Gas: Beat the bloat*. Brigham and Womens. https://www.brighamandwomens.org/patients-and-families/meals-and-nutrition/bwh-nutrition-and-wellness-hub/special-topics/gas-beat-the-bloat

8 home remedies to relieve bug bites. (2018, May 1). Home Pest Control. https://www.homepest.com/blog/8-home-remedies-to-relieve-bug-bites#:~:text=Plants%20%26%20Herbs&text=Three%20are%20particularly%20helpful%20for

Elecampane: Health benefits, side effects, uses, dose & precautions. (2021, June 11). RxList. https://www.rxlist.com/elecampane/supplements.htm

11 all-natural (backed by science) hangover cures that actually work. (n.d.). EZ Lifestyle. https://ez-lifestyle.com/blog/11-all-natural-backed-by-science-hangover-cures-that-actually-work

Essential benefits of Chinese medicne and acupuncture for heart palpitations explained. (2020, September 21). Makari Wellness. https://makariwellness.com/acupuncture-for-heart-palpitations/

Fennel. (2021, June 11). RxList. https://www.rxlist.com/fennel/supplements.htm

Fenugreek: Uses, side effects, interactions, dosage, and warning. (n.d.). WebMD. Retrieved February 7, 2023, from https://www.webmd.com/vitamins/ai/ingredientmono-733/fenugreek

Feverfew. (2020, December). NCCIH. https://www.nccih.nih.gov/health/feverfew#:~:text=Feverfew%20is%20promoted%20for%20fevers

Five herbs that can naturally heal back pain. (2022, May 4). Premier Health Chiropractors. https://premierhealthmn.com/5-herbs-that-can-naturally-heal-back-pain/

Fletcher, A. B. (2020, January). African American folk medicine: A form of alternative therapy. ProQuest: *ABNF Journal, 11(1)*. https://www.proquest.com/openview/fa7a70cc5fa7c535d43e38b35a66de68/1?pq-origsite=gscholar&cbl=32975

Frank, C. (2017, September 6). *Gingivitis: 4 effective home remedies*. Medical News Today. https://www.medicalnewstoday.com/articles/319268#treating-gingivitis-at-home

Frothingham, S. (2018, July 12). *Skin allergy home remedy*. Healthline. https://www.healthline.com/health/skin-allergy-home-remedy

Galan, N. (2019, February 26). *8 herbs and supplements to help treat depression*. Medical News Today. https://www.medicalnewstoday.com/articles/314421#herbs-and-supplements

Geck, M. S., Christians, S., González, M. B., & et al. (2020, July 31). Traditional herbal medicine in Mesoamerica: Toward its evidence base for improving universal health coverage. ResearchGate: *Frontiers in Pharmacology*, 11:1160. https://www.researchgate.net/publication/343338937_Traditional_Herbal_Medicine_in_Mesoamerica_Toward_Its_Evidence_Base_for_Improving_Universal_Health_Coverage

Ginger: Overview, uses, side effects, precautions, interactions, dosing and reviews. (n.d.). WebMD. Retrieved February 7, 2023, from https://www.webmd.com/vitamins/ai/ingredientmono-961/ginger#:~:text=People%20commonly%20use%20ginger%20for

Glass-Coffin, B. (2004, March) Mesoamerican healers. ProQuest: *American Anthropologist; Oxford* 106(1), 192-193. https://www.proquest.com/openview/dee53e65846d90fdc69827c61a322012/1?pq-origsite=gscholar&cbl=40961

Goldman, R. (2018, September 20). *11 effective earache remedies*. Healthline. https://www.healthline.com/health/11-effective-earache-remedies#compresses

Goldman, R. (2020, September 30). *What are the benefits of ashwagandha?* Medical News Today. https://www.medicalnewstoday.com/articles/318407

Granader, J. (2021, November 8). *Spices and herbs for PCOS: Natural PCOS treatment*. Allara Health. https://allarahealth.com/spices-and-herbs-for-pcos-natural-pcos-treatment/

Great plantain: Uses, side effects, interactions, dosage, and warning. (n.d.). WebMD. Retrieved February 7, 2023, from https://www.webmd.com/vitamins/ai/ingredientmono-677/great-plantain

Grieve, M. (n.d.). *Elder*. Botanical. https://www.botanical.com/botanical/mgmh/e/elder-04.html

Griffin, R. M. (2021, March 20). *What Is chamomile?*. WebMD. https://www.webmd.com/diet/supplement-guide-chamomile

Griffin, R. M. (2022, November 6). *Cinnamon*. Nourish by WebMD. https://www.webmd.com/diet/supplement-guide-cinnamon

Guadagna, S., Barattini, D. F., Rosu, S., & Ferini-Strambi, L. (2020, April 21). Plant extracts for sleep disturbances: A systematic review. *Evidence-Based Complementary and Alternative Medicine, 2020*, 1–9. https://doi.org/10.1155/2020/3792390

Harley, J. (2020, January 16). *10 best natural home remedies for IBS*. Mindset Health. https://www.mindsethealth.com/matter/10-best-natural-home-remedies-for-ibs

Harvard Medican School. (2021, February 15). *Herbal remedies for heartburn*. Harvard Health Publishing. https://www.health.harvard.edu/diseases-and-conditions/herbal-remedies-for-heartburn#:~:text=-Catnip%2C%20fennel%2C%20marshmallow%20root%2C

Hawthorn: Uses, side effects, interactions, dosage, and warning. (2019). WebMD. https://www.webmd.com/vitamins/ai/ingredientmono-527/hawthorn

Herbal medicine FAQs. (2016, November 13). American Herbalists Guild. https://www.americanherbalistsguild.com/herbal-medicine-fundamentals

Herbs and supplements for nausea. (n.d.). Complementary and Alternative Medicine | St. Luke's Hospital. Retrieved February 7, 2023, from https://www.stlukes-stl.com/health-content/medicine/33/002581.htm

Hsu, E. (2020, October 1). The history of Chinese medicine in the people's republic of China and its globalization. *East Asian Science, Technology and Society*, *2*(4), 465–484. https://doi.org/10.1215/s12280-009-9072-y

Hui, H., Tang, G., & Go, V. L. W. (2009, June 12). Hypoglycemic herbs and their action mechanisms. *Chinese Medicine*, *4*, 11. https://doi.org/10.1186/1749-8546-4-11

Khalsa, K. P. S. (2009, July 13). The practitioner's perspective: Introduction to ayurvedic herbalism. *Journal of Herbal Pharmacotherapy*, *7*(3-4), 129–142. https://doi.org/10.1080/15228940802142746

Korean ginseng oral: Uses, side effects, interactions, pictures, warnings & dosing - webmd. (n.d.). WebMD. Retrieved February 7, 2023, from https://www.webmd.com/drugs/2/drug-734/korean-ginseng-oral/details#:~:text=Ginseng%20has%20been%20used%20for

Kubala, J. (2020, October 5). *The 10 best herbs to boost energy and focus*. Healthline. https://www.healthline.com/nutrition/herbs-for-energy#2.-Sage

Lang, A. (2022, April 8). *Horsetail: Benefits, uses, and side effects*. Healthline. https://www.healthline.com/nutrition/horsetail

Linden: Health benefits, side effects, uses, dose & precautions. (2021, June 11). RxList. https://www.rxlist.com/linden/supplements.htm

Lubeck, B. (2022, October 19). *The health benefits of olive leaf extract*. Verywell Health. https://www.verywellhealth.com/the-benefits-of-olive-leaf-extract-89489

Luck, M. (2022, August 10). *5 herbal solutions for PMS*. Annex Naturopathic Clinic. Retrieved February 7, 2023, from https://citynaturopathic.ca/herbal-solutions-for-pms/

Marshmallow effectiveness, safety, and drug interactions. (2021, June 11). RxList. https://www.rxlist.com/marshmallow/supplements.htm

McCulloch, M. (2019, April 4). *Goldenrod: Benefits, dosage, and precautions*. Healthline. https://www.healthline.com/nutrition/goldenrod

McDermott, A. (2017, March 22). *Can You Use Herbs to Treat Acne?* Healthline. https://www.healthline.com/health/beauty-skin-care/herbs-for-acne#research

McDermott, A. (2018, October 5). *5 herbal remedies for constipation*. Healthline. https://www.healthline.com/health/digestive-health/herbal-remedies-for-constipation#5.-Slippery-elm

McDermott, A. (2022, July 5). *12 natural remedies to reduce eczema symptoms*. Healthline. https://www.healthline.com/health/natural-remedies-to-reduce-eczema-symptoms#coconut-oil

McGrane, K. (2020, June 12). *What are licorice root's benefits and downsides?* Healthline. https://www.healthline.com/nutrition/licorice-root

Meadowsweet: Health benefits, side effects, uses, dose & precautions. (2021, June 11). RxList. https://www.rxlist.com/meadowsweet/supplements.htm

Menopause & herbs. (2022, March 18). Jean Hailes for Women's Health. https://www.jeanhailes.org.au/health-a-z/natural-therapies-supplements/menopause-herbs#:~:text=The%20types%20of%20herbs%20used

Meyers, A. (2021, August 3). *Restore gut health with 6 herbs and nutrients*. Amy Myers MD. https://www.amymyersmd.com/article/restore-gut-health-herbs-nutrients/

Milk thistle. (2021, June 11). RxList. https://www.rxlist.com/milk_thistle/supplements.htm

Mishra, S. (2023, February 16). *25 remedies to treat edema naturally + signs, causes, & types*. Stylecraze. https://www.stylecraze.com/articles/effective-home-remedies-for-edema/

Motherwort. (2021, June 11). RxList. https://www.rxlist.com/motherwort/supplements.htm

Mullein. (2021, June 11). RxList. https://www.rxlist.com/mullein/supplements.htm

Nall, R. (2019, April 14). *7 home remedies for chickenpox*. Healthline. https://www.healthline.com/health/home-remedies-for-chickenpox#sugar--free-popsicles

Naser, S. (2023, January 31) *10 natural remedies for diarrhea + causes, symptoms, and prevention tips*. . Stylecraze. https://www.stylecraze.com/articles/home-remedies-to-get-rid-of-diarrhoea/

Nickleson, L. (2017, October 16). *13 natural remedies you need to grow for winter colds*. Juice PLUS+. https://www.towergarden.ca/blog.read.html/en/2017/10/natural-herb-remedies.html

Nordqvist, J. (2017, December 13). *Everything you need to know about rosemary*. Medical News Today. https://www.medicalnewstoday.com/articles/266370

O'Sullivan, C. (2005). *Reshaping herbal medicine: Knowledge, education and professional culture.* Elsevier Health Sciences. Google Books https://books.google.com/books?hl=en&lr=&id=z0Yu9k68SzAC&oi=fnd&pg=PA99&dq=herbalism&ots=wx6o3znkzw&sig=TUx53NVYVK70Ltc0_DVK68nsc1g

Oregano: Uses, side effects, interactions, dosage, and warning. (2019). WebMD. https://www.webmd.com/vitamins/ai/ingredientmono-644/oregano

Peppermint. (2021, June 11). RxList. https://www.rxlist.com/peppermint/supplements.htm

Petre, A. (2019, April 12). *What is saw palmetto? Prostate health and other uses.* Healthline. https://www.healthline.com/nutrition/saw-palmetto#:~:text=Saw%20palmetto%20is%20a%20supplement

Petre, A. (2020, June 18). *Goldenseal: Benefits, dosage, side effects, and more.* Healthline. https://www.healthline.com/health/goldenseal-cure-for-everything

Phan, R. (2023, January 17). *The health benefits of holy basil.* Verywell Health. https://www.verywellhealth.com/holy-basil-4766587

Pine. (2021, June 11). RxList. https://www.rxlist.com/pine/supplements.htm

Poulakou-Rebelakou, E., Karamanou, M., & George, A. (2015). The impact of ancient Greek medicine in India: the birth of Unani medicine. *Acta Medico-Historica Adriatica.* 2015;13(2):323-8. https://pubmed.ncbi.nlm.nih.gov/27604201/

Poulson, B., Horowitz, D., & Trevino, H. M. (n.d.). *Kelp.* University of Rochester Medical Center. https://www.urmc.rochester.edu/encyclopedia/content.aspx?contenttypeid=19&contentid=Kelp#:~:text=Kelp%20may%20improve%20sensory%20receptors

Rahimi-Madiseh, M., Bahmani, M., Karimian, P., & Rafieian-Kopaei, M. (2016). Herbalism in Iran: A systematic review. *Der Pharma Chemica, 8*(2), 36–42. http://eprints.skums.ac.ir/964/

Raman, R. (2020, November 18). *10 herbs that may help lower high blood pressure.* Healthline. https://www.healthline.com/nutrition/herbs-to-lower-blood-pressure#:~:text=That%20said%2C%20there%20are%20several

Randall, L. (2018, July 10). *Allergic rhinitis: 6 herbal remedies to try.* Sinus & Allergy Wellness Center of North Scottsdale. https://www.sinusandallergywellnesscenter.com/blog/allergic-rhinitis-6-herbal-remedies-to-try-sinus-allergy-wellness-clinic#:~:text=Try%20some%20ginger%20tea%20to

Red raspberry: Uses, side effects, interactions, dosage, and warning. (n.d.). WebMD. https://www.webmd.com/vitamins/ai/ingredientmono-309/red-raspberry

Rhiannon. (2020, April 27). *Herbal magic for postpartum healing.* Birth Boss. https://thebirthboss.com/blog-archive/2020/4/27/herbal-magic-for-postpartum-healing

Sage. (2021, June 11). RxList. https://www.rxlist.com/sage/supplements.htm

Self-heal: Overview, uses, side effects, precautions, interactions, dosing and reviews. (n.d.). WebMD. Retrieved February 7, 2023, from https://www.webmd.com/vitamins/ai/ingredientmono-130/self-heal

Silver, N. (2019, June 3). *5 Herbs for Severe Asthma: Are They Effective?* Healthline. https://www.healthline.com/health/severe-asthma/herbs-for-severe-asthma#honey

6 must-use herbs to balance hormones. (2022, March 28). CNM College of Naturopathic Medicine. https://www.naturopathy-uk.com/news/news-cnm-blog/blog/2022/03/28/6-must-use-herbs-to-balance-hormones/#:~:text=As%20already%20mentioned%20above%2C%20Vitex

Slodki, M. (2021, December 15). *Beyond extractive ethics: A naturalcultural study of foragers and the plants they harvest.* University of Ottawa. https://ruor.uottawa.ca/handle/10393/43034

Solomon's seal. (2021, June 11). RxList. https://www.rxlist.com/solomons_seal/supplements.htm

St. John's wort: Uses, side effects, interactions, dosage, and warning. (2017). WebMD. https://www.webmd.com/vitamins/ai/ingredientmono-329/st-johns-wort

Stickler, T. (2020, June 4). *Migraine herbal home remedies from around the world.* Healthline. https://www.healthline.com/health/migraine-herbal-home-remedies-from-around-the-world

Stinging nettle: Uses, side effects, interactions, dosage, and warning. (2010). WebMD. https://www.webmd.com/vitamins/ai/ingredientmono-664/stinging-nettle

Stone, E. (1934). Medicine among the Iroquois. *Annals of Medical History, 6*(6), 529–539. https://www.ncbi.nlm.nih.gov/pmc/articles/PMC7943166/

Street, R. A., Stirk, W. A., & Van Staden, J. (2008, October 28). South African traditional medicinal plant trade—Challenges in regulating quality, safety and efficacy. *Journal of Ethnopharmacology, 119*(3), 705–710. https://doi.org/10.1016/j.jep.2008.06.019

Swift, K. (2011, June 17). *Dealing with jetlag.* Common Wealth Holistic Herbalism. https://commonwealthherbs.com/dealing-with-jetlag/#:~:text=Start%20your%20Red%20Clover%20or

Tattelman, E. (2005, July 1). Health Effects of Garlic. *American Family Physician, 72*(01), 103–106. https://www.aafp.org/pubs/afp/issues/2005/0701/p103.html#:~:text=Garlic

10 amazing herbs for good eye care. (2014, December 1). Arizona Retinal Specialists. https://www.arizonaretinalspecialists.com/blog/10-amazing-herbs-for-good-eye-care/

Thyme. (2021, June 11). RxList. https://www.rxlist.com/thyme/supplements.htm

Top 5 herbs for indigestion. (2022, July 25). Australian NaturalCare. https://ausnaturalcare.com.au/blog/top-herbs-for-indigestion

Turmeric: Uses, side effects, interactions, dosage, and warning. (2019). WebMD. https://www.webmd.com/vitamins/ai/ingredientmono-662/turmeric

Uva ursi: Uses, side effects, interactions, dosage, and warning. (n.d.). WebMD. https://www.webmd.com/vitamins/ai/ingredientmono-350/uva-ursi

Valerian: Uses, side effects, interactions, dosage, and warning. (n.d.). WebMD. https://www.webmd.com/vitamins/ai/ingredientmono-870/valerian

Van De Walle, G. (2019, February 11). *Pau d'arco: Uses, benefits, side effects, and dosage.* Healthline. https://www.healthline.com/nutrition/pau-d-arco

Visser, M. (2017, December 26). *14 must-have supplies for herbalists.* Herbal Academy. https://theherbalacademy.com/supplies-for-herbalists/

Ware, M. (2020, January 3). *The health benefits of cayenne pepper.* Medical News Today. https://www.medicalnewstoday.com/articles/267248

Watt S., & Hayes, E. (2013) Monastic medicine: medieval herbalism meets modern science. *Science in School* 27: 38-44. https://www.scienceinschool.org/wp-content/uploads/2014/11/issue27_monastic.pdf

WebMD Editorial Contributors. (2021, June 16). *Herbs for endometriosis.* WebMD. https://www.webmd.com/women/endometriosis/herbs-for-endometriosis

WebMD Editorial Contributors, & Pathak, N. (2020, September 21). *Elderberry: Health benefits, risks, uses, effectiveness.* WebMD. https://www.webmd.com/diet/elderberry-health-benefits#:~:text=The%20berries%20and%20flowers%20of

White, A. (2019, March 7). *Dry mouth remedies: Home and natural remedies that work.* Healthline. https://www.healthline.com/health/dry-mouth-remedies#remedies

World Health Organization. (n.d.). Catalysing ancient wisdom and modern science for the health of people and the planet. WHO Global Centre for Traditional Medicine. https://www.who.int/initiatives/who-global-centre-for-traditional-medicine/#:~:text=88%25%20of%20all%20countries%20are%20estimated%20to%20use,herbal%20medicines%2C%20acupuncture%2C%20yoga%2C%20indigenous%20therapies%20and%20others.

Wiki Contributors. (2021, August 9). *Herbalism.* Wikidoc. https://www.wikidoc.org/index.php/Herbalism

Yarrow. (2021, June 11). RxList. https://www.rxlist.com/yarrow/supplements.htm

Zimlich, R. (2021, November 11). *10 home remedies for bronchitis.* Healthline. https://www.healthline.com/health/home-remedies-for-bronchitis#home-remedies

THE 5 PILLARS OF WICCA

FOUNDATIONS   **BELIEFS**   **PRACTICE**   **MAGICK**   **RITUALS**

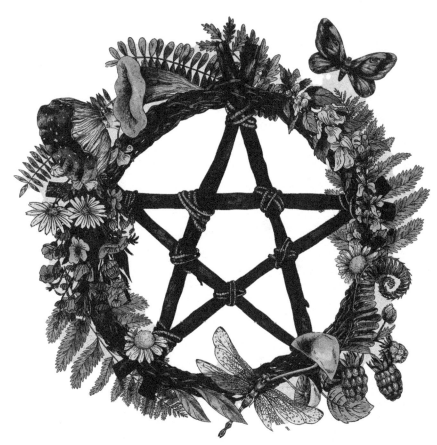

115 TECHNIQUES & TIPS
to Connect to Your Higher Self with the Magick and Rituals of Witchcraft. Find Inner Balance and Harmony by Harnessing the Power and Wisdom of the Craft

INGRID CLARKE

Table of Contents

Introduction 207

Pillar 1: Foundations 209

Chapter 1: What is Wicca? 211
    Old Religion 211
    History and Origin 212

Pillar 2: Beliefs 215

Chapter 2: Deities 217
    The Horned/Sun God 217
    Moon/Triple Goddess 218

Chapter 3: Elements 221
    Spirit or Aether 221
    Air 221
    Fire 221
    Earth 222
    Water 222
    The Elements and Spiritual Direction 222

Chapter 4: Ethics 225
    The Wiccan Rede 225

Chapter 5: Holidays and Festivals 229
    Wheel of the Year 229

Chapter 6: Birth, Marriage, and Death 235
    Birth Rite (Wiccaning) 235
    Handfasting (Marriage) 236
    Handparting (Separation) 237
    Crossing the Bridge (Death) 237
    Afterlife and Reincarnation 237

Pillar 3: Practice 239

Chapter 7: Choose your Practice 241
    Coven Based 241
    Solitary 241
    Hereditary 241
    Eclectic 242
    Secular 242
    Cosmic 242
    Green 242
    Hedge 242
    Kitchen 242
    Hearth 243
    Gray 243
    Augury 243

Chapter 8: Get Initiated 245
    Coven Initiation 245
    Self-Dedication 247

Pillar 4: Magick 249

Chapter 9: Natural Magick 251
    The Elements and Plants 252
    Crystals and Stones 254

Chapter 10: Ceremonial Magick 257
    Components of Ceremonial Magick 257
    Ceremonial Magick Rituals 258
    Ceremonial Magick, the Elementals, and Spirits 260

Chapter 11: Celestial Magick 263
    Constant 1: Prayer 263
    Constant 2: Spirituality 263
    Constant 3: Workings of Celestial Magick 264

Pillar 5: Rituals 265

Chapter 12: Altars 267
    The Wiccan Altar 267
    Setting up An Altar 269

Chapter 13: Tools 271
- Pentacle 271
- Sword or Knife 271
- Wand 272
- Chalice 272
- Boline 272
- Censer and Incense 272
- Besom 273
- Cauldron 273
- Spear or Staff 273
- Bell 273
- Candles 274
- Crystals 274
- Divination Tools 274

Chapter 14: Ritual Wear 275
- Ritual Robes 275
- Cloaks 276
- Pentacle 277
- Other Jewelry 277

Chapter 15: Common Components of Wiccan Rituals 279
- Preparation 279
- Casting the Magick Circle 281
- Calling the Quarters and Invoking the Deities 283
- The Heart of the Ritual and the Book of Shadows 284
- Cake and Ale 284
- Closing the Ritual 285

Chapter 16: Different Types of Rituals 287
- Centering 287
- Cone of Power 288
- Grounding 288
- Shielding 289

Conclusion 291

Glossary 293

References 297

Introduction

When you hear the word "Wicca," what image does it conjure up in your mind? Likely, your vision of Wicca and its practices could be different from another person's. But this does not mean you are wrong. Wicca is varied and multifaceted, making it a practice and lifestyle with which people from numerous backgrounds can adopt and grow a connection. There are countless ways to understand and experience Wicca's essence. And different people may practice it uniquely, which is perfectly fine. Despite the different approaches to Wicca, the basic tenet of interconnectedness remains unchanged.

Wicca brings harmony and balance to one's life, which, during troubling times, is essential. And as inherently spiritual, it raised introspection and questioning how to better connect with oneself and the world. Practicing Wicca helps bring the connection back into your life, whether with the earth, yourself, or others.

This book distills the spiritual principles and practices of the craft that can open your awareness, connect you to the divinity of the world you are living in, and awaken the magick in you. In this book, I will break down the different aspects of Wicca through the five pillars: foundation, beliefs, practice, magick, and rituals. These pillars help shape how we understand and interact with the world.

Daily life contains stress, anxiety, and other negative aspects. These stresses might be caused by work, issues you are facing in your relationship, or troubles you are having with your personal life. In today's modern world, it is becoming easier and easier to detach from our natural environment and ourselves. As we become accustomed to this detachment, it becomes harder to understand our inner natures.

Having suffered severe burnout, my family's Scandinavian roots in neo-paganism drove me to look into different healing techniques. Through my research, I was able to accumulate many teachings and wisdom. Subsequently, I did not only study Wicca but also many metaphysical practices and occult traditions from around the world. And by my exploration and practice, I realized that I was an empath. Now, my mission in life is to share my extensive knowledge and experiences with those who need help and healing. This book will serve as an introduction to Wicca and its practices. The first two pillars will increase your knowledge of Wicca, including its history and modern-day significance, as well as describe its core beliefs and principles. Meanwhile, pillars three to five will talk about Wiccans' different techniques, rituals, ways of worship, and magickal practices.

Throughout this book, we will discuss multiple strategies to help you better understand and align yourself with the elemental nature of the universe. You will find 115 beginner techniques, tips, and strategies to awaken the magick within you and forge a deep connection with your higher self. It's peppered throughout the entire book and it's intentionally designed this way to serve as your guide along each step of the process. I have practiced all the methods discussed in this book, which have empowered me to find ways through any challenges and provided me with a means for self-development and positive change. It is essential to remember that the only way to enact changes in your life is to take charge, and the techniques you will learn in this chapter will enable you to do so. The end goal of this book is to help you with your journey of spiritual awakening and help you to get in touch with your higher self and find your divine purpose. By tapping into your intuition, Wicca offers a path for stirring up celestial magick within yourself. And with this book, you will gain a blueprint for activating the power of divine magick and opening yourself up to its wonders.

Despite the challenges in gaining knowledge about Wicca and its practices, this book makes it accessible for anyone interested in uncovering its mysteries. Regardless of the struggles you are dealing with in your life, the timeless wisdom of the craft will provide a different point of view on how to approach life's complexities. Alongside this awareness, you will uncover inspiration, beauty, and revelations as you rewrite your destiny and uncover the mysteries of the unknown. With proper usage of what you will learn here, you can create a new place for yourself and comprehend the enigma. Hence, by the end of this book, you will have begun your self-discovery journey; all that remains is to access divine power within yourself.

Accordingly, each chapter of this book will give you a better understanding of Wiccan beliefs and conventions, as well as steps and strategies for those looking to walk the Wiccan path and create better connections with their inner self, others, and the world. Likewise, this book will teach you how to open your mind to possibilities and enhance your life. Now, let us dive into the first pillar of Wicca and learn about its foundation.

Pillar 1
Foundations

Wicca is an ancient religion practiced for thousands of years and can be traced back to old Pagan traditions. Today, it is a modern neo-Pagan spirituality based on honoring the natural world, respecting all life forms, and finding the balance between the dark and light to reach a divine understanding. Pillar 1 seeks to explain Wicca and how it has evolved throughout history so you can make more informed decisions when exploring this path.

1

What is Wicca?

Before we can get into the fundamentals or traditions of Wicca, let us take a step back and look at what it is. Subsequently, Wicca is the largest neo-Pagan religion, also called modern Pagans, with followers known as Wiccans, who typically identify themselves as witches. Before the 1950s, Wiccans kept their practices hidden— only coming to light in England and other Western countries. Anyhow, their followership is a few hundred thousand individuals. And although there are no direct ties to Christianity, Wicca was highly influenced by European religions. Now that you have a fundamental definition of Wicca let us dive into the old religion, history, and the prevalence of Wicca in the modern day.

Old Religion

Many religions throughout history have had figures known as witches, some of whom were evil figures, and in others, they were healing and good creatures. There is a long history of old religions that, although not responsible for the creation of the Wiccan religion, is connected to it because Wiccans associated themselves with witchcraft and called themselves witches. Christianity has a long history with witches, although it is seldom a positive one.

The general ideals around witchcraft and witches have changed during the modern day, with it being used in films as a trope of good and evil and a means of resolving social tensions, especially in feminism. However, pre-modern Western civilization held a lot of irrational fear around witchcraft. This fear often stemmed from religious practices claiming witchcraft was the devil's work. Inevitably, the fear sired a hostile mentality towards those identified as witches.

From there, witch hunts started in the 11th century and continued into the 18th century. With the propagation of witchcraft as heresy and devil's work by Christianity and other religions resulted in those accused receiving persecution. As fear continued to grow and fester around the ideas of witches, by the 14th century, it was commonly believed that all people that were witches used a form of malevolent sorcery and were evil.

Witches continued to be regarded with trepidation and linked to the devil. Even the meaning of their rituals, such as the sabbats, was twisted, and it was believed that they gathered to perform orgies and other sexual acts in the name of Satan. It also became a belief that they could transform, had familiars, and kidnapped and murdered children. Think back to the tale of "Hansel and Gretel." It was written long before the creation of Wicca and portrayed a witch that would lure children in and eat them. Although these are ideas of fantasy, they stuck so much fear into people that laws were created to punish those that were witches and allowed for witch hunts to occur. Notably, witch hunts were rarely about capturing those already regarded as 'witches.' But instead, it focused on tracking down those suspected to be hiding.

The Salem Witch Trials also showed religious intolerance, fear, and political control, with numerous women accused of witchcraft being hanged. Altogether, these trials led to the execution of 19 individuals of all ages. However, there was no proof that these people were witches, but rather it is theorized that family feuds, religion, politics, and fear were the cause of the accusations and executions. One person accusing another of their bad fortune was enough to raise suspicion about them being witches. People's fear of witches became so ingrained in the culture that indictments and prosecutions occurred in villages, law courts, and courts of Appeal in Protestant and Roman Catholic communities. Studies have shown that approximately 110,000 people were on record of being tried as witches, and about 40,000 to 60,000 of these trials resulted in executions.

Law and religion played equal parts in witch trials and hunts, and over the years, cultures developed numerous ways to determine whether someone was a witch. The first way was to prick them. If they felt no pain, they were a witch, as the devil had desensitized them to it. A devil's mark, often an oddly shaped mole, was also looked for. Meanwhile, some throw people into lakes and ponds.

Interestingly, it was believed that if an accused person sunk in the water during a trial by ordeal, it was indicative of their innocence as the water was seen to be accepting them; witches would not prevail. These signs were mainly used in local and village trials, while more extensive trials, such as those held before kings, inquisitors, and bishops, resulted in fewer convictions and milder sentences. This is likely due to a heavier influence on the law than religion, although both still played a part in both trials.

Witchcraft and witches have also been linked back to ancient civilizations, as it was believed that magick and religion were needed to appease, manipulate, and protect against evil spirits. These civilizations thought that evil spirits were universal, so magick was necessary. It could also be used for evil at the time. Sabbats have often been compared to the rituals performed in the worship of Dionysus, as people would gather outside and perform many rituals, including sacrificing animals, feasting, drinking, and orgies.

History and Origin

The origins of Wicca can be traced back to a British civil servant by the name of Gerald Brosseau Gardner. He spent most of his career traveling throughout Asia, and during his time there, he learned about many indigenous religions and traditions. He also invested much of his time reading the writings of British occultist Aleister Crowley and other esoteric literature.

Gardner returned to England in the 1930s and joined a British occult community, which claimed they had located a group of witches near New Forest in 1939. Gardner claims that he and the occult group communicated with the New Forest group of witches, and the information they learned from them was the basis on which Wicca was formed. In 1951, the archaic witchcraft laws were repealed, which enabled Gardner to form his coven, publish *Witchcraft Today*, and create the Gardnerian Wicca religion with Doreen Valiente, who served as a high priestess.

Gardner formed not all Wiccan practices, beliefs, and rituals; instead, he helped to jumpstart other occultists to develop their Wiccan traditions throughout the 1950s and '60s.

Most Wiccans claimed they were practicing pre-Christian witchcraft. However, historians disputed this as more studies of modern witchcraft continued. In the 1960s, Wicca emerged as a general term for religion, yet, there were various forms, including Alexandrian. During the first two decades, most Wiccans were initiated into covens, but as time continued, more and more people initiated themselves into Wicca. Many forms of Wicca were created during its emergence, which we will discuss later in this book. The beauty of Wicca comes from the varied ways you can practice it.

Wicca in the Present

Although Wicca was never at the scale of Christianity in terms of followers, it gained popularity throughout America and western culture. Numerous books started to be published in the 1970s and '80s, telling people how they could initiate themselves into Wicca. Although covens are few and far between in the present day, individual Wiccans are still practicing. It is unknown how many people are still actively practicing Wicca, as many initiated themselves and practice solitarily rather than in a coven. In the present day, Wicca, or witchcraft, is more known as a trope in film, television, and books than as a religion.

As Wicca was traveling through America as a religion, it also grabbed the public eye as it became the subject of many films and television series, including *Buffy the Vampire Slayer*, *Charmed*, and *The Craft*. However, many of the portrayals of Wiccans in popular media have caused people to fear those who practice Wicca or have gone on to create false tropes and representations of its ideals. Teenage Wiccan culture was heavily portrayed in the media, often warning young teenagers of the dangers of practicing, which has resulted in a decrease in initiates over the years. Because of the negative portrayals of the Wiccans in mainstream media, many tried to rebrand themselves as traditional witches, but this insinuated that they partook in non-Wiccan occultism and rituals.

Wicca and witchcraft, over time, have started to become used interchangeably. However, it is important to note the difference. Witchcraft has been connected to many religions throughout history, but Wicca has only existed for less than 100 years. Wicca is said to be derived from witch practices; the name Wicca is etymologically connected to the word witch, which is why followers call themselves witches. Yet, this is not concrete proof that the New Forest witches were accurate, which many historians have tried to prove and disprove.

Now that you know the foundations of Wicca, its history, and it in the modern day, it is time to move on to the second pillar and learn all about the beliefs of the Wiccans. Remember that there might be some variation between the different types of Wicca in terms of faith. Still, they all stem from spiritual empowerment and connecting with oneself and the world around you. The first aspect of Wiccan beliefs that we will discuss is deities.

Pillar 2
Beliefs

There is power in understanding, and with learning comes growth. Now, we will explore the tenets of Pillar 2 about Wiccan's beliefs. And through understanding its various components, we can form a more meaningful connection to this ancient spiritual practice.

In Chapter 2, we will learn about the Horned God and the Moon or Triple Goddess. Meanwhile, Chapter 3 will teach us about the five elements: earth, air, fire, water, and spirit or aethyr. Next, Chapter 4 will explain the Wiccan rede, a code of morals for Wiccans.

Then we will move on to Chapter 5, covering both greater and lesser Sabbats, which include religious holidays like Samhain and Yule and seasonal phenomenons such as Spring Equinox and Summer Solstice. And finally, Chapter 6 reveals rituals surrounding birth (wiccaning), marriage (handfasting), separation (handparting), death (crossing the bridge), and afterlife/reincarnation.

We have much to learn before us on our journey into the deep wisdom of this sacred practice; let us begin!

2

Deities

Undoubtedly, the gods and goddesses worshiped in Wicca are among the prominent declarations of faith for devotees of this religion. Unlike Christianity, which only worships one god or deity, Wicca is similar to Ancient Greece or Rome, as there are two central deities. However, the ancient Greeks, Romans, and other cultures worshiped many different gods as they served as symbols for various reasons, such as the harvest, youth, changing of seasons, and fertility, amongst many other things. Whilst Wicca and neo-Paganism have two central deities— the Horned God and the Triple Goddess. In this chapter, we will discuss the origins of each of these deities and their purpose within Wicca.

The Horned/Sun God

Although the Horned God has become tightly linked to Wiccan practices and neo-Paganism, the name was first used in the early 20th century to describe anthropomorphic gods that took on the image of antlered or horned animals. And looking throughout history, many religious beliefs have incorporated horned deities.

The word "witch" is typically believed to be feminine, while "warlock" is masculine. Yet, within the context of Wicca, the distinction between a witch and a warlock has no gender implications. In truth, some followers of witchcraft chose to refer to themselves as witches regardless of gender since warlock was seen as a derogatory word. Nevertheless, the Horned God in Wicca represents the masculine side of Wicca. Likewise, Wicca is known as a duotheistic theology system, which means that masculine and feminine are equal within the system, and both are needed. Depictions of the Horned God differ depending on the source. Some sources show him as having horns or antlers, while the rest of him is human. Other depictions will show him as having an animal head and a human body, thus representing the union between the divine and animals. In this instance, the animal is often a representation of humanity.

Wiccan beliefs also associate the Horned God with the life cycle, nature, hunting, the wilderness, and sexuality. He is also considered a dualistic god, representing two aspects of something: day and night, light and dark, and summer and winter, along with others. As he is associated with the life cycle, his duality can also be connected to life and death.

The Horned God is the consort of the Triple Goddess, but they are both equals within the religion. He is considered masculine, and she the feminine. Often, they serve to represent opposites. Wiccans, like other religions, tend to organize the world in terms of masculine and feminine energy. Anything masculine, such as hunting and the wilderness, is associated with the Horned God.

Although Wiccan believed that the gods and goddesses were both equally important, recent developments have seen a far greater emphasis on the feminist influences of the Goddess, a reflection of feminism's growing mark. Meanwhile, the Horned God is a fundamental part of Wicca worshippers' Wheel of the Year celebrations, symbolizing the cycle of seasons. During the year, he is said to impregnate the Triple Goddess during the spring, die as winter approaches, and is then reborn by the Goddess with the new year.

Aside from that, the Horned God is often compared to Hades, the Greek God of the underworld, as they reside over hell. The Horned God was also Summerland's protector, the realm in which souls awaited reincarnation. Remarkably, the death of the Horned God in the Wheel of the Year resembles Persephone's story, where she stayed in the underworld with Hades before her triumphant return as a harbinger of spring. Unlike other religions, the Horned God's relation to death does not cause fear within followers; instead, he is considered a comforter and consoler to those who have passed and are waiting to be reincarnated.

Moon/Triple Goddess

Wicca is not the only neo-Paganism religion that is practiced. In many of them, the Triple Goddess is a deity, or at least a deity archetype in the religion's practices. The Triple Goddess is often referred to as a Moon Goddess, but her representation as a triunity, a combination of three figures, is the most common. These representations tied to the Triple Goddess include the female life cycle (the maiden, the mother, and the crone), three realms of the world (heaven, earth, and underworld), and the phases of the moon, hence why she is often referred to as a Moon Goddess. Yet, Wicca did not create this figure like the Horned God. While most commonly associated with Wicca, the Triple Goddess has a long religious history extending beyond its modern context.

The origins of a Triple Goddess started during ancient history, including ancient Greece with the Graces, the Horae, and the Moirai. It is also connected to the Hindu religion with the representation of Tridevi. The goddess Hecate, in ancient Greece, was thought to be one of the first Triple Goddesses due to her presence in art and sculptures during her early worship. Later, the Roman goddess Diana, also known as Artemis in Greek mythology, was depicted as a Triple Goddess. Yet, Hecate is significant for the Triple Goddess in Wicca because she associates with witchcraft. Likewise, she was heavily connected to the moon, and her triple nature was seen to be related to the moon's phases.

Within Wicca, the physical female body is viewed as sacred since it reflects the Triple Goddess, a representation of femininity associated with birth, lactation, menstruation, and female sexuality. This depiction of the Triple Goddess as different areas of a woman's life includes the following distinctions:

- The maiden or child represents birth, new possibilities, youthfulness, inception, and expansion. The maiden is described as a waxing moon if there are connections to the moon.
- The mother represents fulfillment, fertility, sexuality, ripeness, power, and life. This stage is often depicted as the full moon, which could symbolize pregnancy.
- The crone or older woman represents repose, wisdom, endings, and death. This stage is defined as a waning moon.

During the 1970s, The Triple Goddess had a special significance for female followers when feminist movements blossomed. Her image brought solace and liberation to many who sought her out. Although she had a consort, The Triple Goddess was often solitary in the days following his death, a role that transcended what was traditionally viewed as masculine. Thus, she was transformed into an image of self-sufficiency and encouraged Wiccan women to take on more traditionally male roles, especially as more and more coven leaders were becoming women rather than men.

Wicca draws influence from the Horned God and the Triple Goddess, with their combined power representing the five-pointed pentacle symbol. The Horned God is known for his duality, while the Triple Goddess manifests threes; together, they give form to the powerful five-pointed star. Their meaning and how you worship them differ depending on the type of Wicca one is practicing. Still, no matter how you practice Wicca, these two deities are critical for spiritual empowerment and learning to connect with oneself. For female Wiccans, the Triple Goddess is paramount because she is an influential figure they look up to and can connect with at all times. In the next chapter, we will explore the importance of the elements in Wiccan beliefs.

3

Elements

For Wiccans, magick is simple and effective. It is not complicated or convoluted but rather is a part of nature. Thus, when someone can connect with their spirituality and the world around them, they should be able to use the elements as a form of magick. Primarily, Wiccans embrace the foundational elements of air, fire, earth, and water with an extra fifth element, spirit or aether, for their metaphysical practice. This blend of both physical and spiritual components brings their magick to life. And this chapter will explore how each element is vital to Wiccan beliefs and rituals.

Spirit or Aether

Before we talk about the four traditional elements, we must first talk about the influence spirit or aether has on one's ability to perform elemental magick and its effect on a person. One's energy or spirit is essential for performing magick. In Wicca, spells and words are only used to guide focus; the person's spirit performs that magick. One's spirit can also play a large part in influencing the elements. When someone has a light or good spirit, their effect on the elements will be positive, while someone with a dark or negative soul will have a negative impact. For example, with earth, someone who has a good spirit can help the land and even produce gems. But someone with a bad spirit will cause earthquakes and damage. Spirit and energy are present within each of the four other elements, which enables Wiccans to influence them.

Air

Wiccans are deeply connected to air, the first masculine element, and associated with the Horned God and his practices. This warm and moist element is symbolic of spring. Although air is intangible, it is seen as a powerful element more influential than tangible substances like water and earth. During rituals involving air, wands and staffs symbolize this element, and incense and smudge sticks are used as part of the ceremony. These air spells are typically connected to healing or purification.

Fire

Fire is considered one of the most spiritual elements and is on the masculine spectrum. Although it has no physical form like water or earth, it creates warmth and light and is believed to have powerful transformative abilities. Likewise, it is a warm and dry element associated with summer. Candles are one of the most commonly used tools for fire magick, along with burning spells and rituals. Meanwhile, red and gold gems, such as red jasper, tiger's eye, rubies, and bloodstones, are used in fire magick along with herbs and spices, such as allspice and cinnamon. Lastly, fire magick is associated with power, creativity, strength, love, and passion.

Earth

Earth has strong ties to the goddess, making it a common element used in the practices of Wicca. Salt, onyx, and aventurine are often used within these rituals to draw upon the prosperity and abundance associated with earth magick. This is mainly due to its connection with the Triple Goddess and the earth's fertility. Yet, not only does earth bring about life and new beginnings, but also death and rebirth. When we die, we return to the earth; our decomposition sustains new generations of life. Lastly, winter months are connected to earth as an element as they can be described as cold and dry.

Water

Water is another feminine element and is considered superior as it has more motion and activity than the element of earth, which is known for being sturdy and stable. This is why it is one of the most prominent magick in Wicca. But what makes it unique is its ability to interact with our senses. Associated with fall, this cold, moist element closely connects emotions, water's undulating waves are often likened to tears shed in both times of sorrow and joy, symbolizing the deep emotional currents it embodies. Symbols like water lilies or aloe plants, alongside gems like amethyst, aquamarine, and opal, are often integrated into this magick.

The Elements and Spiritual Direction

The elements are not only used for elemental magick, but according to Selena Fox, a high priestess of the Circle Sanctuary coven, they also serve as a "framework of spiritual symbology, teachings, and practices" (*Wicca manual, n.d.*) that Wiccans have. Elements are a framework, as each element is associated with different sacred directions. The rituals you practice can differ depending on which element you are influenced by the most. People can also have times when they are more connected to one element over others. However, the majority of Wiccans try to connect with all five elements. Here are each of the directions that the elements are associated with:

- Earth is associated with the north.
- Air is associated with the east.
- Fire is associated with the south.
- Water is associated with the west.
- Spirit is associated with the center because each human holds their spirit.

The pentacle is a symbol that represents Wiccans' ability to bring spirit to the earth or the elements. The five elements are often placed on the pentacle as a way of showing how each of the elements is essential for different areas of one's life, and unity of all five is needed for spiritual empowerment and wholeness. Here are how the elements are arranged on the pentacle and which areas of one's life they influence:

- Earth influences physical endurance and stability and is placed on the lower left corner of the pentacle.
- Fire influences daringness and courage and is placed in the lower right corner of the pentacle.
- Water influences intuition and emotions and is placed on the upper right of the pentacle.
- Air influences thoughts, intelligence, and the arts and is placed on the upper left of the pentacle.
- Spirit is placed on the top point of the pentacle and represents oneself and the divine.

People who are physically active and fit will likely be more connected to the earth than the other elements.

The elements play a large part in Wiccan beliefs and practices. Wicca enables people to connect with themselves and nature, understanding the importance of the elements in our lives and acknowledging the damage or healing we can do to nature. In the next chapter, we will start to dive deeper into Wiccan beliefs as we explore their ethics and the Wiccan rede.

4

Ethics

As with any religion, there are ethics that followers must identify with. Typically, the ethics associated with a religion is what draws people in. Although there are different ways to practice Wicca, those doing it for good all follow the same moral codes outlined in the Wiccan Rede and the Rule of Three. In this chapter, we will explore the Wiccan Rede, the Rule of Three, and their importance to Wiccan ethics and beliefs.

The Wiccan Rede

The Wiccan Rede is essential to the beliefs and practices of the Wiccans. It outlines the moral standards associated with Wiccans and other neo-Paganism religions. The word rede is derived from the words advice and counsel. Wiccans often seek out the Wiccan Rede during hard times. It is believed that the first iteration of the Wiccan Rede was publicly recorded by Doreen Valiente in 1964. The first form of the Wiccan Rede was only composed of eight words which varied in different forms. The original Wiccan Rede read: "An ye harm none, do what ye will" (*Wiccan rede*, 2022).

In 1974, a longer Wiccan Rede, which would become the one officially recognized, was published and is as follows:

Bide the Wiccan Laws, we must In Perfect Love and Perfect Trust.
Live and let live. Fairly take and fairly give.
Cast the Circle thrice about to keep the evil spirits out.
To bind the spell every time, let the spell be spake in rhyme.
Soft of eye and light of touch, speak little, listen much.
Deosil goes by the waxing moon, chanting out the Witches' Rune.
Widdershins go by the waning moon, chanting out the baneful rune.
When the Lady's moon is new, kiss the hand to her, times two.
When the moon rides at her peak, your heart's desire seeks.
Heed the North wind's mighty gale, locked the door,
and dropped the sail.
When the wind comes from the South, love
will kiss thee on the mouth.
When the wind blows from the West,
departed souls will have no rest.

When the wind blows from the East, expect the new and set the feast.
Nine woods in the cauldron go, burn them fast and burn them slow.
Elder be the Lady's tree, burn it not, or cursed you'll be.
When the Wheel begins to turn, let the Beltane fires burn.
When the Wheel has turned to Yule,
light the log, and the Horned One rules.
Heed ye flower, Bush and Tree, by the Lady, blessed be.
Where the rippling waters go, cast a stone, and truth you'll know.
When ye have a true need, hearken not to others' greed.
With a fool, no season spend, lest ye be counted as his friend.
Merry meet and merry part, bright the cheeks and warm the heart.
Mind the Threefold Law, you should,
three times bad and three times good.
When misfortune is enow, wear the blue star on thy brow.
True in love ever be, lest thy lover's false to thee.
Eight words the Wiccan Rede fulfill: An ye harm none, do what ye will. (The Wiccan Rede, n.d.)

The Wiccan Rede is much like all religions' fundamental Golden Rule. The majority of Wiccans, no matter which type, follow the Wiccan Rede. However, a small group of Gardnerian Wicca chooses to use the Charge of the Goddess, specifically the following line as their moral code: "Keep pure your highest ideal, strive ever toward it; let naught stop you or turn you aside, for mine is the secret door which opens upon the door of youth" (*Wiccan rede*, 2022).

The Charge of the Goddess is fundamental to all Wiccans and their practices; however, it typically is not used as a moral code. This poem is used during many rituals. During that time, the priest or priestess leading the ceremony became a representation of the Triple Goddess. The Charge describes how the Triple Goddess will guide and teach the Wiccans. It is essential to their practice and beliefs, despite the Wiccan Rede being the standard moral code.

There is often debate around the meaning of the Rede, with some Wiccans believing it to be a commandment, while others believe it to be advice. There is no statement of what precisely the Wiccans Rede means, and it is left to the individual's interpretation of what to make of it. The common understanding is that the Wiccan Rede tells followers to do good for others and themselves. Another interpretation of the Wiccan Rede is to not only seek the simple wants of life or what other people want you to do but always follow your true will. Unlike other religions, there are no guidelines for what will harm and what will not, leaving it entirely up to interpretation. Some Wiccan sects take the Wiccan Rede to mean not harm yourself. This sometimes also extends to animals and plants but will disregard other people. Overall, the interpretation of the Rede is up to the Wiccan. Still, it is commonly understood that it encourages people to take responsibility for their actions and not to harm another person or thing.

The Rule of Three

Occultists, Neopagans, and Wiccans follow the tenet of the Rule of Three, which states that the energy a person puts into the world will return to the person three times. The Rule of Three pertains to both positive and negative energies, which can help to deter Wiccans from practicing dark magick. Although some

Wiccans call the Rule of Three karma, they are not the same concept. However, they both encourage a person to do good, and good will be done to them in return.

Some Wiccans do not take the Rule of Three literally. Instead, they believe energy will return to them as often as possible until they learn the lesson they need. The ideas of the three also relate to the Triple Goddess. Although not all Wiccans adhere to the Rule of Three, some believe it was created to mimic Christianity.

The Rede and Rule of Three are two fundamental Wiccan beliefs that different sects can variably interpret. By looking at these practices, it is evident that speeches and poems are often reinterpreted, with their resulting practices reflecting these shifts in understanding. In the next chapter, we will discuss the numerous holidays and their significance to Wicca.

5

Holidays and Festivals

Deities and magick are essential parts of the Wiccan belief and practice. As we know, the Triple Goddess and Horned God are beings integral to the Wiccan religion, and a part of their worship is through holidays and festivals. Like any religion, holidays and festivals are vital parts of their practice. Historically, religions had numerous festivals that served many different purposes. Looking at the ancient Greeks had festivals that were meant to appease Demeter so that people would have healthy crops and abundant harvests. They had gathered for Dionysus, and they would worship him through drinking, feasting, and having sex. There were festivals for the transition of children from childhood to adulthood. As with past religions, Wiccans have many festivals and holidays. Although nowadays, when we think about holidays, Christmas and Halloween are likely to come to our minds, the festivals and holidays which the Wiccans practice are not the same. In this chapter, we will explore many of them and what their purpose is.

Wheel of the Year

The Wheel of the Year is a symbol used to show the eight sabbats in which Wiccans participate throughout the year. A thousand years ago, Celts celebrated the festivals present on the Wheel of the Year that Wiccans use today. However, there is no proof of an ancient Wheel of the Year used during the ancient times, as some Wiccans try to claim. The names of the festivals the Celts celebrated differ from those of the Wiccans.

The passing of time and life is captured in the Wheel of the Year. It is a reminder that nothing is ever-lasting but also an affirmation of eternal return and rebirth. And although the seasons change and people die, everything comes around again. This goes along with the Wiccan belief in rebirth or reincarnation. Even if someone's physical body might die, their soul is reborn into a new body. Despite modernization changing ideas around time being linear, the Wheel of the Year and its celebrations allow them to connect with nature and accept their time as it is.

Greater or Eight Sabbats

Through the eight sabbats, Wiccans can honor their connection with nature. Represented by the Wheel of the Year, these seasonal celebrations provide an opportunity to reflect on our place in the world and come together in harmony. Although you might think, why are there eight celebrations when there are only four seasons? This is because they mark the beginning and middle of each season. Despite many Wiccans practicing in solitary rather than in a coven, the greater sabbats keep time for everyone to get together and connect with other Wiccans and nature. The cyclical nature of time represented in the eight sabbats allows Wiccans to reflect on what they have gained and lost in the past year. Reflecting on gratitude and looking toward the future, but also reflecting on the past, allows Wiccans to find balance and harmony in their lives.

Samhain (October 31)

Although each of the sabbats falls on a day or a couple of days to which the Wiccans hold significance, Samhain is one of the most important. For Wicca, Samhain marks the beginning of a new year, like the New Year's Day that most people celebrate on January 1st. The name Samhain means summer's end and is especially important because it occurs on the last day of the season of light and marks the beginning of the darkness. Yet, misconceptions persist that the season of darkness is inherently evil, particularly in light of Halloween. But this is incorrect; darkness and light to Wiccans are not symbols of good and evil but necessities. One cannot have light without regenerative darkness. Symbols of light and dark, the Horned God and the Triple Goddess, are neither good nor bad. Instead, they emphasize our interconnectedness with nature and remind us that there is a balance between two opposite forces.

Samhain was celebrated throughout history as ancient sites in Ireland, Wales, Scotland, and Britain all showed gathering sites for Samhain. While non-Wiccans do not typically observe Samhain, many of its older practices resemble today's Halloween traditions. Bonfires on Halloween and many practices of mischief night have been traced back to the practices of Samhain. As the bonfires were lit, sacrifices such as crops and animals were burned, which is a protective measure against evil spirits. And nowadays, people will burn bonfires to symbolize this meaning.

During this festival, Wiccans took a moment to reflect on the past year and honor those who had been lost and their ancestors. Wicca, along with many other cultures, believed that the veil between the lands of the living and dead was the thinnest on Samhain, which allowed the dead to traverse the land of the living easily. Although this might have been frightening for some, Wiccans believed it allowed ancestors and departed loved ones to communicate with the living. One custom for this was to make the favorite meal for those who had died. However, spirits being able to cross the veil also meant that those who felt as though they were wronged could seek compensation or retribution.

Meanwhile, traveling at night on Samhain was warned against as it was believed that non-human spirits, such as fairies and sprites, lived in the spirit world and could cross over into the human realm to seduce and abduct mortals that were not being careful. And to protect their identity, people use masks and costumes to ward off spiritual beings that seek to do them harm.

Yule, The Winter Solstice (December 20-25)

Yule is the sabbat celebrating the shortest day of the year, the Winter Solstice. This day is significant to the Wiccans as it represents the renewing nature of life's cycles because the length of the day only prolongs after this festivity. Pagans use Yule to celebrate the birth of a Sun God. And for Wiccans, this same date marks the reincarnation of the Horned God at the hands of the Triple Goddess. So, on Yule, Wiccans take special notice of the evergreen tree, decorating it in honor of the Sun or Horned God and leaving gifts for him. Among Wiccans, the evergreen stands for life's strength and ability to endure despite changing seasons.

Alongside the evergreen tree, a bonfire is lit to burn the Yule log. Once again, a bonfire is present during the season of darkness to resemble rebirth and new beginnings. Each year, a piece of the Yule log is saved for the next year, and as people sang around the fire, they would throw holly into it. The holly was meant to symbolize the challenges that they have been experiencing and how they will not weigh them down but help them to grow.

Now, let us discuss the two figures in Wicca: The Oak King and Holly King. The Yule celebration is to show the Oak King coming back into power over the Holly King. These two figures stand for light and darkness. As the days become shorter and there is less light, the Holly King rules, and the Oak king rules when the days are longer. The exchange of power between these two shows the continuity of life.

Imbolc (February 1-2)

Sitting halfway between the Winter Solstice and Spring Equinox, this festival is a time to celebrate purification and rebirth. Imbolc means in the belly, which signifies fertility, promise for the future, and hope. The Celtic goddess Brigid is often symbolized during this festival, as she was the goddess of fertility, poetry, medicine, sacred springs, and the forge. Some Wiccans will make dolls in the goddess' likeness by weaving cornstalk. Making these gifts in her honor was meant to represent continuity, luck, and fertility. February 2nd is relevant even to non-Wiccans, as in Western society, Groundhog Day occurs. Wiccans would celebrate Imbolc in the hope of an early spring.

Ostara, The Spring Equinox (March 20-23)

The promise of hope, birth, and fertility is met when Wiccans celebrate Ostara, also known as the Spring Equinox. In history, Ostara has been sacred to Pagans. Still, their celebrations were kept secret, and very little is known about how Pagans would celebrate Ostara before Jacob Grimm brought it to light. Eostre, the Germanic goddess of spring and fertility, inspired the holiday's name. Like Persephone, Eostre was said to rise from the earth on the equinox, bringing spring with her. Different myths say that she either sleeps during the months before or is pregnant and gives birth as she leaves the earth. The Triple Goddess is depicted as becoming impregnated by the Horned God around this time. This sabbat emphasizes renewal and rebirth, yet little is known about how Wiccans commemorate it. Evidence suggests that feasting, which may sometimes include a rabbit, was part of the festivities.

Beltane (April 30 - May 01)

Beltane is a festival that occurs in the middle of spring and celebrates fertility, light, and the coming of summer. Bel, the Celtic god, is believed to be the inspiration for the name as it comes from the phrase "Bel's Fire," which means bright fire. Bonfires are essential during this festival, as fire is associated with passion. During this festival, people are meant to indulge in their desires and set aside their inhibitions.

During ancient Pagan rituals, dancing around a tree and wrapping ribbons around a maypole were performed. A young woman would also be picked to become the May Queen, who was meant to stand in for the fertility goddess Flora.

This festival signifies the increase of light in the world as nature continues to awaken. However, this also means unseen awakening entities within the spirit realm. Although fairies were typically seen as being safe, they were also known to be mischief makers. The ritual of placing a rowan branch in the house's ceiling was performed by the head of the home, as well as a cleansing, which involved carrying a lit candle from the front door to the back door, to the corners of the house, and from the hearth to one side of the main rooms. The walking around symbolizes the creation of a net with eight points.

Litha, The Summer Solstice (June 20-22)

As the year's longest day draws near, it is marked by the celebration of the Summer Solstice or the Litha sabbat. This celebration makes the official transition of power from the Oak King to the Holly King. After this day, the days start to become shorter. Dancing, bonfires, feasting, honey cakes, and fresh fruits are traditional at this festival. However, this festival is celebrated as light triumphing over darkness, despite knowing that darkness would slowly overtake light again after that day.

At the Summer Solstice, individuals protect themselves from unseen dangers, like spirit entities. It is believed that these mystical forces began to stir during Beltane and are at their peak when summer arrives, causing harm to those who do not take preventive measures. To protect oneself from such external forces, rituals are conducted all day long at Litha Sabbat, and sun wheels made of stalks are crafted as a symbol of this celebration. If one was married on this day, protection rituals were especially performed on the couples to ensure their marriages were happy and healthy.

Lughnasadh (August 1)

This festival is named after the Celtic god of truth and order, Lugh. Known as a harvest festival, Lughnasadh focuses on the passing of summer and the coming of fall. The Horned God's death is seen as approaching, and he would return to Summerland and the underworld until the Triple Goddess brought him back. During this festival, fruits and vegetables would be harvested; the first offered to the gods and goddesses.

Harvest, fall, and death also link to the god Lugh and the myth of him and his foster mother, Tailtiu. She was one of the first Celtic gods, and her tale depicts her dutifully and selflessly slowing the land of Ireland to prepare it for its people; as a result, she died from exhaustion. To honor her, Lugh would hold an annual feast on her death, which became Lughnasadh.

Common activities during this sabbat include archery, horse racing, fencing, racing, boxing, and wrestling matches. These activities are funeral rituals to honor Tailtiu, but they also were used as a final celebration of summer.

Mabon, The Autumn Equinox (September 20-23)

Mabon, the celebration of the Autumn Equinox, completes the wheel of the world and is used as a time for reflection and giving thanks. Unlike many other sabbats, the name is a modern invention, first being named in the 1970s. It has been observed that nearly every ancient civilization had a figure that would descend into the underworld as a marking of autumn and winter approaching and then reemerge at the beginning of spring. Depending on the religion, a god or goddess would be seen as dying on this day and returning to the underworld. For Wiccans, this would be the Horned God. Other examples include Persephone from ancient Greece.

During the Mabon sabbat, Wiccans and Pagans will celebrate the second harvest and the coming of winter. Giving thanks for the crops they had been able to harvest that year was especially important during this sabbat. Celebrating the gifts, they could gather from the forest also comes with the acknowledgment that the soil was dying for the winter seasons.

Esbat

Aside from the greater or eight sabbats, there are other festivals and celebrations known as Esbats that Wiccans participate in. Every month, when the full moon rises, people meet and celebrate together in groups or by themselves for Esbats. These gatherings are an opportunity to take part in initiations and healing magick. The thirteen lunar months of the year are all marked by Esbats, making each full moon a special occasion.

Wiccans often observe Esbats during the full moon. Yet, specific covens or practitioners may also choose to celebrate them at new moons. Esbats are essential as covens or individuals will draw power from the moon, allowing others to feel empowered during these times. During new moon Esbats, rituals are performed for healing, personal growth, and initiation into new ventures. They are the most intimate among the celebrations, and outsiders are rarely invited.

Gods and goddesses are still honored during Esbats, although not as much as with sabbats. Traditionally, during an Esbat, a circle would be cast. But if a coven or singular person does not do this purifying, alternative purification methods, such as smudging, are performed in specific areas. Doing this marks the place as sacred. Bowls of water and moon candles are essential to the rituals performed during an Esbat. More on Wiccan rituals will be explored later in the book.

As you have learned, there are numerous festivals, holidays, and rituals that Wiccans partake in throughout the year, and this does not include any personal ones that a coven or person might practice, including those around birth, marriage, and death, which will be discussed in the next chapter.

6

Birth, Marriage, and Death

Each religion and person have a way of celebrating or grieving. And within Wicca, there might be different ways that different types of Wiccans perform rituals. Besides celebrating Sabbats and Esbats, there are numerous other rituals; Wiccans participate, either in a coven or individually, including birth, marriage, separation, death, and the afterlife. In this chapter, we will look at how Wiccans perform rituals of wiccaning, handfasting, hand parting, crossing the bridge, and afterlife and reincarnation.

Birth Rite (Wiccaning)

If you are a part of the Pagan community and have a child, you will likely hear whether you will have a wiccaning ceremony for your child. You can also be new to the Pagan community and hear whether you will have a wiccaning ceremony for yourself. It is important to remember that not all Pagans are Wiccans; you can be part of the Pagan community but not be a Wicca. The wiccaning ceremony welcomes an infant, child, or new person into the Pagan or Wiccan community. It is often compared to baptism for Christians.

Pagans who do not identify as Wiccan go through their welcoming ceremony called saining. You do not need to go through a wiccaning to be a Wiccan, nor do you need to perform this ceremony for your children. It is entirely up to you as a person or parent whether you want to have a wiccaning.

Saining is very similar to wiccaning, and during this, charms will be made for the child, and rituals to perform to ensure they remain safe and healthy throughout their lives. In ancient wiccaning and saining practices, there are writings of children being passed through a hole carved from stone, and the act was meant as a protective measure from fairies and other creatures in the spirit world. Protection from fairies was critical because Pagans believed that fairies would come to the mortal realm and kidnap babies, leaving a changeling in its place. A wiccaning or saining ceremony emphasizes the protection of children. Presenting a person or child to the gods and goddesses is traditional for a wiccaning ceremony.

It is important to remember that partaking in a wiccaning ceremony for yourself or your child does not mean you are locked into anything. A wiccaning is just a matter of welcoming you or someone else into a spiritual community where you will hopefully be able to grow and flourish.

Handfasting (Marriage)

Handfasting is a marriage ceremony that has existed for thousands of years and is present in numerous cultures; however, it is believed to have Celtic origins. Its origins are heavily tied to nature and spirituality and where the phrase "tying the knot" comes from when discussing marriage.

The history of handfasting predates Christianity, and since many people could not afford to buy gold rings for their spouses, a handfasting ceremony was a much more affordable option. Despite the ritual being nothing more than a ribbon, an old fabric, or a cord tied to the hands of two people as they exchange vows, it still felt deeply spiritual. Typically, the couple would keep their hands tied together until midnight. If they overcome their hardships while connected, their union will succeed. Yet, nowadays, the couple would typically only stay tied together for the ceremony.

The rope and fabric used in a handfasting ceremony carry different meanings. But it will be up to the couple to decide which symbols to impart. When selecting the colors, factors are considered, such as:

- past, present, and future
- dreams, adventures, and hopes
- promises you are making to one another
- personality
- special individuals in your life

Wiccans are the only community to practice handfasting. But if you are part of a coven, the coven leader will typically perform the handfasting ceremony. Several parts go into this ceremony, and they usually go in the following order:

- music and processional
- welcoming the guests and statement of intention
- first reading
- second reading
- presentation of cords or ribbons for handfasting
- ritual in which couples' hands are bound
- vow exchange
- declaration of marriage
- closing statement
- recessional and music

How your handfasting ceremony goes might differ depending on whether you are part of a coven, if you are also performing other rituals, or wish to include anything else in the ceremony. Alongside the ceremony, the couple and guests might partake in a tradition known as jumping a besom broom, which signifies the building of a home and hearth together.

For Wiccans, in particular, there are two stages of marriage. The first is betrothal, which lasts a year. At this time, the couple is given a chalice, and after the year, the couple performs the handfasting ritual. The chalice is also shattered during this ritual, and the couple is given the pieces.

Handparting (Separation)

Not everyone is meant to be married, and Wiccans recognize this; thus, they have hand parting rituals. Handparting is the rite that formally ends a handfasting, cutting the symbolic and spiritual ties established during the ceremony. This ritual also emphasizes that, although there is no longer emotional love between the couple, there is still a friendship. Wicca does not punish divorce as their marriage vows are as long as love shall last. There being no punishment or discrimination of divorce makes it much easier for a couple to separate, making their relationship outside of marriage much healthier.

If a couple is legally married, they will still need to undergo a civil divorce, and the handparting ceremony can occur any time before or after this happens. For Wiccans, handfasting can equate to marriage, but to be legally married, one would need to have a civil marriage and, thus, a divorce. If a couple does not have a civil union, the handparting ceremony equates to divorce.

Who attends this ceremony is wholly on a case-to-case basis. Some couples will want only a priest or priestess present, while others will wish to have parents, loved ones, and children if the situation is amicable.

The handparting ceremony will occur at an altar that can be set up in someone's home or the officiant's office. It will be covered in cobalt blue, black for wisdom, red for healing, and other cloth that might be meaningful to the couple. The shards of the chalice and the cords from their handfasting should be present during the ritual. Gods and deities are called on to oversee the ritual, and the couple will discuss the lessons they learned from the marriage. The goal of this ceremony is for the peaceful separation of the parties so that they may respect their former partner and the relationship they had.

Crossing the Bridge (Death)

As you can tell throughout this chapter, Wiccans have numerous rituals for different aspects of life, and one of the final ones is the crossing the bridge ritual performed at a Wiccan's death. Other Wiccan groups will perform this ceremony differently, but they all honor the death of a Wiccan with a crossing the bridge ritual. Some common rituals include a spiral dance representing the cycle of life or a reenactment of a god or goddess descending into the underworld. Storytelling, feasting, and drinking are also common funeral rites of Wiccans. The stories would typically reflect the life of the person who has passed on. Emphasis on life and death is essential during this ritual as it leads to the next aspect of Wiccan beliefs: the afterlife and reincarnation.

Afterlife and Reincarnation

As we learned in an earlier chapter, the Horned God is the ruler of the underworld, and Summerland is the realm where spirits wait to be reincarnated. Concepts of the afterlife and reincarnation are not new, as each culture and religion have its own. Depending on the culture, the aspect of a reborn human will differ, whether mind, soul, or consciousness. Although the afterlife and reincarnation are present within the Wiccan practices, not all Wiccans believe in them. Wiccan traditions are meant to make the most out of your life rather than dwelling on what will happen afterward. Depending on the Wiccan, some believe that humans can only be reincarnated into new human bodies, while others acknowledge that you could be reincarnated into an animal. When spirits were within Summerland, a medium could contact them.

Feri Wicca is one type of Wicca that has ideas about the soul and what happens afterward. It adopted the Hawaiian notion, which states human beings have three souls. This can connect back to the ideas of three with the Rule of Three and the Triple Goddess.

We have discussed numerous Wiccan beliefs, including deities, the elements, ethics, holidays and festivals, and numerous rituals that occur throughout a person's life. We have completed Pillar 2, and it is time to discuss Pillar 3, which is all about Wiccan practices, starting with the numerous ways you can practice Wicca.

Pillar 3
Practice

Many of us are drawn to Wicca for the freedom it offers. We each have our journey, and sometimes we must figure out which path to take. That is why Pillar 3, covering the practices of Wicca, is so essential; it focuses on what kind of practice you could pursue. Thus, this section will discuss Chapter 7, about choosing your practice, and Chapter 8, about getting initiated.

In Chapter 7, we explore the different types of practices within Wicca. You can choose from coven-based, solitary, hereditary, eclectic, hedge, secular, cosmic, green, kitchen, hearth, gray, or augury practices. Whichever one calls out to you will best fit your spiritual path.

Then, in Chapter 8, we will look at getting initiated into a particular tradition through coven initiation. There are two rites; the rite of dedication and the rite of passage. Through these rites comes transformation and an initiation into a new way of being in the world that may bring greater understanding and connection to yourself and deeper ties with others who are also on that path.

7

Choose your Practice

Depending on the type of religion you practice, there can be many different branches of that religion from which you can choose to practice. As we have learned, Wicca was formed by Gardner but did not force all Wiccans to practice the same way he did. Within Wicca, there are numerous ways you can practice because the primary goal of Wicca is connecting with yourself and nature; however, you choose to do so. As Wicca reached different parts of western culture, it was introduced to many people who adapted it to best suit them. This chapter will discuss some of the most common ways that Wicca is practiced.

Coven Based

When Wicca was founded, the primary way that it was practiced was through covens. Gardner formed one of the first covens at the beginning of Wicca, and as it exploded, it was the primary way witches practiced Wicca. A coven is a group of witches that gather to perform rituals and rites. For the sabbats, esbats, and rituals discussed in the previous section of this book, covens would gather for those. The number of witches within a coven would vary, and witches did not need to be related to form a coven. Three or more is considered a coven. The strength of a coven was not determined by the number of witches that were a part of it. Instead, it was about their connection, nature, and power. Three powerful witches could be stronger than a coven of 10.

Solitary

As Wicca is not as popular as it used to be, it can be hard to find a coven, so many Wiccans decide to practice solitarily. A Wiccan might want to work alone as well. Not having a coven can give a witch some freedom because instead of following the coven's practices, you can combine different practices to do the best for you and allow yourself to make the deep connections you want.

Hereditary

Not all witches are born as such. Many Wiccans, especially when it was just created, were likely a part of another religion and decided to practice Wicca because they agreed with its core values and practices more. Hereditary witches are those that inherit their magick from their families. Many people born into Wiccan families likely identify in some regard as hereditary witches. These witches probably do not have rituals and practices solely based on their status as hereditary but are part of another type of Wicca.

Eclectic

Eclectic witches identify as Wiccan, but their practices and beliefs are not strictly Pagan. Instead, they adopt aspects of other religions and philosophies into their practices. Whether in a coven or not, the ideologies and religions you embrace will vary. There are no concrete rules to eclectic Wicca, which is why many Wiccans choose this type of practice.

Secular

Unlike other witches who rely on religion and spirituality to tap into their magical abilities, secular witches do not bind their power to any faith or mysticism. This means that they are free to practice their craft without the constraints of adhering to Wiccans' particular set of beliefs. Likewise, these witches are often distanced from the Wiccan tradition or any other faith-based practice and define themselves independently.

Cosmic

Cosmic witches focus on the stars, astronomy, and astrology as integral parts of their practice. The moon is a fundamental part of their rituals in all its phases, as it is with other Wicca forms. These aspects of cosmic witchcraft, which are present in many Wiccan rituals, add to the power of their practice. Usually, these witches use incantations and moon cycles for protection against celestial happenings. They have an affinity for star signs and birth charts in their craft. Likewise, they change energies using their extensive knowledge of the star signs and help people better understand themselves and the cosmos' influence on them.

Green

Green witches are those that specialize in healing, nature, and nurturing. Their power, rituals, and tools all come from the earth. Plant, flowers, and herbal preparations are commonly made by these witches and are a primary source of ingredients for different spells. These witches hold nature in the utmost regard and respect it above all else. Plus, they play a large part in sabbats around harvesting, healing, and fertility.

Hedge

Hedge witches share much in common with green witches, but while the latter dedicate their magick to nature, hedge witches can practice various forms of magick. Also, they often practice alone, and like eclectic witches, they do not limit themselves to one belief system. Instead, they can incorporate numerous spiritual and religious approaches in their work. Likewise, these witches keep everything basic and straightforward, as they often do not have the support of other coven members. They also focus their abilities on herbal remedies, the elements, and nature. The freedom that hedge witches have makes it viable for someone who is drawn to nature but does not want to be a part of a coven like most green witches are.

Kitchen

As the name suggests, kitchen witches focus their energy on the kitchen. They mix magick into their cooking and baking, utilizing herbs for their metaphysical properties. Every ingredient has been carefully chosen to ensure the best outcome for each dish, not just for flavor but also to unlock the potential of its magical qualities. When there are celebrations and festivals, kitchen witches prepare meals to share with the coven and external community. Depending on the purpose of the gathering, they will make different dishes.

Hearth

Hearth witches are similar to the kitchen and green witches but are centered around the home. These witches concentrate their abilities on rituals and objects around the house, including ritual cleansing, herbalism, and candle magick. They also have a vast knowledge of protection spells as they take it into their hands to protect the house.

Gray

White and dark magick is used through Wicca, with different types of witches leaning one side over the other. Yet, gray witches like to straddle the line between the two as they use whichever is best for the situation they find themselves in. Curses and hexes are typically considered dark magick, and while most witches will not use them, gray witches will if they think it is necessary. Although these witches use both forms of magick, they are not evil. Instead, they use dark magick to redirect bad energy and seek justice. They use their magick to call on unseen forces to help them correct unfair circumstances and injustices.

Augury

Augury witches can use their power to decipher omens, typically from the behaviors of birds, animals, and the weather. These witches are generally able to use divination as well. They might also call themselves prophets. Besides that, they could use the movement of birds, animals, or the weather to determine auspices, of which there are five different kinds:

- **Ex caelo = from the sky:** does not involve birds but looks toward thunder and lightning for the omens of the gods.
- **Ex avibus = from birds:** not all birds or animals were symbols of gods communicated. There were traditionally two ways augury witches could interpret, through song and their movement while flying. Common birds used for these practices included ravens, owls, hens, and crows.
- **Ex tripudiis = from birds feeding:** chickens were generally used for this practice. Augury witches would throw food at chickens; depending on how they reacted, it would be a good or bad omen.
- **Ex quadrupedibus = from quadrupeds:** omens were taken from animals that walked on four legs, such as a dog, fox, wolf, or horse.
- **Ex diris = from portents:** these are the least likely to be used as they are not from weather or animals but are essentially any action that seems to be abnormal.

These are just a few of the many Wiccan practices you can choose from. You can even select a few different ones and decide which rituals, forms, and practices you want. No matter where you are drawn, there are so many other Wiccan practices that you can adopt. The next part of Pillar 3, after you have chosen your practice, is getting initiated into Wicca. You might be surprised to learn that there are multiple ways to begin.

8

Get Initiated

Now that you know the history of Wicca and its foundations and have chosen which Wiccan practice you would like to focus on, it is time to get initiated into Wicca. Initiation into Wicca is different from the wiccaning we talked about earlier. Being welcomed into the spiritual side of Wicca through a wiccaning does not imply any commitment to practicing Wicca. Yet, one way to become initiated is by performing a ritual where you are devoted to it. But this does not mean someone is forced to stay within Wicca; you can leave Wicca and a coven whenever you desire. There are two ways that you can become initiated into Wicca: coven initiation or self-dedication.

Coven Initiation

During the start of Wicca, taking part in a coven initiation was how the majority became Wiccan. This is because very few people would know about Wiccan practices without being part of the community unless they were looking for it. Unlike larger and more widespread religions, information about Wicca was not easily accessible like it is today, making coven initiation the go-to. Coven initiations do not occur as much today as many Wiccans practice solitarily rather than as part of a coven. This is because the number of Wiccan covens has significantly decreased since its beginning. However, there are still a few covens, however small they may be. To take part in a coven initiation, there are two rites in which you have to partake. The first is the rite of dedication, and the second is the rite of passage. It is important to note that although all covens have these two rites, there can be different ways of performing them. And each coven might have various rites or rituals that need to be completed by initiated members to become fully integrated into the coven.

Rite of Dedication

The rite of dedication is used to signify when someone wants to join a coven. After Wiccans performed this dedication, they start to train with the coven. Depending on the coven, how long the training period goes on will differ. The meaning of this dedication to the person and the coven will vary based on the circumstances. Some covens might take it very seriously, while others might not as much. The training after the proper ritual is performed can also be considered part of the rite as initiates learn the rules and skills of the coven. During the dedication, a witch is learning to embody all the coven stands for.

Going through a rite of dedication can change someone's curiosity about Wicca and its beliefs to a commitment to learning the practices and developing their own identity. Under the lunar light, this is an opportunity for initiates to connect with nature and have the direct attention of the gods while dedicating themselves to Wiccan teachings.

Rite of Passage

After someone has gone through the rite of dedication, they can go through their rite of passage. The rite of passage into a coven usually occurs a year and a day after their rite of dedication. Typically, it is a ceremonial event in which the person or people performing it must execute different tasks or rituals to complete the rite. Across the ages and in many other societies, rites of passage have been observed. The extent of this ceremony and everything that goes into it will differ depending on your coven. For such, the rite of passage's cultural, social, and psychological significance may vary. Going through this process allows a person to gain acceptance into society. As for Wiccans, this means that the witch or witches performing the ceremony will be initiated into the coven upon completion.

Depending on whether you are born into Wicca or find it later in life, your rite of passage will be different. For those born Wiccan, their rites of passage are likely connected to bodily milestones like puberty or entering adulthood. However, when you find Wicca later in life, your rite might be based on how long you have been practicing. The type of rite of passage you perform will differ from coven to coven. For any rite of passage, the goal is to purify the person and prepare them to start the next part of their life as a Wiccan. The purification that is performed allows individuals to communicate with the supernatural and connect with nature. For someone not born into Wicca, the cleansing of this rite can symbolize the shedding of your past life and the beginning of your new one as a Wiccan.

Social transformations, like coming of age or being inducted into a coven, are also part of the rite of passage. Here is a breakdown of the different rites of passage you might experience.

Life Cycle Ceremonies

Each coven will have different life cycle ceremonies. These rites of passage are linked to biological milestones in a person's life, including birth, childhood, and transitioning into adulthood. Depending on the coven you are in and their practice, you could go through numerous life cycle ceremonies, and there could be different rites for different sexes. Depending on the type of magick they use and their practices, the events and what is performed can differ significantly.

Social Transformation Ceremonies

Social transformation also encompasses the life cycle ceremonies as people transition from one stage of their life to another. These transitions also cause their social status and roles to change. Ceremonies outside those connected to life cycles do not have a connection to biological milestones but occur as someone's social role transforms. An example of a social transformation as a rite of passage would be someone being initiated into the coven as a new Wiccan, or it could be when someone's role in the coven is changed, such as a new coven leader being put into power.

Religious Transformation Ceremonies

Sacrifices and offerings are very common during these ceremonies to symbolize everything a person is giving up and what they are willing to give. Someone who is not a Wiccan, being initiated into a coven, would experience a religious transformation during their rite of passage.

Self-Dedication

Wicca today is very different from what it was even 20 years ago. Covens were much more prominent then and accessible to people looking to be initiated into Wicca. However, finding covens is much more challenging nowadays, especially ones publicly looking for more initiates. Meanwhile, self-dedication became much more recognized, allowing you to practice the way you want and not need to follow the rules of a coven. As we discussed, covens would perform the rites and rituals for a proper initiation, but you must execute them alone during self-dedication. You cannot initiate yourself into Wicca because this would mean there would be other witches performing the ceremony; this is why it is called a dedication rather than an initiation.

Although it is not necessary for you to perform a self-dedication ceremony, doing so is an excellent way of solidifying your relationship with the gods, goddesses, nature, and the Divine. When and how you choose to dedicate yourself to Wicca will depend on you. Some people like to study for one year and a day and then devote themselves; others will choose specific times in the year or the month to do so. It is entirely up to you how you choose to dedicate yourself to Wicca. Yet, even if you can decide when and how to commit yourself, it is essential to take time because it is a significant part of your spiritual journey. Here is an example of a simple self-dedication ritual that you can change to fit your needs better.

The Wiccan practice of self-dedication is traditionally performed in a state of nudity. For instance, being naked during the ritual represents a sincere vulnerability and openness to the divine forces and the self. Likewise, it is believed to remove any barriers that may hinder the practitioner's connection with their inner essence, as well as with the natural world and the divine energies. However, if being naked is impossible, alternative conditions are provided for the ritual. These conditions include ensuring that the area is free of distractions, private, and quiet. Both options aim to create an environment conducive to focused and uninterrupted ritual practice. To complete this ritual, you will need blessing oil, salt, and a white candle. Begin by grounding yourself through meditation. Allow your mind to relax, and do not focus on anything mundane. Once settled, pour salt onto the ground and stand in it. Have the white candle close enough to feel its heat when you light it. Look into the flame of the candle and think about your motivations as you follow this script to complete your self-dedication:

Stand by the altar and say: *"I am a child of the gods, and I ask them to bless me."*

Dip your finger into the blessing oil, and with your eyes closed, anoint your forehead. Some people trace a pentagram on the skin with the oil. Say: "May my mind be blessed so I can accept the wisdom of the gods." Anoint the eyelids (be careful here!) and say: *"May my eyes be blessed, so I can see my way clearly upon this path."*

Anoint the tip of your nose with the oil, and say: *"May my nose be blessed, so I can breathe in the essence of all that is Divine."*

Anoint your lips, and say: *"May my lips be blessed, so I may always speak with honor and respect."*

Anoint your chest, and say: *"May my heart be blessed, so I may love and be loved."*

Anoint the tops of your hands, and say: *"May my hands be blessed so that I may use them to heal and help others."*

Anoint your genital area, and say: *"May my womb be blessed so that I may honor the creation of life."* (If you are male, make the appropriate changes here.)

Anoint the soles of your feet, and say: *"May my feet be blessed so that I may walk side by side with the Divine."*

If you have specific deities you follow, pledge your loyalty to them now. Otherwise, you can use *"God and Goddess"* or *"Mother and Father."* Say: *'Tonight, I pledge my dedication to the God and Goddess. I will walk with them beside me and ask them to guide me on this journey. I pledge to honor them and ask that they allow me to grow closer to them. As I will, so it shall be"* (Wigington, 2018c).

This is just one way you can perform the self-dedication ritual. Because it is you and you alone performing it, you can change it however you want. What matters is that you are fully allowing yourself to become dedicated to Wicca and that this ceremony best suits your desires for your experience as a Wiccan. Do not let others dictate how you dedicate yourself to Wicca. The self-dedication ritual I gave you above is simple. If you want something more extravagant, make it so; if you are going to keep it as simple as possible, do it. You can include other rituals in this as well.

Whether a coven initiates you or you go down the path of self-dedication, you are now a full member of Wicca. Now that you have chosen your practice and are a full member, it is time to dive into Pillar 4 and discuss the various forms of magick.

Pillar 4
Magick

In pillar 4, we will explore Wiccan's magick, an ancient, mysterious, and powerful practice with many layers. Also, we will delve into three different chapters about natural magick, ceremonial magick, and celestial magick, each of which has unique aspects to explore.

Starting with natural forces in chapter 9, we will learn how to perform rituals and spells using plants, herbs, animals, crystals, and more. Then we will soon uncover the core elements of ceremonial magick in chapter 10 and techniques for summoning spirits. And finally, in chapter 11, celestial magick will be discussed on how it relates to the divine.

As we explore pillar 4, more of its components will be unveiled. Now, let us dive deeper into the mystery that awaits us in the upcoming chapters.

9

Natural Magick

There are three different kinds of magick that a Wiccan can use. The first kind that we are going to talk about is natural magick. As the name sounds, this magick draws on the natural world. Wiccans believe there are two worlds, the natural and the spirit, and to draw on these worlds requires different magick. Natural magick is used for the human world and uses different plants, herbs, animals, crystals, and other natural forces to perform various rituals, potions, and spells.

Although the word magick is attached to the name, much of natural magick is drawn from natural sciences, such as alchemy, astronomy, astrology, chemistry, and botany. And even if Wicca is modern in its invention, natural magick has been around since the Renaissance. When using natural magick, many different flowers, herbs, fruits, and crystals are used, which people call upon for their magick properties. Depending on the purpose of your magick, the substances you use will change. Throughout this chapter, we will learn about natural magick materials, practices, and rituals.

The Elements and Plants

We learned earlier in this book the importance of elements for Wiccans, and now we have come back full circle. The elements are a central part of natural magick, and in the next chapter, they will also play a large role in ceremonial magick and summoning spirits. You might wonder why the elements and plants are together in one category. You might assume that plants would naturally fall under the category of earth. Still, following the writings of Agrippa in the 17th century, different parts of the plant are associated with other elements: the roots to earth, the leaves to water, the flowers to air, and the seeds to fire (Ball, 283). The thickness of the roots and being buried in the earth connects them to the element of the earth. Then, the leaves are connected to water because they contain juices. Meanwhile, flowers are connected to the air because of their subtlety. And the seeds are connected to fire, an element associated with passion and reproduction because this is how the flowers spread and grow.

Depending on the area that a Wicca lived, their access to different plants would be varied, but here are some of the most commonly used plants and their magickal properties.

Acacia

Acacia is also known as gum Arabic or Arabic gum and is associated with money, platonic love, spiritual and psychic enhancement, and protection. It can be used in many different ways, including incense. Augury witches, or those specializing in divination, used acacia to promote a meditative state, allowing them to interpret omens and messages more clearly. Protective elements of this herb make it helpful in storing ritual tools to ensure they are not corrupted or stolen by someone. This herb will also be prepared with oil to anoint censers and candles to help boost their spiritual and psychic abilities and protect them.

Bergamot

Bergamot is an herb that is traditionally used for burning during rituals to promote success. Bergamot was burned as it was believed to strengthen its power, versus if it was crushed and used in a potion. The burning aspect of this ritual and its strength can be related to modern-day aromatherapy, as burning would release the scent of bergamot, enhancing its ability. This herb is associated with money, prosperity, improving memory, promoting a better night's sleep, stopping inference, and protecting one from illness and evil. One can burn a bit of bergamot near their bedside for sleep benefits. Getting a better night's sleep is shown to improve memory as well. If you do not have access to fresh bergamot, using essential oil can give you some of the benefits it is associated with.

Berries

A multiple of berries are used in natural magick during rituals, but their primary use did not lie in their magickal abilities. Instead, it was left as an offering for gods, goddesses, and spirits. Strawberries are commonly used because of their bright coloring. How ripe and bright a berry determined the wealth of the crop, and the best-looking ones were made as an offering. Appeasing the gods, goddesses, and spirits with fruit helped ensure continued protection and fertility of the land.

Bluebells

Bluebells were used for many reasons, but one of the most common was to determine how psychically polluted the world was becoming. It was believed that bluebells would disappear as the world became more polluted. However, bluebells were known to be connected to witches, and people would no longer plant them, especially during witch hunts. Traditionally, it is said that witches could hear bluebells ringing if they had a visitor, which is why they would be planted near the door.

Deadly Nightshade

Poisonous plants are also used in natural magick, and deadly nightshade is one of the most commonly used. During ancient times, it was used as a preparation for anesthetics and poisons. For witchcraft, deadly nightshade is soaked in fat from an animal to create a cream that was said to promote astral projection. Astral projections could be used to help decipher messages from the gods. Nowadays, this type of potion is not used because the astral projections witches claimed to have are now known to be hallucinations caused by the deadly nightshade.

Eyebright

Another herb that is connected to divination and clairvoyance is eyebright. This plant was used to create an eyewash that would help to develop a witch's ability to perform telepathy. To make this eyewash, you will need about two handfuls of eyebrights, a heatproof bowl, a bottle, and boiling water. Follow these steps to create your eyewash:

1. Add herbs and water into the bowl.
2. Stir the mixture until the herbs are coated and allow to infuse for a minimum of 10 minutes. The longer you let it infuse, the more powerful the mixture will be.
3. If you choose to, this is the time to invoke a spirit or deity.
4. Once the water has cooled, pour it into a bottle.

To use, rinse your eyes with the wash and perform the desired rituals.

Ginger

Ginger root is typically dried and ground into a powder to be used in spells and rituals. The herb is aromatic and used to spice rituals and spells and get results quicker. It was believed that putting ginger in food offered to the gods would make effects happen faster and stronger.

Lady's Mantel

Alchemy is one of the natural sciences used in natural magick, and lady's mantel was one of the herbs used in alchemy. It was believed that glassy beads of liquid that accumulated on the leaves of this herb overnight were used to create the philosopher's stone because the fluid was infused with the herb's magickal properties at a concentrated level. Likewise, the stone was believed to have healing properties that could prolong life, cure disease, and turn metals into gold. Witches using natural magick could try to remake the philosopher's stone.

Mugwort

Dream pillows and incense meant for divination typically had mugwort in them, the herb believed to aid in prophecy. However, its potency and power meant that it was used with caution, so it was only used as an infusion sparingly.

Vervain

Vervain also went by enchanter's herb and was used primarily to protect against negative energy and evil spells and purify sacred places and items, including homes, temples, altars, and tools. This herb dates back to ancient times, with the Egyptians, Greeks, and Romans using it for its magickal properties.

Crystals and Stones

Like plants, not all crystals and stones are linked to the earth. And so various types of crystals and stones correspond with different elements, making it essential to know which crystal is associated with which element when planning spells or rituals. Looking at each element, here are the crystals associated with them:

- **Air:** Clear stones and crystals. Yellow-tinged crystals are found to be okay, but they should be as clear as possible. Quartz is very commonly used. Imperfections in the crystal do not matter. As it is associated with air, imperfections or flaws are often compared to clouds in the sky.
- **Fire:** Stones and crystals associated with fire typically range in colors like orange, red, and black. Those crystals linked with volcanoes signify the fire that originated from within the earth.
- **Water:** Blue-green and blue stones and crystals are to be used for water. Pebbles found near water that are white or gray can also be used. These stones and crystals do not need to be polished. Besides that, pieces of salt or sandblasted glass can also be used.
- **Earth:** Green and brown crystals and stones are recommended. As all stones and crystals are products of the earth, you want to make sure you distinguish them as being for the earth.
- **Spirit:** Purple stones and crystals, such as amethyst, are often used to represent the fifth element. Amethyst is considered one of the best crystals because it's a transmitter and receiver of spiritual and psychic energy.

To use stones and crystals for natural magick, there are a few things you need to understand and know about them. Stones and crystals have a way of speaking to witches to draw their attention. Yet, you might be drawn to them because of their shape or appearance. But as a Wiccan, you must trust your intuition and listen to which stones and crystals are calling you. When picking a suitable stone or crystal, ensure that you can comfortably hold it and fit it into your pocket. Once you have found the perfect stones or crystals for your needs, you must learn their story and how to use them properly. Different stones and crystals have other uses; it is up to you to determine those.

First, you must consider how the stone or crystal came to be in your possession. Ask yourself what it might have been before you picked it up. Was it larger and weathered over time, or was it broken off a larger piece? What has the stone or crystal experienced to get to you? When thinking about these questions, use your imagination first. But you will soon find that as your relationship with the stone and crystal grows, it will start giving you information and telling you its story. Your crystal's journey can be used to help you find the way through your own life.

After discovering its story, it is time to consider how and why you connected with it. Crystals and stones are packed with energy. They were once a gaseous material compacted into shape by energetic forces. The forces and energy within the crystals and stones can send out vibrations that can call to you, forming a connection.

Stones and crystals can have many benefits for the users, which you need to be aware of. The best way to ensure your crystals and stones are perfect for the natural magick you are trying to use is to understand the benefits you can get from them. Here are some of the benefits your stones and crystals can give you:

- **Can be used as an energizer:** Establishing a relationship with a crystal or stone can act as a mental and physical stimulant. When feeling exhausted, down, or disconnected, rubbing the stone can bring back feelings of stability and renew any lost connections, allowing you to tap into its energies again.
- **Can help you ground yourself:** Your stone or crystal can be used as a foundation for your journey. It can help ground you and support you in pursuing your goals effectively. Likewise, they can always remind you that we are all from the same earth, which is something to be grateful about.
- **Connect you to eternal wisdom:** We do not always recognize how much time and unseen forces go into the formation of stones and crystals. But for a crystal or stone to reach you, it can take some time, like how we exist on earth because of numerous decisions and hidden powers coming together.
- **Protection from harm:** Challenges coming in harm's way occur in everyone's lives, and your stone and crystal can help you work through your challenges. Your crystal and stone can help to remind you that you have the strength to weather the storms you are facing and stand tall against adversity. Many crystals and stones are believed to be able to protect against evil as well.
- **Can be used as a meditative aid:** Your stone or crystal can help you reach a peaceful state of mind, aiding your meditation.
- **A reminder that you are a part of a larger whole:** Your crystal or stone is one minuscule part of a larger whole. No matter where your crystal or stone originated, it was once a part of a larger whole, the same way you are. You are one part of your coven or one part of your family. You are one part of the world in itself. You can also make your stone or crystal a repository for your desires and dreams, which you can use to reflect on what you want from life.

Here are some common crystals and their known properties:

- **Clear quartz** helps to balance energy and amplify it, as well as aid in concentration and memory.
- **Rose quartz** helps enhance connections, restore trust and harmony in relationships, provide calm and comfort, and encourage respect, love, faith, and self-worth.

- **Obsidian** helps to remove emotional blockages, helps with finding one's true self, and promotes compassion, strength, and clarity.
- **Jasper** empowers the spirit, protects against negativity, promotes quick thinking, confidence, and courage, and supports you through times of stress.
- **Citrine** encourages warmth, optimism, motivation, and clarity, encourages creativity, supports concentration, and helps you release negative emotions.
- **Amethyst** helps rid of negative thoughts, promotes healthy choices and willpower, aids sleep, and allows for serenity, spiritual wisdom, and humility.
- **Turquoise** helps balance emotions and supports spiritual groundedness and good luck.
- **Bloodstone** encourages the circulation of energy and ideas, promotes creativity, idealism, and selflessness, and reduces aggressiveness, impatience, and irritability.
- **Ruby** restores energy levels and vitality, supports intellectual pursuit, brings recognition of truth and self-awareness, and promotes sensuality and sexuality.

Preparing a Circle with Stones and Crystals

Later in the book, we will discuss how to prepare magick circles, but one of the many ways is to use stones and crystals. You will want to arrange the different crystals and the elements they represent in the right spiritual direction. Here are some examples of crystals you can use for your magick circles:

- **North:** emerald, olivine, salt, moss agate, and black tourmaline
- **East:** imperial topaz, pumice, citrine, and mica
- **South:** obsidian, ruby, garnet, lava, amber, and rhodochrosite
- **West:** chalcedony, lapis lazuli, jade, sugilite, aquamarine, and moonstone

Depending on the circle size, you will put 7, 9, 21, or 40 stones in the circle, starting and ending at the beginning of the northern side. The number is significant because they serve to enhance your power. Some will also use ribbons or cords for their circle, which the stones can be placed on the inside or outside. The purpose of the ritual will also play a part in the direction of your crystals or stones. For rituals that send your power outwards, the points of your stones and crystals will face outwards, and protective ones will have the points inwards.

Natural magick can be potent, but it can also be nurturing and allow you to connect with yourself and nature on a level you did not think was possible. Many people are unaware of how much power the earth has because they do not open themselves to it. In the next chapter, we will discuss the second type of magick that someone can practice: ceremonial magick.

10

Ceremonial Magick

When someone says they practice ceremonial magick, this could mean they are performing a variety of different magicks because it is an encompassing term that can refer to various rituals and techniques. Traditionally, this magick requires the witch to use accessories that aid their magick. And like natural magick, it has been used for centuries and is believed to be originated during the Renaissance period. But they still have differences, as ceremonial magick requires both natural and external elements. Ceremonial magick is also used to summon gods and spirits. Throughout this chapter, we will discuss the numerous components of ceremonial magick, techniques, and the spirits that might be summoned.

Components of Ceremonial Magick

The components used in natural magick are all nature-based, including the elements, plants, crystals, and stones. Yet, for ceremonial magick, you need to use artificial ingredients, which help to enhance the user's magickal ability. Users will use four pieces: grimoires, magickal formulae, magickal weapons, and vibration of god names.

Grimoires are magick textbooks that every witch using ceremonial magick will carry. These grimoires contain spells, rituals, and instructions on creating amulets and talismans, summoning gods and spirits, and performing spells appropriately. Depending on the witches and covens, grimoires are believed to be imbued with magickal abilities. But covens and solitary witches use grimoires differently. Often, a single grimoire is kept by the leader of a coven. Or, by chance, they may present one to a witch when they come of age. Meanwhile, solitary witches who have access to a grimoire can choose what they do with it.

Magickal formulae, or 'words of power,' are individual words believed to possess supernatural or invocation abilities. These words encapsulate the levels of understanding and principles necessary to achieve a specific spell or ritual. Although they do not often fit into the context of sentences, they are meant to communicate abstract ideas. And while a single word or sentence may have little meaning, breaking it down into individual parts can give it much greater significance. Likewise, groupings of letters signify deeper sequences with witches, hinting at historiographic data, psychological stages, and spiritual hierarchies. By themselves, the magickal formulae are useless, but with the user's ability to meditate on its meaning and internalize it before using it, it becomes powerful.

During rituals and spells, crafted magickal weapons are in use. These weapons help to direct a person's magick. They can also symbolize the user and their psychological elements and metaphysical concepts.

Some of the magickal tools witches use include altars, wands, pentacles, swords, daggers, crowns, robes, and lamens. Depending on the user, the meaning these weapons can have can change.

The last commonly used component for ceremonial magick is the vibration of god names. Invocation of deities is very common in ceremonial magick; to do so, users will use a vocal technique known as vibration. Rather than tools, this component is a series of steps, breathing, and thinking patterns. Crowley, a leading teacher of ceremonial magick, described the proper techniques as follows:

> *A physical set of steps, starting in a standing position, breathing in through the nose while imagining the name of the god entering with the breath, imagining that breath traveling through the entire body, stepping forward with the left foot while throwing the body along with arms outstretched, visualizing the name rushing out when spoken, ending in an upright stance, with the right forefinger placed upon the lips (Ceremonial magick, 2021).*

Many Wiccans use this technique in a much simpler version, as they will say the god's name in a drawn-out, long fashion and uses nasal passages, which give the sound and feeling of vibration.

Ceremonial Magick Rituals

Any form of magick that a Wiccan can use has different techniques and purposes and often can be paired with one another. Usually, a witch will employ different types of magick during the same rituals. Then, other witches combine the two to have a more powerful spell. Although the following techniques are said to be ceremonial, they have versions that can be performed with natural magick. It is important to note that how a Wiccan performs the following rituals can differ from clan to clan. There is no set way to practice them.

Banishing

Banishing rituals are performed as a means of eliminating evil, often unseen forces, that are a threat to Wiccans. Often, banishing rituals are used during festivals to protect against fairies and sprites. Remember when we talked about fairies stealing human babies or spirits crossing into the mortal realm to exact revenge? Banishing spells would be used in these situations, along with protection ones. At sabbats, esbats, and other sacred gatherings, many banishing rituals begin the ceremony, ranging from simple to complex practices. Some will rely heavily on natural magick and invoke the elements; others will use the planets, adjacent spaces in astral worlds, or the zodiac signs. But there are limits to banishing rituals as they will not work in an infinite space, so one must be defined with a magick circle or within a singular room.

Purification

Like banishing, purification is typically performed to prepare oneself and space for other spiritual and magickal work. During ancient times, purification was often performed in arduous methods that would last for days, weeks, months, or even lifetimes to remain purified. These purification techniques included sexual abstinence, fasting, diets, excessive cleaning of oneself, and complicated prayers. Although in the present day, these extreme purification practices are no longer used as shorter ones have replaced them. Symbolic purification is also heavily used before ceremonies, including washing oneself and putting on fresh robes.

Consecration

Consecration is a ritual vital to ceremonial magick because it is used to dedicate magickal instruments and spaces for a specific purpose. Wiccans perform consecration rituals on the magickal objects to show their intent and ensure they are not used for dark purposes. Spirits or gods would often be invoked to bless the things as well.

Invocation

Invocation is the act of identifying and bringing forth a spirit or deity. Depending on the Wiccan practices you are using, there are multiple deities or spirits that you could invoke, all of them having different purposes. Crowley and many other Wiccans also believed in the ability to invoke one's secret self or holy guardian angel, which allowed someone to get to know their true selves and their will. There are multiple ways to invoke a deity or spirit, but the magick user must identify with the spirit or deity they are trying to summon. Identifying with the spirit or deity allows for a connection to form, which makes invoking easier. Summoning the spirits of someone you know can be easier because a living link is there; for deities, it can be more challenging because you rely on a spiritual connection, and sometimes gods do not want to answer. However, the same goes for some spirits. They might not want to respond at first.

There are three main categories that invocations can fall into including:

- **Devotion:** This invocation method has someone identifying with the spirit or deity from a place of surrender and love. Users will give up irrelevant and often illusionary parts of themselves that are suppressing them from their full potential.
- **Drama:** Connection with the deity or spirit is created through sympathy and often is invoked through dance or acting. However, this invocation can be complicated as it requires the user to completely lose themselves in their actions and embody the spirit or deity.
- **Calling forth:** The Wiccan using this form, rather than letting go of parts of themselves, will call on their innermost desires, connecting them to the spirit or deity.

Besides the other forms of invocation, assuming the form of a deity or spirit is another option. This entails picturing oneself in the shape of the god or spirit that one wishes to invoke. Each deity represents something, and the user needs to be able to embody this. Typically, Wiccans position themselves in a way associated with the deity or spirit they are trying to summon as if it were enveloping their body. Sometimes, this method also uses the vibration of god names.

Evocation

Invoking and evoking, although they seem alike and perform similar tasks, are quite distinct. Evoking is the act of calling upon a deity, spirit, or entity to request their presence, services, guidance, or knowledge. Hence, the focus is on establishing a connection or communication with the entity and seeking their help or insights. Meanwhile, invoking involves drawing the energy, essence, or presence of a deity or spirit into oneself or a specific space. Subsequently, its purpose is to connect with and merge with the energy or consciousness of the entity to bring about transformation, guidance, inspiration, or spiritual communion. However, not all Wiccans participate in both practices; evoking typically calls upon gods and spirits to supply services or advice. When asking for help, gods are rarely summoned; usually, it is spirits or other entities like demons. Yet, deities can be evoked for information-gathering purposes. It is believed that Wiccans can call forth up to 72 infernal spirits with an evocation ritual that often involves drawing a triangle to give the spirit or god a place to enter.

Eucharist

Originally derived from the word "thanksgiving," Eucharist is now used by Wiccans and other magickal communities to signify the transformation of regular food or drink into holier sacraments. Then, these sacred sacraments are consumed by the coven or an individual. Many kitchen, green, or hearth witches partake in eucharist rituals as they infuse food and drink with magickal properties. Depending on the type of eucharist rituals, the divine properties allow the consumer to embody a deity.

Divination

Divination is used mainly for gathering information and obtaining a guide from the spirit world. It is important to note that divination and fortune-telling are different. Fortune-telling is more about telling the future, while divination is more about looking toward the past and gathering information. Divination is meant to help the Wiccan to gain insight into the decisions they need to make. Many different divinatory techniques can be used based on the type of Wicca or coven you are in. Western Wicca and occult methods of divination include:

- **Astrology:** using divination to learn of the influence heavenly bodies have.
- **Tarot:** the use of a deck of 78 cards, each of which has its meaning, and the user will pick a few cards and determine a message from them.
- **Bibliomancy:** choosing random passages from books and reading them to gain meaning.
- **Geomancy:** the Wiccan will make random marks on the earth or on paper to form 16 patterns and determine meaning from this.

Although divination is accepted, it is not infallible due to the subjectivity of each Wiccan's interpretation.

Ceremonial Magick, the Elementals, and Spirits

Ceremonial magick is renowned for calling upon and summoning spirits, often with the assistance of the elements, to target specific types of entities. Although ceremonial magick does not require the use of the elements, they can be drawn on to help enhance rituals. Each element is associated with a different spirit, and they are as follows:

- **Earth spirits = gnomes:** These spirits are often called upon because of their vast knowledge about the earth's power and locations of riches. They are often called the guardians of earth's treasures as they live underground, guarding them. These spirits embody earthen qualities and are said to be able to dissolve into tree trunks or the ground to hide. Other spirits that are associated with earth include brownies, dryads, earth spirits, elves, pans, and satyrs.

- **Fire spirit = salamander:** Out of all four elements, fire is regarded to be the strongest. Yet, many believe that physical fire could not exist without aid from salamanders. Although no particular species of salamander has been assigned as the spirit of fire, many representations mean that they are around a foot tall or just small-looking balls of lightness or 'sparks.' Salamanders are also believed to reduce in size or amplify themselves and are considered naughty creatures. But much like other spirits, they are influenced by the thinking of humankind and can be dangerous when out of control.
- **Air spirits = sylphs:** These spirits are believed to live at the top of mountains and are changeable and volatile. They also vary in size and work through the winds and gases in their area. While often depicted with wings, they can also be seen in human form. Sylphs have been associated with helping humans with creativity, which is why many people will go to high and windy places to work.
- **Water spirit = undines:** These spirits are known to be graceful and beautiful, residing in oceans, waterfalls, and lakes. They take care of the plants growing beneath the surface, displaying a human form, sometimes naked or encased in an almost transparent material similar to water. Sizes can differ depending on their energy levels. And while they may be emotional, they are also said to be friendly.

Ceremonial magick is truly amazing and can be used to learn so much more about the natural world and the unseen world. Embracing your magick, you can learn much more about yourself and the world thanks to ceremonial magick. In the next chapter, we will discuss the third type of magick Wiccans can practice: celestial magick.

11

Celestial Magick

To top off the three types of magick a Wiccan can practice, there is celestial magick. As it sounds, celestial magick deals with the divine. Still, it can be tough to give a concrete definition because depending on the coven or type of Wiccan you have, celestial and the divine can have different meanings and figures. Celestial magick focuses on learning the interactions gods have with mortals and the earth and invoking gods in the hope of causing earthly changes. The beliefs and methods used in celestial magick will change depending on the person performing it. It can be one of the most personal of the three magicks adapting to each user's values. Although it varies based on the user's beliefs, there are a few constants no matter the Wiccan's beliefs or values, which we will discuss throughout this chapter.

Constant 1: Prayer

The first constant in celestial magick is the method in which a Wiccan or other users communicate with deities: prayer. Prayer forms a pseudo-telepathic link, synergy, or emanation, enabling a connection between the Wiccan and the god of their choice. Different prayers might be used for various deities. Often, celestial magic is used to seek guidance, aid, or hand over daily worries and stresses to the gods. But when using it, a person needs to know the specific deity they are trying to communicate with, or they could connect with one that is more sinister or will not be of help. Besides that, celestial magick is also used with special ceremonies to please the spirit being called upon and protect the practitioner from other forces that might cause harm. Some common ceremonial rituals used with celestial magick include purification, offerings, blessings, sanctification, and asking for favors. However, there is still a high chance of failure when attempting to ask an entity to stop doing something, which can result in the anger of deities with unforeseen consequences, something Wiccans do not want to risk.

Constant 2: Spirituality

Celestial magic's second tenet is the spiritual nature of the divine, to whom Wiccans pray instead of one another. These Wiccans are considered heavenly because their prayers are directed towards non-physical beings with power and intelligence over the earth, such as stellar, ethereal, infernal, or celestial. Among other divine beings, astral deities are the only one that lives amongst the stars. Meanwhile, other spirits that can be called upon often live in an undefined space or multiple plains as their importance, meaning, or influence shifts. As we learned earlier in this book, the Horned God changes locations throughout the year to signify the different seasons.

Though summoning and celestial magic may appear the same, there is a notable contrast between them: the type of spirit involved and the power of the Wiccan. While performing a summoning ritual, the Wiccan controls the spirit. If something starts to go wrong, the Wiccan can maintain control and send the spirit back to where it came from. But in celestial magick, the Wiccan cannot act arrogant, restrict, nor control the deity they communicate with. Instead, they must be humble in asking for help or guidance, as demanding something of a deity will only anger them.

Constant 3: Workings of Celestial Magick

The third constant of celestial magick is the skills and abilities which celestial Wiccans need to have knowledge and practice. One of the essential skills that Wiccans need to perform celestial magick is divine intervention. Although more mundane or inhuman spirits are not assumed to have high levels of intelligence, deities allow celestial Wiccans to ask them to complete much larger goals rather than a simple task or two. Giving the care of problems into the hands of the deity can ensure they are done faster, and the Wiccan no longer needs to worry about something. Depending on the problem, deities can also be sure to check up on situations and keep the coven safe.

Another skill that celestial Wiccans have is protection from deities. If a celestial Wiccan feels that they are in trouble or that their coven is in grave danger, they can seek the protection of a deity. Many deities use the world's energies to make changes that the celestial Wiccans have asked of them. Deities can also adapt to circumstances and observe situations, making decisions based on what is happening. However, it is important to remember that a deity is not bound to listen to you, and although your goals might be met, they might not be as you thought they would be.

The third skill that these witches have is overpowering lesser spirits. Not all Wiccans can conquer lesser spirits, which is why celestial Wiccans and their abilities can be of great value to a coven. A celestial Wiccan can ask for a deity to lend them their strength, which can help them to vanquish demons or dispel troublesome spirits. However, a deity must be willing to give some of its power to the user.

Celestial magick can be one of a coven's most advantageous powers, often with the leader seeking this magick to protect the coven from danger. The intelligence of the deities can be a great tool as they have lived much longer and experienced much more than the person. However, celestial Wiccans must tread lightly because not all deities are friendly or willing to help. Now that you know the three types of magick that Wiccans can use, it is time to move on to the fifth and final pillar: rituals.

Pillar 5
Rituals

Rituals have been part of the Wiccan tradition for centuries, providing structure and guidance to those who practice their faith. In this chapter, we will explore some of the common components found in rituals, and different types of altars, tools, and ritual wear used when performing these ceremonies.

We will begin by looking at altars—what they are, what items you typically find on them, and where you should locate them in a room and decorate it. Then, we will also discuss the various tools that make up a witch's arsenal, from the pentacle to the cauldron, and how they function within a ritual. Finally, we will examine which clothing fits a Wiccan ceremony and how a ritual is properly carried out from start to finish.

Once we have gone through all these topics, you will better understand the rich symbolism behind each component of ritual work and be ready to apply them in your journey as an individual or with others around you. So, let us dive into this fascinating topic and discover more about the rituals of Wiccans!

12

Altars

Various components go into a single ritual or spell, the first being the altar. Altars are a common element among different belief systems, including Wicca. The altar used can have different purposes, but most rituals will have some form of altar. For Wiccans, the primary use of an altar is to be a physical structure meant to honor deities, ancestors, and other spirits, or they are also meant to hold the ritual object that will be used. Altars also serve as the focal point of celebrations, so an altar will be in the center of one of the eight sabbats, esbats, or any other celebration that a Wiccan might have. For covens, this might be a permanent altar in the center of the coven grounds. There are also often small altars inside witches' homes, or they will make them perform spells in the house. Throughout this chapter, we will discuss the typical Wiccan altar and various ways you can set one up.

The Wiccan Altar

Depending on the type of Wiccan a person is, the look and location of an altar can vary. Altars belonging to covens may be located outdoors, in a designated building, or within the leader's home, which is used for rituals with the entire coven. Furthermore, many spells are based on particular locations, prompting Wiccans to have small altars in their houses.

Variations in the appearance of a Wiccan altar also depend on the available space. For solitary Wiccans with limited space, a double-duty altar is ideal as it allows them to use it for rituals, spells, and regular activities. Often, double-duty altars are kept in small sizes that can be neatly tucked away when not in use. Desks and tables work best for this purpose. As regards its shape, it is entirely up to the Wiccan and their space. Yet, most Wiccans prefer circle-shaped as it allows movement while mimicking the sacred circle made before rituals. Natural materials, such as wood or stone, are also chosen because they can connect a Wiccan to nature, especially if they do not have access. And so willow and oak are often selected for altars.

Transforming a space in your house into an altar can be done by performing rituals that imbue it with magickal energy. This is particularly helpful for future ceremonies and spells you may wish to do. Meanwhile, wood and other natural products are recommended, as nature typically holds more power for magickal practices. As you get closer to nature, the more potent the outcome of your rituals and spells will be. But if you have access to a natural area that provides security, feel free to use a large stump or flat rock as an altar.

Types of Altars

Different altars can affect the power of your rituals and spells. With so many options, the type you have can make a difference. Yet, altars that contain more natural products are more powerful than those made of artificial products. Here are some different kinds of altars you can create, especially if you do not have access to natural spaces.

Box Shrine

These shrines are relatively small and can be designed to honor a singular god, goddess, or deity. Often, these shrines or altars are created in suitcases, which can be great if you are trying to connect to a past relative with some connection to the briefcase. However, not all carry-ons are made with natural material, so if you are planning to make this kind of altar, having links to other Wiccans, such as a relative, can give it the little boost of power that it needs. These altars are also transportable, which is a nice feature if you travel somewhere to perform the rituals. Also, if you do not feel safe having your altar open when people visit, this form allows you to close it up and out of sight.

Shrine

Unlike traditional box shrines, Wiccan shrines are typically fixed in a dedicated room for rituals and prayer. The complexity, ranging from simple to extravagant, is entirely up to you. Besides, anything from a simple to an elaborate shrine altar can be used as a point of focus to revere a god, goddess, spirit, or deity. To create one, you need items representing what you worship, relevant tools such as incense or centers, and decorations. Flowers or natural objects can also add the right touch of nature if the shrine is crafted from non-natural material like plastic.

Adding more objects to the altar or shrine will make it more susceptible to magick. And if you have a specific purpose for a ritual, you can add crystals, herbs, and candles. There are often occasions in which a Wiccan decorate their altar more heavily. Samhain, or the beginning of the Wiccan year, and the time in which the veil between the spirit and human world is thinnest, make their altars or shrines much more elaborate, such as with lots of pictures of passed family members. Some also move the shrine to the central area of the house so that the entire family can get together and feast. But other people only decorate their altars decorated during sabbats or other celebrations.

Tabletop Altar

Tabletop altars are just as they sound; they are made on the top of a table. Many people hosting rituals in their homes may create a temporary altar on the top of a table in a big room for the entire group. These altars are also often made when someone has a shrine that cannot be moved, but they want the ritual celebration to be in another house room that is more fitting.

Ritual Altar

Ritual altars are typically the most complicated to construct, as they are designed for meaningful rituals during sabbats and esbats. Essentially, they require a wide range of tools, including a wand, athame, pentagram, candles, incense, and any other objects you may need for a ritual. Due to their size, usually much larger than regular permanent altars, it requires more space to arrange all the elements correctly.

Working Altar

Not all altars are built for magickal rituals; some exist to honor gods or loved ones. Prayers can be said at these altars, but no magickal practices may occur there. Working altars, however, are those that are made to carry out magick-related tasks. Likewise, these altars should be kept uncluttered and contain only the necessary objects so the magick can avoid accidentally diverting them elsewhere. Also, make sure you customize your altar suited to your abilities and the rituals and spells you plan to work with. And remember, altars set up for daily magick differ from those meant for sabbats, esbats, and celebrations as they are more simplistic yet effective. Meanwhile, festivity altars require more elements to be included in them due to the complexity of their purpose.

Often, a witch can have multiple altars that serve different purposes. They can have one for magickal rituals and spells, one for prayer and honoring deities or spirits, and another for rituals performed during sabbats and esbats.

Setting up An Altar

Depending on which type of altar you are putting together, there are plenty of ways to craft one, but let us assume that you are making an altar on a piece of furniture you already own. To start, cover the altar with fabrics or scarves of different colors. When deciding on the colors for your ritual, you may choose meaningful shades or whatever's easiest to find if you are in a pinch. Many people often change the fabrics with the seasons to mimic the year cycle. Depending on the ritual being performed, different textiles might be used. The decorations might also go through the same changes as the fabric. Still, it is entirely up to the Wiccan who decorate the altar. An example of decoration you might see being rotated is holly berries and fir leaves during Yule. On top of seasonal or ritual decorations, you can use your favorite crystals, stones, images of deities, or any other item.

When deciding on a layout for your altar, you have many options. Some are more intricate, while others are quite simple—it all depends on your performing ritual. But generally speaking, the altar is split down the middle. The left side represents the Triple Goddess and has tools that align with her and the elements of earth and water. While on the right side symbolizes the Horned God and includes those tools associated with him and the elements of fire and air

Another layout has objects meant to represent the Triple Goddess and the Horned God in the center of the altar and the tools required for the ritual in order of element: earth in the north, the air in the east, fire in the south, and water in the west.

Some Wiccans also decorate their altars eclectically, which means they intuitively decorate the altar, allowing their consciousness to find patterns and places they resonate with. But whether it is elaborate or basic, how you design your altar is totally up to you. The amount of space available also plays a huge role in arranging it. Thus, your options may be more restricted if there is little space.

Where to set up your altar is totally up to you. Pick the spot that feels right, even if it is inside your home, outside, or anywhere you feel connected. And if you have a grimoire that outlines specific directions on constructing an altar for particular rituals, you may follow those instructions. But you could also follow your intuition if it does not provide further direction. After you set up your altar, it is time to gather all the tools you will need to participate in your rituals and spells, which we will learn about in the next chapter.

13

Tools

Setting up the altar can be considered laying the foundations for your ritual, and now it is time to start building up that foundation using various tools. However, remember that not all magick requires magickal tools, and not all tools will be used during a ritual. Natural magick very rarely uses artificial tools but relies on nature. Some rituals in natural magick, especially more extensive rituals performed by covens, use tools to help direct the magick. Meanwhile, ceremonial and celestial magick depend on them much more heavily. Yet, tools are not always used to direct magick; they are often used to honor gods, goddesses, or deities. Here are the most commonly used magickal tools and items used by Wiccans.

Pentacle

A pentacle is a consecration tool that is placed on an altar. Typically, pentacles have a magickal symbol or sigil engraved on them. Although the emblem engraved on them might be different for some Wiccans, it is commonly a circle with a pentagram inside. The pentacle symbolizes the earth element, often used for evoking blessings and energizing items. Likewise, it acts as an indicator of things that have been blessed and provides a means to charge them up with spiritual power.

Pentacles are the most commonly used tools in almost any ritual or spell a Wiccan might perform. They can be made from any material, including clay, wood, metal, or wax. But the more natural the material, the better, as it will be easier to infuse with magickal abilities. In ceremonial magick, pentacles serve as protective talismans. Creating your pentacle can be an empowering experience, allowing you to pour your magick and energy into it in a way you would not be able to with a purchased one. But if making one is not an option, plenty of ready-made versions are available.

Sword or Knife

Ritual swords or knives, known as athames, are utilized in Wiccan rituals, with Gardnerian Wicca highly dependent on them as they represent the element of fire. These double-edged daggers usually come with a black handle, sometimes decorated with etchings. Wiccans can also opt for either crafting or purchasing their athames. But it is important to note that they are rarely used for cutting or directing magick. And for many Wiccans, using an athame to draw blood is seen as defiling the tool, so it usually needs to be destroyed afterward.

Wand

Wands can take many forms, with some representing fire and others symbolizing air. But Gardnerian Wicca holds to the latter. Materials used to make wands range from rock and wood to metal and even crystals. To further personalize their wand, they may add engravings of runes, stones, or crystals that are meaningful to them. For many practitioners of natural magic, wands can be a helpful tool for amplifying and channeling their energy. These can be made more effective by adding crystals to the wand. However, not all crystals are suitable for embedding into wands.

Having a dual purpose, wands direct magick and energy and summon spirits. In many Wiccan traditions, these methods are interchangeable. Meanwhile, fairies and other elemental spirits were historically said to be scared of iron and steel, so wands made from natural materials are generally preferred for summoning. In contrast, metal ones are employed for containment. Although athames can sometimes serve the same purpose, wands are still considered stronger and more suitable for handling spirits. Typically, witches who do not rely on athames resort to using a wand for summoning.

Furthermore, wands are a phallic symbol representing male power, virility, and energy. Rituals for the Horned God will often have wands in them to honor him. Invoking deities and consecrating spaces are also performed using wands.

Chalice

Chalices or goblets are cups used to represent the element of water. In some traditions, the chalice is not used as a tool but as a representation of the Triple Goddess' womb. But even during rituals that are not exclusive to the Triple Goddess, a chalice or cauldron is typically present to symbolize the feminine energy and representation of a womb. Likewise, at symbolic rituals of the Great Rite, chalices and athames stand for femininity. Some popular materials for these items include pewter and silver.

Boline

Bolines are another type of knife that can be used during rituals. These knives traditionally have a white handle and a curved blade in the shape of a crescent moon. Unlike the athame, bolines have practical uses, including cutting herbs, harvesting crops, inscribing candles with sigils or symbols, and cutting ritual cords. Although these tools might not be used during the actual ritual, they are used for physical preparation. Moreover, they represent two distinct realms: the human plane and the spiritual plane. For the physical plane, bolines are used, while athames are for the spiritual one.

Censer and Incense

Burning incense is a common practice to create a calming atmosphere, especially during religious ceremonies. Different fragrances can evoke the gods, goddesses, and deities associated with different times of the year. Furthermore, censers are containers that hold and release incense smoke during prayer.

Besom

Besoms, a term for a broom, is used to clean out ceremonial spaces before a ritual is performed. By sweeping, the Wiccan who does this duty removes the negative energy. And so before a ritual, it is essential to clean away negative energies that can otherwise affect the outcome. This purifying tool is connected to the element of water, and besoms, like wands, are phallic symbols often used in fertility dances. During handfasting ceremonies, a couple will also jump over a besom as part of the ritual.

Cauldron

When witches come to mind, two of the first images likely to appear are a besom and wands. The third image commonly associated with witches is a cauldron, which can be used in place of a chalice, particularly in female-oriented rituals. Cauldrons are seen as feminine and symbolic of water, making them an essential part of many rituals and often placed on an altar filled with liquid. Plus, it has relevance in honoring the Triple Goddess in feminine-focused rites. Meanwhile, in Celtic mythology and tradition, cauldrons are associated with the goddess Cerridwen, who has prophetic abilities and is the cauldron keeper of inspiration and knowledge and resides in the underworld.

Cauldrons have numerous magickal uses, including burning offerings, incense, and candles, blending herbs, representation of the Triple Goddess or any other goddesses, and using for moonlight scrying when filled with water. Using a cauldron for culinary purposes is not recommended, as the primary purpose of a cauldron is for practicing magick. Rather than cooking, a cauldron is better utilized in rituals and spells. But if you want to prepare food in a cauldron, have one for magickal purposes and one for food. Often, kitchen witches have multiple cauldrons, but it is essential to remember that cast iron cauldrons intended for cooking must be adequately seasoned.

Spear or Staff

Seax-Wicca tradition uses a spear to represent the god Woden, who takes the place of the Horned God. While not all Wiccans use a spear, their uses of one can differ. In contrast, the staff is more regularly incorporated into Wiccan practices. Although the staff is not essential for Wiccans, many use it to symbolize their authority and power. Representations differ based on culture, but men are often represented by staff. In some, they convey air; in others, fire. When in a coven, the high priest or priestess will carry a staff as a physical embodiment of their power.

Bell

According to folklore, intense noise, such as bells, is thought to ward off evil spirits. So, to keep malicious spirits away, witches often hung bells around their homes and utilized them in outdoor rituals. In particular, witches hoped to repel mischievous entities by ringing bells during outside ceremonies. Likewise, the vibrations caused by bells are often believed to be a power source. Other than bells, you can also use a ritual rattle, sistrum, or singing bowl. The sounds of these tools are also thought to bring harmony during ceremonies.

Candles

Candles are a popular tool for Witches, representing the element of fire. They can be carved and shaped into figures to pay honor to gods or goddesses. Although sometimes used in rituals, they are most frequent in casting spells, as it is said that these objects accumulate one's energy. And once lit, this stored energy combined with magick is released as its flame burns away.

Many Wiccans prefer to make their candles for ritual and spellwork since they believe this increases the item's magickal power. Moreover, crafting a candle can be both a spiritual and an empowering experience as it allows you to pour your energy, magickal abilities, and intentions into its creation. Yet, other Wiccans believe that making a candle does not make a difference; the intent behind burning a candle is what gives it more power. Different colors and aromas are also often used in rituals and ceremonies throughout the year, each having a special meaning and purpose.

Crystals

As we have learned in previous chapters throughout this book, crystals are very common in Wiccan traditions, no matter the type of Wiccan you might be. Natural magick uses crystals often; however, they are also used in other magick and many Wiccan traditions. Different traditions also use various crystals, and which ones you choose are essential because they represent different elements and attributes. When selecting a new crystal or stone, purify it before you use it for magickal rituals and spells.

Divination Tools

Not all Wiccans use divination. However, those that do have specific tools designed exclusively for clairvoyance. There are many different divination tools, but having only one or two items is all you need. There is also no need to keep them on your altar constantly. But one of the most commonly used divination tools is tarot cards.

Remember, you do not need to pile on every tool under the sun when performing a ritual, nor do they not all necessarily have to be present on your altar. Use only the tools necessary, and there is no need to overdo it. Hence, if you do not need any staff for a ritual, there is no point in having them around. But now that you have your altar and what you need, the next aspect of a ceremony you need to have is your ritual wear, which we will discuss in the next chapter.

14

Ritual Wear

What a Wiccan chooses to wear for their ritual is solely up to them. Although, many traditions could be followed from the practices of witches, which were said to have inspired the practices of Wicca. During its beginnings, it was popular for those taking part in rituals to go skyclad or even nude. However, for modern Wicca, this is rarely how people conduct rituals. Depending on whether you are part of a coven or practicing solitarily, the ritual wear you have might differ. In a coven, different attire might be required for ritual practice. But if you practice alone, it is your choice whether to stick with tradition. Here are some of the most commonly worn ritual wear that Wiccans use.

Ritual Robes

Taking on a robe is more than just putting on the physical garment; it is about preparing for the ritual, embracing ancient customs, and connecting with those who have come before. The primary purpose of wearing ritual robes is to distinguish oneself from the mundane and enhance your magick. Many take a cleansing bath before donning their ritual robes to ensure they are as pure as possible. Traditionally, Wiccan robes should go without anything else underneath, allowing one to embody their nature fully; however, this is your choice.

For those in a coven, the color of their robe can indicate their rank within the group. However, not all covens are like this. Likewise, if you are practicing solitarily, you can have multiple robes of different styles and colors for specific rituals or during different seasons. Colors that are associated with each season include blue (spring), green (summer), brown (fall), and white (winter). Usually, many Wiccans opt for white or earthy tones to harmonize with nature and avoid black due to its negative symbolism. Despite this, you do not need to feel obliged to stick to traditional seasonal fabrics, but still, pay attention to the type of fabric and color you wear.

When crafting or purchasing a robe, one thing to bear in mind is the presence of candles and fire during rituals. Due to this, having a robe made of materials that cannot catch fire is essential for safety. The design of your robe can also be as intricate or simple as you prefer.

Wiccans who create their robe put in the extra effort to make them meaningful by customizing and filling them with their energy and magickal abilities. But even for those inexperienced with sewing, creating a robe is doable, as patterns are available in-store and online. For a good design in stores, look for one under costumes. Historical and Renaissance are also categories you can look for robes. Here are sewing patterns you can find online that are perfect for creating ritual robes:

- **Simplicity 4795**: For those participating in a passion play, an angel-designed ritual robe is an ideal choice for Wiccans. Although slight alterations to the sleeve length might be needed, it is an easy pattern for beginners to follow.
- **Simplicity 3616**: Though it is a campy wizard costume, the robe is perfect for a masculine version of a ritual robe. Just be sure to discard the long white beard and trim.
- **Simplicity 3623**: This is a Scottish-themed costume with a masculine underdress under the skirt and bodice and an uncomplicated pattern that works well for a ceremonial robe.

These three patterns are all beginner friendly and simple. But if you want a more elaborate robe and are an advanced sewer, try the McCall 4490; it is a perfect Renaissance-style dress that can be used as a ritual robe.

Buying a pattern is not necessary, either. You can make one without it. There are a few supplies that you will need, including a sewing machine, six feet of cord or light rope, measuring tape, scissors, thread, your fabric of choice, and tailor's chalk. Follow these steps to make a robe without a pattern:

1. Get help from another person to take your measurements properly. Outstretch your arms and measure the length from wrist to wrist. Write this measurement down with the letter "A" next to it.
2. Measure the distance between the nape of your neck to the area even with your ankle, and write this down with the letter "B."
3. Fold your material in half and cut out a T shape using the measurements you got for "A" and "B." Do not cut along the fold.
4. Measure out the center of measurement "A" and cut a hole for your head. Make sure it is not too large or will slide off your shoulders.
5. Sew on the underside of the arm, leaving the end of the T open for hands. Sew from the armpit to the bottom. Turn the robe inside right, trying it on to make adjustments.
6. Add a cord around the waist. If you are practicing solitarily, you can create this cord for yourself. Depending on whether you are in a coven, this cord might be provided to you at initiation and as you progress through different levels of training.
7. If you would like, add trim, beading, and other designs to the robe to make it more personal. Magickal symbols can also be sewn into robes.
8. Before wearing your robe, be sure to purify it.

Cloaks

Cloaks can be crafted or purchased. And since they do not provide sufficient body coverage with only a clasp, ties, or button at the neck, they are commonly worn over a robe during colder months. Yet, some more lavish versions do come with hoods and sleeves attached. However, sometimes you do not need a cloak if the ritual takes place indoors.

For both cloaks and robes, there is no need to go out and buy an expensive one. You can use clothing you already have and remake them into a robe or cloak. If your family practices Wicca, you can use their cloaks and robes.

Pentacle

We talked about pentacles in the last chapter because they are a common tool used by Wiccans. To recap, pentacles are a consecration tool and often hold blessed items. When placed on an altar, they are usually made of stone, wood, clay, metal, or other natural materials. There are several ways to wear a pentacle, including jewelry or sewing it into your garments.

When performing rituals or evocation, identifying yourself as a Wiccan can be essential for the deities you are trying to summon. Wearing a pentacle on your person during rituals is a way of declaring yourself as a Wiccan. However, during specific times, such as Samhain, wearing any markers of you being a Wiccan should be avoided because it will attract spirits and fairies that want to try to play tricks on you.

Other Jewelry

There is no specific jewelry that a Wiccan must wear; this is a highly personal part of the ritual wear of Wiccans. In covens, it might be required not to wear jewelry, so they are as close to skyclad as possible while wearing a robe. Any jewelry worn during rituals is typically magickal, containing runes or symbols that are meaningful to the person. Yet, some ritual jewelry may differ as each can boost the spell's power and Wiccan's abilities. Any jewelry that enhances one's energy can be worn during a ceremony.

Many Wiccans also craft special pieces with crystals they feel connected to, wearing them in everyday life and during rituals to benefit from them. Meanwhile, others may opt to create jewelry honoring gods or deities. But it is an entirely personal process. If you are out and shopping for jewelry, focus on how you feel when you pick a piece. For such, when you touch a piece of jewelry and feel a buzz of energy, that is a sign that this is for you and is boosting your energy.

Overall, what you wear during a ritual is very personal, especially when practicing solitarily. Although it is best to wear a robe during ceremonies, there are no strict rules. Aside from that, you can also make your robes, cloaks, and jewelry personal, boosting your energy. We have the altar, the tools, and the ritual wear you need, and now it is time to explore the standard components of a Wiccan ritual.

15

Common Components of Wiccan Rituals

Depending on the type of Wicca you practice, how rituals are performed can differ, but the bare bones of a ritual, no matter the form of Wicca you practice, are similar. Think back to celestial magick and the commonalities it has, despite there being so many different types. The same goes for Wiccan rituals. Many types of ceremonies can be performed, and each kind of Wicca can do them differently. There are several types of rituals and spells that Wiccans can perform, and they have different purposes and meanings. We will learn more about the kinds of rituals in the next chapter, but first, let us know the essential components that all Wiccan rituals have.

Preparation

Before starting any spell or ritual, preparation is necessary. For spells, a witch may need to have their ingredients and tools ready. Consecrating those tools, garments, and even the Wiccan is essential for a successful ritual. Neglecting proper preparation can have a serious impact on ritual success as well as one's ability to cast magick.

The primary purposes of consecration are to purify objects used in the ceremony and to cleanse them of any dark energy that could have gathered. This is essential, as these tools must interact with the Divine, and if there is dark energy, it can damage rituals. As with an empty room, unwanted energy can accumulate over time, like dust, so it is essential to clear it out before performing any new ritual. Hence, this is why consecration must always take place between practices.

Although consecrating your tools before a ritual is optional, it is still a great practice to develop, especially if you use a pre-owned tool. With consecration, it is also possible to know what types of energies have been used or what kind of magick has been performed with your tool. Likewise, before using any brand-new tools, purify them once. After that, performing a consecration occasionally should be enough for upkeep.

How often you choose to consecrate your tools is entirely up to you. Yet, it would be best to do it as often as possible to ensure dark magick or energy is not messing with your rituals. You can also cleanse the space where your altar and tool are to reduce how much consecration you need to do.

Different people may perform a consecration differently. And as there are many variations in this process, one thing remains the same: getting to know the four elements is an integral part of the ritual. When performing a consecration, there is no wrong or right way to do it as long as the tool is connected with the four elements. So, your ceremony can be as detailed or minimalistic as you would like. Once the four elements have blessed the tool, it is considered purified.

For the consecration ceremony, you will need a cup of water, a white candle, a small bowl of salt, and incense. Each of these items represents a direction and an element:

- Salt (north and earth)
- Incense (east and air)
- Candle (south and fire)
- Water (west and water)

At this point, some Wiccans will cast a circle before their consecration, but this is not necessary. After you have gathered the materials and have your tools, cast the circle if you decide to. Place each of the items in their proper spot and light the candle and incense. Here is an example of how you might perform the consecration.

Grab the tool you are consecrating, and start by facing north. Pass the item over the salt and say the following words:

"Powers of the North,
Guardians of the Earth,
I consecrate this wand of willow (or knife of steel, amulet of crystal, etc.)
and charge it with your energies.
I purify it this night and make this tool sacred" (Wigington, 2019a).

Turn to face the east, and pass the item or tool through the smoke of the incense and say the words:

"Powers of the East,
Guardians of the Air,
I consecrate this wand of willow
and charge it with your energies.
I purify it this night and make this tool sacred" (Wigington, 2019a).

Face the south and pass the item over the fire. Be extra cautious here because many items are flammable. Say these words as you pass the item over the fire:

"Powers of the South,
Guardians of Fire,
I consecrate this wand of willow
and charge it with your energies.
I purify it this night and make this tool sacred" (Wigington, 2019a).

Turn to face west and pass the item over the water, saying the words:

> *"Powers of the West,*
> *Guardians of Water,*
> *I consecrate this wand of willow [or knife of steel, amulet of crystal, etc.]*
> *and charge it with your energies.*
> *I purify it this night and make this tool sacred"* (Wigington, 2019a).

Last, face the altar and hold your item up to the sky and say the following words:

> *"I charge this wand in the name of Old Ones,*
> *the Ancients, the Sun and the Moon, and the Stars.*
> *By the powers of the Earth, of Air, of Fire, and Water*
> *I banish the energies of any previous owners*
> *and make it new and fresh.*
> *I consecrate this wand,*
> *and it is mine."* (Wigington, 2019a).

Taking a shower before dressing in your gown is an excellent method to consecrate the person. This consecration ritual being performed is mainly for tools. Consecrating your robes can also occur in this manner, but avoid getting the garment too close to the candle's fire.

In some Wiccan traditions, some will immediately use their recently consecrated tool to bind it. Using the newly purified tool in a ritual right after is also believed to increase its strength.

Casting the Magick Circle

Depending on the ceremony and tradition, you might cast a magick circle before consecration or after. There is no right or wrong way of doing it. Magick circles are performed before every ritual, whether you are in a coven or not. Although casting a magick circle is not absolute, there are no definite rules that need to be followed for witchcraft; however, casting a magick circle can help boost your magick's power and ward off evil spirits and energy while you are working.

Just as with the consecration ritual, there are multiple ways to cast a magick circle that can change based on what tools and materials you have on hand or how much time you have. You will not need to do an elaborate magick circle for quick rituals, but a simple one. Many people use four candles to represent the direction and chant as they light each one. A person might also include an item representing the four seasons and elements, but this is unnecessary. In the sample casting of a magick circle I share with you, you will have different colored candles symbolizing the elements.

To cast a magick circle, you will need the following:

- A besom
- A green candle to represent the north
- A yellow candle to represent the east
- A red candle to represent the south
- A blue candle to represent the west

- Incense
- Salt, pine branches, or flowers
- Bowl of water
- Bowl of salt

Cleanse the area you are performing your ritual with a besom first. This way, you will rid the area of any dark energy that has gathered since the last ritual you had. Once you have cleansed the room, it is time to set up the candles, starting in the north. Set each candle up, going clockwise. If performing some form of dark magick, you will go counterclockwise.

Depending on the type of ritual, you will either have the candles inside the circle or outside of it, as we talked about in an earlier chapter. Ensure that your altar is inside the circle. Have a bowl of salt and water on the altar as well. Light incense and candles before grabbing your wand or athame from the altar and place the point at the bowl of water and say,

> *"I consecrate and cleanse this water so it may be purified and fit to dwell within the sacred circle.*
>
> *In the name of the Mother Goddess and the Father God [or the names of specific deities], I consecrate this water"* (How to Cast a Wicca Ritual Magick Circle, 2021).

When you say these words, imagine you are blasting away all the negative energy that might be contained in the water. Move the point of your dagger or wand to touch the bowl of salt and say:

> *"I bless this salt that it may be fit to dwell within the sacred circle.*
>
> *In the name of the Mother Goddess and the Father God, I bless this salt"* (How to Cast a Wicca Ritual Magick Circle, 2021).

After blessing the water and salt, hold your athame or wand at waist height and slowly walk around the circle clockwise. As you walk around the circle, charge it with your magick energy. Imagine your energy stretching and forming a sphere, half above the ground and half underground. Remember that spirits and otherworldly beings can appear from anywhere, including beneath. Say these words as you walk around the circle:

> *"Here is the boundary of the circle.*
> *Naught but love shall enter in.*
> *Naught but love shall emerge from within.*
> *Charge this by your powers, Old Ones!"* (How to Cast a Wicca Ritual Magick Circle, 2021).

Take the salt and sprinkle it to form a circle, starting and ending in the north. If you are using flowers or branches, place them to form a circle. Repeat the process with the incense and water, sprinkling it around the circle's parameter. At this point, the circle is sealed, but you can take it further if you wish.

The circle is now complete, and with the spirits of the elements invoked, it helps to grow your power, and you can now perform any spell or ritual or evoke or invoke any deity you would like.

Calling the Quarters and Invoking the Deities

Calling the quarters goes by many names, including calling the elements or the guardians of the watchtowers. This ritual can be viewed as a supplement to the casting of a magick circle; invoking the four elements and spirits is used to amplify the power of this kind of secret circle. Getting in touch with the quarters or invoking deities can be done without a specific method. Everyone is free to choose the most meaningful and powerful approach; there's no one right way. Besides, all you need is an athame or wand, nothing else. Still, if you would like, you can also put a tool associated with each element in the appropriate cardinal direction, marked by the candles you used for casting the magick circle.

Once you have placed each of the tools, if you choose to, in each cardinal direction, it is time to start summoning the spirits. There are numerous ways to imagine the elements and their spirits. You might imagine the spirit forms we discussed earlier in the book or just an embodiment of the element. Either will work.

Holding your wand or athame toward the north, imagine a green mist rising from the candle, forming a spirit or trees, and say the words:

"O Spirit of the North,
Ancient One of Earth,
I call you to attend this circle.
Charge this by your powers, Old Ones!" (How to Cast a Wicca Ritual Magick Circle, 2021).

Move to the east, visualizing a yellow mist becoming a spirit or whirlwind, and say the words:

"O Spirit of the East,
Ancient One of Air,
I call you to attend this circle.
Charge this by your powers, Old Ones!" (How to Cast a Wicca Ritual Magick Circle, 2021).

Move to the south, visualizing a red mist becoming a spirit or flames, and say the words:

"O Spirit of the South,
Ancient One of Fire,
I call you to attend this circle.
Charge this by your powers, Old Ones!" (How to Cast a Wicca Ritual Magick Circle, 2021).

Last, move to the west, visualizing a blue mist becoming a spirit or wave, and repeat the words:

"O Spirit of the West,
Ancient One of Water,
I call you to attend this circle.
Charge this by your powers, Old Ones!" (How to Cast a Wicca Ritual Magick Circle, 2021).

Visualization is key to calling the quarters or summoning a deity because you have to connect with them. They are in the spiritual plane, so you must use your third eye and visualization skills to make the initial connection. Your power will then help to form the connection. For specific deities, there will be different ways to summon them. Symbols and different words might be used for other deities. If you have a grimoire, it will likely outline the different ways your specific Wiccan type invokes or evokes a deity.

The Heart of the Ritual and the Book of Shadows

After you have prepared the ritual, cast the circle, and summoned the element, spirits, or deities you need, it is time for the heart of the ritual, which will be the main ritual you want to perform. You can do various things, including grounding, centering, or shielding, which we will learn about in the next chapter.

The Book of Shadows is a sacred text for all Wiccans, but not all Wiccans have access to it. This book is said to contain instructions for many magickal rituals. Many grimoires that Wiccans come across were derived from the Book of Shadows. Gerald Gardner wrote the first and most famous Book of Shadows, which initiated the craft in the 1950s. Although he was the first person to write the book, he allowed others to copy it and change it to fit their needs better. It was believed that a Book of Shadows would work for only the owner. That is why when other Wiccans read Gerald's version and tried to use the same spells, not all of them worked. They needed to be changed to fit the user better. So, new spells are created, and existing rituals are modified when needed, showing no fixed and rigid way of executing magic. This flexibility allows for much more freedom in practice rather than a restrictive approach.

However, not all Wiccans have access to a Book of Shadows, and it is often believed that there were two versions, one for covens and one for personal use. The personal version of the Book of Shadows will be different for everyone and have various spells, rituals, and recipes.

Eclectic witches have different meanings when it comes to the Book of Shadows. To them, it is a personal journal, not a traditional text. In this journal, a witch would record the result of spells and rituals, how they worked or did not, and any other magickal information they came across during their lifetime. While a Book of Shadows to other witches might be passed on from teacher to student, or copies made for covens, for eclectic witches, they were not typically passed on. An eclectic witch must learn, discover their magick, and create rituals.

Cake and Ale

Throughout many religions, it is a common and sacred act to share food and drinks during different rituals and ceremonies. The same goes for Wiccans. If you practice in a coven or solitary, you will offer ale and cakes to the gods and goddesses and eat them yourself. All participating members would consume the cake and ale in a coven during the ceremony.

Before the casting of the magick circle, cake and ale are prepared and placed on the altar. A chalice will hold the ale being served, and a special plate is often used for the cake to sit on. These dishes are to be used for the cakes and ale alone and for no other purpose, as they could corrupt the food or magick. There is no specific type of cake or ale that is served. Consecration occurs on the cake and ale before being offered. Some people consecrate the food with the tools, while others do it right before offering it to the gods. But be sure to offer the food to the gods before handing it out to everyone else and eating it yourself. Remember, consuming ale and cake without offering some of it to the deity is considered disrespectful by Wiccans.

Closing the Ritual

We are now at the end of the ritual, and although you will always have a connection to the deities you invoked, you have to revoke them, allowing them to leave the circle. Use these words or something similar to revoke a spirit or ritual:

"Lady of the Moon, of the fertile Earth and rolling seas,
Lord of the Sun, of the sky and wild,
Thank You for Your presence in our circle today.
Stay if you will, go if you must,
But know that you are ever welcome in our hearts.
We bid you hail and farewell" (Wright, 2022b).

After you have revoked the deity, goddess, or god you have summoned, you must also revoke the elements. When invoking, we started in the north, but to revoke, you will begin in the west and work counterclockwise. Use your hands, athame, or wand, standing westward, and say:

"Powers of the West: powers of Water;
Thank You for Your presence in our circle today,
For sharing your deep mysteries and intuition,
Hail and farewell, powers of the West" (Wright, 2022b).

Turn toward the south and say:

"Powers in the South; Powers of Fire;
Thank You for Your presence in our circle today,
For sharing your inspiration and courage,
Hail and farewell, powers of the South" (Wright, 2022b).

Turn to the east and say:

"Powers of the East; powers of Earth,
Thank you for Your presence in our circle today;
For sharing your stability and growth,
Hail and farewell, powers of the East" (Wright, 2022b).

Last, turn toward the north and say:

"Powers of the North; powers of Air,
Thank you for your presence in our circle today;

For sharing your wisdom and knowledge
Hail and farewell, powers of the North.
Finish the ritual with a final declaration, such as:
The circle is open but never broken!" (Wright, 2022b).

You have officially ended your ritual at this point. Remember that this is just an example of what might occur in a Wiccan ritual and how it can be performed. Wiccan rituals are unique for each person, so there is no pressure to follow exactly what I have shown you. Feel free to tailor it to fit your practice. A lot goes into a singular ritual, but it is worth it in the end because you connect with yourself and nature and make changes. Now that we know of the basis of many Wiccan rituals, it is time to explore the last part of Pillar 5, which is the types of rituals that Wiccans perform.

16

Different Types of Rituals

Every new Wiccan should be aware of a few essential rituals. However, it is impossible to cover them all due to the sheer number and variety. Nevertheless, understanding these fundamentals is key to successful practice. Throughout this chapter, we will talk about four essential rituals all Wiccans need to know, including the centering, cone of power, grounding, and shielding.

Centering

Many Wiccan rituals use energy manipulation, and the start of any energy work is centering. Although there is a common idea of what centering is across the different kinds of Wicca, how someone centers themselves can differ. But to effectively use energy and your magick, you should begin centering yourself. Previous experience with meditation, although it is not needed to learn how to center, can make it much easier because meditation and centering use similar techniques. Practicing meditation outside of rituals can also make it easier to center during a ritual.

To center yourself, find a spot where you will be left undisturbed. If you have children, find a time during the day when you would not be disturbed, such as when they are in school or have a time when they go outside to play. Even if you live alone, make sure there are no disruptions. Turn your cell phone on mute, lock the doors, and turn off the television. You can choose to sit or lie down. Many will opt to sit because lying down might make them too relaxed and lead to them taking a nap. Take deep breaths, in through the nose and out through the mouth. Repeat the process, keeping your breaths even.

Once you have relaxed, it is time to visualize your energy and the energy around you. If you are having difficulty doing this, rub your hands together and hold them close, ensuring they are not touching. At first, you might not feel anything, but you should eventually feel the charge between your palms. This energy should feel like there is some resistance between your hands as you try to bring them back together.

Now that you know what the energy feels like, you can start manipulating it. Focus on the feeling of the energy and then visualize it moving and expanding. It will take some time to master centering, but once you do, you should be able to manipulate energy so that it bends to your will. Centering is not about producing new energy but harnessing what you already have. Visualize bringing your energy forward and forming a ball. Repeat this process to get yourself more familiar with the process. As you continue to practice, it will become more natural, and you can manipulate your energy better.

Cone of Power

The cone of power ritual is all about gathering and directing energy and magick. Both coven and solitary witches can perform this ritual. Naturally, covens produce more power and energy as several witches come together. Meanwhile, a solitary witch can also perform this ritual but would not experience as much energy increase. The cone of power ritual is primarily used as an energy-boosting ritual which allows for spells and other rituals to be more powerful as energy is gathered and released. One of the primary reasons why it is visualized as a cone is that it aligns with the body's chakras. The root chakra, located at the base of our spines, is believed to be the base of the cone, which then tapers as chakras move upwards toward the head. There are various names that someone might use for the rituals, and they might also imagine it as a different shape. But what is important to remember is that many Wiccans use this ritual daily. First, let us discuss how this ritual would be performed with a group.

A magick circle would be cast, and the members who were partaking in the ritual would be inside the circle. The people inside will form a circle, creating the base of the cone of power. Depending on the coven, the witches might join hands, or they might visualize the energy rising from each person, forming a cone. Likewise, the witches inside the circle will chant and sing; as they do this, their power will rise and form a cone of power above them. And based on the coven and the magickal systems being explored, the energy gathered might expand past the cone's apex and float into the world. After enough power has been collected, the coven's leader will complete the ritual, sending the energy toward the group's magickal purpose, including protection and healing. The rest of the ritual would continue, as discussed in the previous chapter.

As we have learned, covens are not nearly as popular as they were at the beginning of Wicca, with most Wiccans nowadays practicing solitarily. Depending on the Wiccan you ask, some say that an individual cannot raise a cone of power by themselves, while others say they can. The process can be done the same way a group would, but only one person exists. How one accumulates enough energy to form a cone can differ depending on the person, with some methods working better than others. Some methods for gathering energy include chanting, singing, drumming, and physical exercise.

Grounding

Connecting with the earth through grounding helps access its healing power and ease anxiety and stress. This method allows you to release energy while drawing upon the earth's power without depleting your own. Earthing helps you, in a sense, recharge your batteries so you have more energy to handle any stressful situations that may come your way. Many natural magick users use grounding because of their inherent connection to the earth.

To ground yourself, sit or lay down with your palms face down. Grounding yourself outside is easier because it allows you to connect with nature physically. You do not need to go into the forest or anything, just into your yard or park. However, if you do not have a safe space in nature to do this process, then doing it inside will be alright. You can either have your eyes closed or open. Imagine your energy traveling through your body, your hands, and then down into the earth. You can also imagine your power traveling from the base of your head, down your spine, and deep into the earth. Where you imagine your energy traveling from will be rooted to where you think it originates. If you think it comes from your head, imagine traveling from there. Or if you feel it in your gut, imagine it traveling from there, into your hands, and then into the ground.

Expelling your energy into the air can help you to find balance and ground your energies. But you need to be cautious and remember that you will not be able to draw onto this magick like you would from grounding it into the earth. Also, discharging magick into the air allows other people to absorb it, which could leave them in a similar position as you are. If you cannot get onto the ground easily, you can also practice grounding by having your bare feet touch the floor or ground and imagine your energy down your body, into your feet, and then into the ground.

Sometimes this is not enough, especially when you first start practicing Wicca. You can try grounding with something tangible, including crystals, phrases, and pots of dirt. As a Wiccan, you likely already have a crystal that you have connected to. When feeling overwhelmed, stressed, or anxious, hold onto your crystal and let it absorb your energy. Create a phrase, simple or complex, that you will say when imagining your energy leaving the body. This can be a great way to finalize the process. Lastly, you can keep a pot of dirt close by, and when you need to expel some energy, place your hands in the soil and feel your energy transferring to it.

Shielding

Shielding is the last of the essential rituals that all Wiccans need to know, as it protects against mental, magickal, and psychic attacks. Likewise, it creates an energy barrier around yourself that others cannot penetrate. However, you can also push magick and energy outside of the barrier. The shielding process is very similar to grounding, but instead of pushing energy outside your body, you will envelop your body with energy. Focus on the ball of energy you form when centering and imagine it expanding around yourself.

Visualize your shield as being reflective. This will repel negative energy and influence back to the person who sent it. Your shield can also be similar to a tinted window, as it will let good things in and keep harmful things out. Shielding techniques can be essential if you are affected by other people's emotions or if you find interacting with specific people exhausting.

These are four essential rituals that all Wiccans need to know when it comes to practicing Wicca appropriately. And now that you have learned them, you have reached the end of this book and know the five pillars essential for Wicca. Before we part ways entirely and you start your Wiccan journey, let us recap what we have learned throughout this book.

Conclusion

When you started exploring Wicca, you might have had a rough time. You might still be going through troubled times, questioning how to connect with yourself and the world more. Stress and anxiety are normal, but Wicca, its practices, and beliefs can all help you get through these challenging times. In the modern day, it has become much harder to connect with oneself, others, and nature as we become more enthralled with technology, but Wicca can help you to connect with yourself, nature, and the divine.

Throughout this book, we learned about the five pillars of Wicca, which are essential for learning and practicing Wicca, and these include the following:

1. **Foundation:** the history and origins of Wicca and Wicca in the present day.
2. **Beliefs:** the deities of Wicca, including the Triple Goddess and the Horned God, the importance of the elements, ethics, holidays, birth, marriage, and death rites.
3. **Practice:** the many different types of Wicca and how to get initiated.
4. **Magick:** natural, ceremonial, and celestial magick.
5. **Rituals:** what is needed for a ritual, how a typical one is performed, and some essential rituals to know.

You have learned how varied and multifaceted Wicca is. It can fit into any lifestyle and help you to align yourself with nature and the universe. The rituals, celebrations, and many Wiccan techniques, such as grounding and centering, can help with self-development and better coping with stress and anxiety. These are essential things to know about Wicca.

Learning about the five pillars of Wicca and starting to practice the Wiccan practices you connect with helps you to harness your intuition and awaken the divine magick inside yourself. Remember that we are all part of the earth, and it is about opening yourself up to the divine to connect with the earth on a deeper level.

Now you have all the information you need to start practicing Wicca and connecting with yourself. I have given you all the tools and information you need, and now it is time for you to take the next step. I know it can be scary to try something new and connect with yourself, but it is time to make positive changes in your life. So, get out there, start putting energy into the world, and rekindle your relationship with yourself!

Glossary

Augury Witches: Wiccans and witches that use their abilities to decipher omens, typically from the behavior of animals.

Beltane: Occurs on April 30th and May 1st and celebrates light, fertility, and the coming of summer. This celebration represents the continued waking up of the earth as more light is brought from the sun. A young girl is often picked to become the May Queen, a stand-in for the Celtic fertility goddess Flora.

Celestial Magick: Magick focused on interactions with the gods in hopes of making earthly changes.

Ceremonial Magick: Magick used to summon gods, goddesses, deities, and spirits. Contains rituals, including banishing, purification, consecration, invocation, evocation, eucharist, and divination.

Cosmic Witches: Wiccans and witches that specialize in astronomy, astrology, and reading the stars. Use spells and moon cycles to protect celestial events and use birth charts and star signs in their practice.

Coven: A group of witches that practice Wicca together, including performing rituals, attending sabbats, esbats, and training.

Coven-Based Witches: witches that practice within a coven.

Crossing the Bridge: The ritual performed during the funeral of a Wiccan. Depending on the Wiccan type you are, how this ritual is performed will differ, but they all honor death. Spiral dances, which represent the cycle of life, are across-the-board.

Eclectic Witches: Are individuals who practice Wicca and identify as witches but adopt other non-Pagan beliefs, philosophies, and practices.

Esbat: Celebrations and festivals that occur during the full moon. These celebrations are not as big as sabbats, and although gods and goddesses are still honored, they do not play a big part. In one year, there are 13 full moons in which the Wiccans will practice.

Gray Witches: Witches that practice white and dark magick, often seeking justice for wrongdoings and redirecting dark magick to appropriate places.

Green Witches: Witches that specialize in healing, nurturing, and nature. They use plants and flowers to make herbal preparations.

Green Witches: Wiccans that specialize in nature, nurturing, and healing. Their tools, rituals, and power are all connected to nature.

Handfasting: The marriage ceremonies that Wiccans have. It is not a Wiccan invention, as it has existed for thousands of years. How the ceremony is performed will differ depending on the person. Still, the primary aspect of tying the couple's hands with colorful ribbons, different fabrics, and cords is always performed. The duration of how long they are tied will vary depending on the people. Handfasting does not equate to legal marriage.

Handparting: The separation or divorce ritual occurs when a married couple no longer wants to be together. Wiccans do not punish divorce; they perform these ceremonies to cut spiritual and symbolic ties. These rituals are supposed to promote continued respect between the partners.

Hearth Witches: Witches are similar to green and kitchen markers, but their practices are centered around the entire house, where they perform protection rituals, herbalism, cleansing, and candle magick.

Hedge Witches: Similar to green witches. However, they do not bind themselves only to the practices of Wicca. Their magick allows them to connect with the elements and create herbal remedies.

Hereditary Witches: Witches born into their powers, typical of later-generation Wiccans.

Horned God: The central male deity of Wicca, who is depicted as a male with horns or antlers or a figure with a male body, but the head of a horned animal. He represents Wicca's male aspects and is the Triple Goddess's consort. He is also a dualistic god, representing two aspects: day and night, light and dark, summer and winter, and life and death. He is associated with the life cycle, hunting, nature, sexuality, and the wilderness.

Imbolc: Is the midpoint celebration between winter and spring and occurs on February 1st and 2nd. This festival celebrates purification and rebirth. Fertility is a big focus of this celebration, as the name Imbolc means in the belly.

Kitchen Witches: Witches that focus their abilities in the kitchen and use herbs in their baking and cooking to extract their medicinal properties.

Litha: Is the celebration of the Summer Solstice and the year's longest day. Celebrations occur between June 20 to 22. As the spirit and human worlds are fully awakened at this time, protection rituals are very commonly used as dark spirits become more powerful.

Lughnasadh: Is the midpoint celebration between summer and fall, occurring on August 1st. The first harvested fruits and vegetables are offered to the Horned God and the Triple Goddess. The Horned God's annual death is known to be approaching, and he is to return to the underworld and Summerland.

Mabon: The celebration of the Autumn Equinox and occurs between September 20-23. This celebration marks the descent of the Horned God into the underworld, where he would not return until after Yule.

The second harvest occurs at this time in preparation for winter. This celebration emphasizes reflecting and giving thanks as the soil begins to die in the coming winter months.

Natural Magick: Uses various plants, earthen materials, crystals, alchemy, botany, chemistry, and astronomy.

Ostara: The celebration of the Spring Equinox and occurs between March 20-23. Hope, birth, and fertility are essential to this celebration. The Triple Goddess is said to have become impregnated by the Horned God during this time. Older Pagan generations kept their celebration during this time secret.

Rite of Dedication: A ritual to declare someone's interest in joining a coven. They can start to train with a coven after this rite.

Rite of Passage: A ritual that fully introduces a Wiccan into a coven. Often Wiccans will need to perform various tasks during this rite, typically occurring a year after the rite of dedication.

Sabbat: Seasonal celebrations occur at the turn of the season and in the middle of each season. The eight, or greater, sabbats are depicted on the Wheel of the Year. Usually, witches celebrate Sabbats in a coven and by those practicing solitarily. Solitary witches that know each other will often come together to celebrate the sabbats. The sabbats represent the cyclical nature of life and the seasons. They focus on reflecting on the past and looking toward the future.

Samhain: Celebrated on October 31st and marks the beginning of the Wiccan year. The name means summer's end, and the veil between the mortal and spirit worlds is the thinnest during this time. The transition from summer to fall signifies the end of the light season and the beginning of the dark season. Bonfires are essential for this celebration to mark the continued perseverance of light through the dark season.

Secular Witches: Wiccans and witches that do not equate their powers to religion or spirituality. They do not follow the rules or morals of Wicca and sometimes do not identify as Wiccan.

Self-Dedication: A non-mandatory ritual that solitary Wiccans can perform to dedicate themselves to Wicca, its beliefs, and practices.

Solitary Witches: Wiccans that practice by themselves and without a coven. This is the most common way that Wicca is practiced today.

The Rule of Three: A tenet that many Wiccans follow, which says that what you put into the world will return to you three times. Some interpret this rule as meaning energy will return to them in the form of lessons, often in threes. This pertains to both good and bad energy.

The Wheel of the Year: Is a symbol used to show the eight great sabbats and the 13 esbats celebrated throughout one year. The Wheel of the Year originated thousands of years before the creation of Wicca and was used by Celts.

Triple Goddess: Also known as a Moon Goddess, the primary female deity of Wicca. She represents the magick number three and triunity. She often represents the female life cycle (maiden, mother, and crone) along with the three realms of the world (heaven, earth, and the underworld). She represented the feminine side of Wicca and became a figure for feminism in Wiccan females because she was a symbol of comfort and liberation.

Wicca: One of the largest neo or modern Pagan religions practiced today. It emerged in the 1960s and was created by Gerald Gardner, credited because of his influence on a coven of witches known as the New Forest Group. Gardner's original writings and practices are now known as Gardnerian Wicca. Wicca, as a religion, has no strict rules and individual covens, and people have created their rituals and theories based on the writings of Gardner.

Wiccans: Followers of the Wicca practices and beliefs and identify themselves as witches.

Wiccan Rede: A poem or speech that outlines the moral standards of Wicca and other Pagan religions. It first started as one line: "An ye harm none, do what ye will" (Wikipedia, 2022a). This was later expanded to be much longer. It is fundamentally the golden rule of Wicca and is interpreted by many to mean: do good to others and yourself.

Wiccaning: The birth rite or welcoming ceremony to those looking to be introduced into the Wiccan's spiritual community. This is not a rite that then makes you practice Wicca but is welcoming you to the community. Many Wiccans will hold this rite for their children, but this does not mean they have to partake in Wiccan practices. Wiccaning is often considered to be the Wiccan version of baptism.

Yule: Also known as the Winter Solstice, it celebrates the shortest day of the year with celebrations between December 20 to 25. Although winter is sometimes associated with death, Yule marks renewing the life cycle as the Horned God returns from the underworld and the days become longer. Evergreens are decorated in honor of the god, and gifts are left out for him. Bonfires and the burning of the yule log also occurs.

References

A list of herbs and their magickal uses. (n.d.).Spiral Rain. https://spiralrain.ca/pages/a-list-of-herbs-and-their-magickal-uses

Alexander B. & Norbeck, E. (2020, November 10). Rite of passage. In *Encyclopædia Britannica*. https://www.britannica.com/topic/rite-of-passage/Life-cycle-ceremonies

Augury. (2023, January 6). Wikipedia. https://en.wikipedia.org/wiki/Augury

Ball, P. (2020). *Natural magick: Spells, enchantments, and personal growth* (pp. 282–290). Arcturus.

Beyer, C. (2019, June 5). *What to know about the five classical elements.* Learn Religions. https://www.learnreligions.com/elemental-symbols-4122788

Ceremonial magick. (2022, December 19). Wikipedia. https://en.wikipedia.org/wiki/Ceremonial_magick

Ceridwen. (2019, March 8). *Elemental magick for beginners: Basic principles.* Craft of Wicca. https://craftofwicca.com/elemental-magick-for-beginners/

Classical element. (n.d.). Chemeurope. https://www.chemeurope.com/en/encyclopedia/Classical_element.html#Neo-Paganism

Eclectic paganism. (2021, July 3). Wikipedia. https://en.wikipedia.org/wiki/Eclectic_Paganism

Esbat. (2022, December). Encyclopedia. https://www.encyclopedia.com/science/encyclopedias-almanacs-transcripts-and-maps/esbat

Horned god. (2022, November 14). Wikipedia. https://en.wikipedia.org/wiki/Horned_God

How to cast a wicca ritual magick circle. (2021). The Not so Innocents Abroad. https://www.thenotsoinnocentsabroad.com/blog/how-to-cast-a-wicca-ritual-magick-circle

Lewis, I. M. & Russel, J. B. (2022, October 21) *Witchcraft: The witch hunts.* (2019). In Encyclopædia Britannica. https://www.britannica.com/topic/witchcraft/The-witch-hunts

Magickal tools in wicca. (2022, November 29). Wikipedia. https://en.wikipedia.org/wiki/Magickal_tools_in_Wicca#Cauldron

Mark, J. (2019, January 28). *Wheel of the year*. World History Encyclopedia. https://www.worldhistory.org/Wheel_of_the_Year/

Patterson, R. (2020, February 14). *The art of ritual: Calling the quarters*. Beneath the Moon. https://www.patheos.com/blogs/beneaththemoon/2020/02/the-art-of-ritual-calling-the-quarters/

Rabu. (2022, October 19). *Apparently, there are different types of witches*. CXO Media. https://www.cxo-media.id/art-and-culture/20221019175249-24-176660/apparently-there-are-different-types-of-witches

Rekstis, E. (2022, January 21). *Healing crystals 101*. Healthline. https://www.healthline.com/health/mental-health/guide-to-healing-crystals

Rule of three (Wicca). (2023, January 2). Wikipedia. https://en.wikipedia.org/wiki/Rule_of_Three_(Wicca)

Shade, P. (2022, October 28). *The supernatural side of plants*. Cornell Botanic Gardens. https://cornellbotanicgardens.org/the-supernatural-side-of-plants-2/

Smith, D. (2016, March 26). *Looking into habits of effective wiccans*. Dummies. https://www.dummies.com/article/body-mind-spirit/religion-spirituality/wicca/looking-into-habits-of-effective-wiccans-201046/

Term: Crossing the bridge. (n.d.) Llewellyn Worldwide. https://www.llewellyn.com/encyclopedia/term/Crossing+the+Bridge

The art of handfasting. (2019, November 19). The Celebrant Directory. https://www.thecelebrantdirectory.com/art-of-handfasting/

The Editors of Encyclopedia Britannica. (2022, December 23). *Reincarnation*. Encyclopædia Britannica. https://www.britannica.com/topic/reincarnation

The wiccan altar: The tools of wiccan ritual. (n.d.). Wicca Living. https://wiccaliving.com/wiccan-altar/

The wiccan rede. (n.d.). Web.mit.edu. https://web.mit.edu/pipa/www/rede.html

Tomekeeper. (n.d.). *Celestial magick*. Luna's Grimoire. https://www.lunasgrimoire.com/celestial-magick/

Triple goddess. (2022, December 20). Encyclopedia. https://www.encyclopedia.com/religion/legal-and-political-magazines/triple-goddess

Triple goddess (neopaganism). (2023, January 9). Wikipedia. https://en.wikipedia.org/wiki/Triple_Goddess_(Neopaganism)#Contemporary_beliefs_and_practices

Ward, K. (2022, August 26). *FYI: There are many types of witches*. Cosmopolitan. https://www.cosmopolitan.com/lifestyle/a37681530/types-of-witches/

White, E. D. (2022, September 2). Wicca. In *Encyclopædia Britannica.* https://www.britannica.com/topic/Wicca

Wicca. (2023, January 9). Wikipedia. https://en.wikipedia.org/wiki/Wicca#Five_elements

Wicca clothing and ritual attire. (n.d.). Wicca Living. https://wiccaliving.com/wiccan-clothing-ritual-attire/

Wicca manual. (n.d.). Federal Bureau of Prisons. https://www.bop.gov/foia/docs/wiccamanual.pdf

Wiccan cakes and ale ceremony. (n.d.). Wicca Living. https://wiccaliving.com/cakes-ale-ceremony/

Wiccan handparting. (n.d.). Beliefnet. https://www.beliefnet.com/faiths/pagan-and-earth-based/2001/04/wiccan-handparting.aspx

Wiccan rede. (2022, November 14). Wikipedia. https://en.wikipedia.org/wiki/Wiccan_Rede

Wigington, P. (2018a, May 14). *How to sew a simple pagan ritual robe.* Learn Religions. https://www.learnreligions.com/make-a-ritual-robe-2562742

Wigington, P. (2018b, May 21). *Hold a wiccaning ceremony for your baby.* Learn Religions. https://www.learnreligions.com/what-is-a-wiccaning-2562532

Wigington, P. (2018c, December 30). *How to perform a self-dedication ritual.* Learn Religions. https://www.learnreligions.com/self-dedication-ritual-2562868

Wigington, P. (2019a, January 6). *Consecrate your magickal tools.* Learn Religions. https://www.learnreligions.com/consecrate-your-magickal-tools-2562860

Wigington, P. (2019b, February 9). *Celebrate the full moon with an esbat ritual.* Learn Religions. https://www.learnreligions.com/esbat-rite-celebrate-the-full-moon-2562864

Wigington, P. (2019c, March 22). *What is the cone of power in magick?* Learn Religions. https://www.learnreligions.com/the-cone-of-power-2561490

Wigington, P. (2019d, May 8). *The wheel of the year: Celebrating the 8 pagan sabbats.* Learn Religions. https://www.learnreligions.com/eight-pagan-sabbats-2562833

Wigington, P. (2019e, May 9). *14 magickal tools for pagan practice.* Learn Religions. https://www.learnreligions.com/magickal-tools-for-pagan-practice-4064607

Wigington, P. (2019f, June 25). *How to magickally ground, center, and shield.* Learn Religions. https://www.learnreligions.com/grounding-centering-and-shielding-4122187

Wikipedia Contributors. (2022, December 23). *Book of shadows.* Wikipedia. https://en.wikipedia.org/wiki/Book_of_shadows

Wright, M. S. (2022a, August 3). *Beginning wicca: Types of altars*. Exemplore. https://exemplore.com/wicca-witchcraft/Beginning-Wicca-Types-of-Altars

Wright, M. S. (2022b, August 3). *Wicca rituals: A standard ritual opening and closing for beginning wiccans*. Exemplore. https://exemplore.com/wicca-witchcraft/Wicca-Rituals-A-Standard-Ritual-Opening-and-Closing-for-Begining-Wiccans

THE 4 PILLARS OF SHAMANISM

FOUNDATION

CONNECTION

JOURNEY

SPIRITS

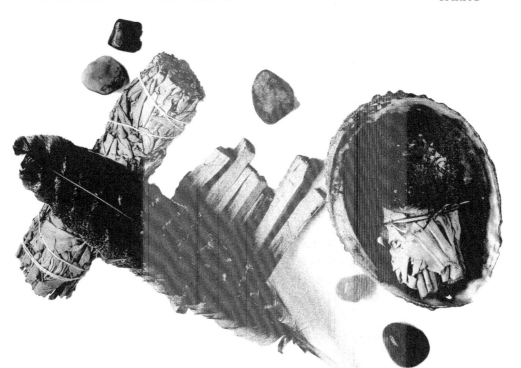

113 BEGINNER TECHNIQUES & INSIGHTS
to Harness Your Inner Power and Intuition With Shamanic Rituals. Find Balance, Harmony, and Healing by Connecting With Your Spirit Guides

INGRID CLARKE

Table of Contents

Introduction **305**

Pillar 1: Foundation **307**

Chapter 1: Understanding Shamanism **309**
    What is Shamanism? 309
    Traditional and Contemporary Shamanism 310
    History 311
    Shamanism in Modern Times 313

Chapter 2: Shamanic Beliefs **315**
    Communicating with the Spirit World 315
    Treating Malevolent Spirit Sickness. 316
    Vision Quests 317
    Entering Supernatural World for Answers 318
    Evoking Animal Images as Spirit Guides 319
    Performing Divination 320

Chapter 3: Shamanic Healing **321**
    Definition 321
    The Benefits of Shamanic Healing 322
    Plant Spirit Medicines 324
    Medicine Wheel and Four Directions 328

Pillar 2: Spirits **331**

Chapter 4: Spirit Guides **333**
    Connecting with Your Spirit Guides 333
    Your Higher Self 334
    Angels and Archangels 335
    Ancestors 336
    Plants 338
    Animals 339
    Deities 340

Pillar 3: Journey 343

Chapter 5: What Is a Shamanic Journey 345
    Soul Flight 345
    Practicing Shamanic Journeying 345
    Gaining Insights Through Meditation and Rituals 346
    Embodying the Practice 347

Chapter 6: Three Shamanic Worlds 351
    Lower World 351
    Middle World 352
    Upper World 353

Pillar 4: Connection 355

Chapter 7: Dreams 357
    What Are Dreams 357
    Out of Body Experience 358
    Lucid Dreams 362

Chapter 8: Trance 365
    Altered State of Consciousness 365

Conclusion 373

Glossary 375

References 383

Introduction

Are you lost and seeking guidance to reconnect with the spiritual side of life? Captivated by shamanism but need help knowing where to begin? This book is the perfect source to help you understand one of the oldest practices that can provide healing on your journey. It contains the knowledge and understanding needed to help you progress.

Surrounded by the rigors of modern life, the impacts of physical and psychological stress plague us daily. To counter this, alternate options are necessary to reach a state of equilibrium. Shamanism provides a way to align with spiritual aspects of the cosmos, unlocking the power of guardian spirits for healing and understanding.

After personally experiencing burnout, I have been devoted to studying different healing practices and gathering insight from metaphysical techniques and occult customs around the world. As an empath, I aim to bring forth the knowledge and understanding gleaned from a lifetime of experiences and in-depth research to those seeking healing. Subsequently, I will introduce the four pillars of shamanism in this book and illustrate how they can shape your viewpoint on portals that connect to realms inhabited by benevolent spirits. Through it all, you will discover how to unlock your consciousness of the sacredness of nature, establish contact with those entities, and communicate with them for counsel and therapy.

In the initial three chapters, you will understand shamanism more deeply, including its history, convictions, and healing capabilities. Chapter four will closely examine the various entities you can associate with, and chapters five and six will investigate the shamanic passage and other realms. Finally, chapters seven and eight will go into further detail on how to travel through a shamanic journey to communicate with your spirit guides and gain wisdom for healing.

With this book, I discovered a clearer understanding of the spiritual dimensions around me and how to find balance. I was given tools to make it through difficult times and remained in harmony with this newfound knowledge. It changed my life for the better, and it can do the same for everyone who needs guidance. Through this book, you can achieve harmony and balance by directly connecting to the spiritual realm. You will find 113 techniques, tips, and strategies to connect with realms inhabited by benevolent spirits. It's peppered throughout the entire book and it's intentionally designed this way to serve as your guide along each step of the process. It will help guide you in unlocking your awareness of divine beings and connecting with them to gain their infinite power for healing, balance, and harmony.

Moreover, this book is designed to give you access to shamanism's secrets and provide an alternate outlook on life. By employing this ancient wisdom, you can activate your inner creativity and use it to bring about meaningful change in your life. With this knowledge, you can see your current struggles from a completely different perspective, aiding you in finding solutions.

Ergo, investigate and discover the shamanic path with this book. Each chapter contains steps and strategies to help you better understand the theories and techniques you can use to make your spiritual journey more fulfilling. Learn how to access the knowledge held by spirits so you can bring your life back into balance and joy with shamanic practice. Unlock the power of divine beings to help restore harmony in all aspects of your life.

Now, set out on an adventure where self-discovery awaits you. All that is required is a willingness to explore and an open heart. Embark on a wonder, magic, and healing journey with shamanic practice. Let the ancient knowledge from spirits guide you to a place of balance and harmony.

Pillar 1
Foundation

Welcome to the first pillar of shamanism, the foundation. Here we will delve into the fundamentals of this ancient spiritual practice, which has been a part of cultures around the world for millennia. The core belief of shamanism is that everything in the world has a spirit, and these spirits can be communicated with to seek guidance and healing. As we explore further, we will investigate the concept of the spirit world and the role of a shaman, who acts as an intermediary between physical and spiritual realms. Finally, we will discuss how shamanic healing can help individuals reach physical, emotional, and spiritual balance. Join us in uncovering the history and traditions surrounding this ancient practice.

1

Understanding Shamanism

For thousands of years, shamanism has been an integral part of spiritual practices worldwide. This practice involves a shift in consciousness and connecting with spirits and natural forces. Although historically associated with remote or indigenous communities, it is now also embraced by many other cultures. People from all backgrounds have come to understand its power in seeking emotional, physical, and spiritual transformation.

What is Shamanism?

In the spiritual discipline of shamanism, healing and spirit-world communication are practiced, as well as an altered state of consciousness or ASC. One may use techniques like drumming or chanting to achieve this altered state. Some rituals employ psychedelic plants or mushrooms to create a uniquely mind-altering experience, which should always be done cautiously. Through these practices, shamans strive to access deep spiritual knowledge and seek to understand the interconnectedness of all life.

The purpose of Shamanism is to assist people in connecting with their deeper selves and unlocking secret knowledge, such as past experiences, future occurrences, and even alternate realms, like heaven. Shamanic healing works on both the physical and spiritual aspects; it can address physical problems while simultaneously aiding in discovering peace within one's mind, making life's troubles more manageable.

To find out if you are a shaman, ask yourself specific questions. A 'yes' response to any of them might mean that you have been practicing shamanic techniques in your life, even unknowingly.

- Do you feel a special bond with animals, even your pets?
- Can you forge deep connections with people, family, and friends?
- Is using plants, herbs, and crystals an easy way for you to help others heal their physical and emotional ailments?

Did you know that contemporary shamans are still around? You could even have one living close to you. Healing is their specialty; these shamans exist across the West and other regions. What sets them apart from traditional shamans is that they employ modern Western medicine and psychology practices as the basis for their healing remedies. Yet, they still draw on many of the same techniques practiced by historical shamans, such as meditation or divination, to gain insight into your body, mind, and soul, which can assist with recovery.

The term 'shaman' originates from the Tungusic languages. As such, a shaman is a spiritual leader who uses their abilities to heal, divine, and connect with unseen realms. Today this practice can still be found among indigenous populations in Siberia, Canada, and other areas. By utilizing spiritual techniques, shamans bridge the gap between physical and nonphysical realities to benefit their communities.

Although shamanism is widely practiced today, its roots can be traced back to traditional Siberian culture. In Siberia, shamans were highly regarded for their ability to enter trance states and explore other worlds. Whenever someone needed healing or guidance from beyond our reality, these shamans were called upon to help. They assisted people transitioning through life-changing events like childbirth or marriage. Likewise, they helped hunters predict success when hunting animals of significance to their tribes, such as bears

However, shamanism is not a religion but an ancient form of spirituality. Paganism, on the other hand, encompasses many different religious beliefs. Unlike the latter, shamanism does not require specific deities or beliefs about them; all it needs is someone with a passion for connecting with their inner self and the natural world. It has been practiced by people from various cultures around the globe, and anyone can participate if they are willing to put in the effort.

Despite common misconceptions, shamans and those practicing witchcraft do not have a unified code of conduct, such as Christianity or Islam. Instead, they typically draw from several traditions to create their unique practice. Paganism and witchcraft are often used interchangeably when referring to this type of magic, yet the two terms have distinct meanings depending on which group uses them. Witches tend to be eclectic and take inspiration from multiple sources rather than adhering to one specific path.

Likewise, shamans are not here to cause harm. Instead, they aim to bring balance into the world through their knowledge, intuition, and healing abilities. Those who have had the experience of participating in a shamanic ceremony as a part of their spiritual practice know that shamans do not engage in any cruel practices; instead, they work with spirit guides that assist them in helping individuals deal with challenging times. Shamans have been around since antiquity and remain so today to provide guidance when needed.

Traditional and Contemporary Shamanism

Shamanism is a distinctive method of engaging with the world through an intimate relationship with nature and other entities. It is done by utilizing altered states of consciousness, usually aided by mind-expanding herbs like peyote. In this way, shamans can access spiritual forces and explore life's deepest questions, such as *'why are we here?'*. This ancient practice offers insight into living in harmony with the natural environment and its inhabitants while continuing to grow spiritually over time. Shamans can leverage their knowledge by connecting with otherworldly beings for rituals known as "soul retrievals," in which a soul that may be stuck somewhere needs saving before it can return to where it belongs.

Chanting and drumming are powerful tools for achieving a higher state of consciousness. These practices allow one to reach the deepest levels of the mind and experience an altered state. The rhythmic repetitions evoke a trance-like atmosphere, facilitating inner exploration. By engaging in this practice, one can delve into esoteric realms rarely accessed by the average person.

Acting as healers, teachers, seers, and leaders, shamans are an integral part of many communities. They serve as a bridge between people and the spirit world, a role that is often revered in Indigenous cultures. Shamanism exists in regions across the globe, from North and South America to Europe, Australia, Asia, and Africa, and is still practiced by non-indigenous populations too. Shamans are valued for their work on behalf of their community members and exemplify spiritual understanding throughout much of the world.

Throughout history, many tribes have deeply rooted traditions passed down orally from one generation to the next. Shamanism is alive today through these oral teachings brought forth in stories. For instance, shamanism has evolved to adapt to current circumstances. While traditional shamanism involves practices that originated in ancient times, modern-day shamanism incorporates new techniques and beliefs that reflect the world today.

Practitioners of contemporary shamanism incorporate various tools and techniques to connect with the natural world and spiritual beings. As such, they use guided meditations, visualization, and energy work. While some practitioners may incorporate traditional shamanic practices into their work, contemporary shamanism is often viewed as more accessible and open to interpretation. Likewise, rather than adhering to strict traditions, contemporary shamans focus on individual growth and fostering a connection with the divine. Modern shamans also work with people of different cultures and backgrounds, as they recognize that spirituality is a universal human experience.

One notable difference between traditional and contemporary shamanism is their spiritual approach. While traditional shamanism focuses on interacting with spiritual entities outside of oneself, contemporary shamanism centers on an individual's personal growth and development. Modern-day shamans may use shamanic techniques like journeying or deep meditation to gain insight, but the focus is often on self-discovery. Additionally, contemporary shamanism can be seen as a more individualistic practice. Meanwhile, traditional shamanism usually involves the entire community. However, traditional and contemporary shamanism share a common spiritual connection and healing goal, even if their methods and approaches differ.

Overall, shamans believe that all beings possess a spirit, from rocks and trees to animals. Through proper interaction with these spirits (i.e., oneness), you can use them to heal yourselves. Also, whether journeying through other dimensions or finding solace in a peaceful walk through nature, embracing shamanism brings your ancestors' practice full circle, connecting to the shamans of centuries past.

History

Shamanism is an ancient spiritual practice passed down from generation to generation. Originating in Siberia and eventually becoming famous worldwide, indigenous peoples have adopted its practices everywhere, from North and South America to Africa and Australia. The term "shaman" comes from the Tungus word "saman," which refers to a person who can enter a trance-like state and communicate with the spirit world. As one of the earliest societies to embrace shamanism, the Tungus people carried on their beliefs throughout Siberia. Today, it is still practiced by various indigenous groups in many corners of the globe.

In each culture, shamanism had fundamental characteristics shared across most shamanic traditions. Among these are the capacity to communicate with spiritual entities, entering a trance state or altered consciousness to access the spirit realm, and believing that all things in existence are linked. Shamans were held in high regard by their communities and relied upon for their insightful understanding of the spiritual world, healing physical and mental suffering, interpreting dreams, and connecting people with the divine. Every civilization has modified these practices to fit its distinct environment, but these common threads remain unchanged.

The ancient practice of shamanism was prevalent among hunter-gatherer societies that lived during prehistory before written records began. This primitive lifestyle relied heavily on the connection with nature; their rites and rituals were integral to this relationship. Shamans utilized various methods to reach a transfigured state and access the spiritual realm—drumming, singing, and consuming entheogenic substances. From here, they could access supernatural entities and capacities to receive healing, knowledge, and guidance.

Across the globe, numerous cultures have shamans. From Native American medicine men and medicine women to Australian Aboriginals' songmen, Norse pagans' völvas, African tribal healers invoking herbs and magic spells, and Japanese Buddhists practicing Shintoism through praying rituals instead of direct contact, all these people have unique methods to communicate with spirits. Shamans were also knowledgeable in the diverse art forms of music, dance, and storytelling, which they used to pass down knowledge and insights to their community. Furthermore, they were considered wise counselors, guiding those who requested their help. By utilizing these different expressions, shamans effectively expressed the wisdom they received from the spiritual realm.

In many ways, shamanism is seen as a predecessor to many aspects of modern life, from religion and science to medicine. By entering altered states of consciousness, shamans employed methods like those used in hypnosis and meditation today. Praying to and conversing with spiritual entities is a ritual in many religions, similar to divination. In terms of healing, natural remedies are comparable to herbal medicine, which is commonly used in modern medical settings.

As the interest in spiritual pursuits grows, shamanism has become increasingly popular. Modern shamans have adapted historical practices to suit their beliefs and customs, including new methods while respecting the tradition's heritage. Those looking for a healing, insight, or a closer relationship with the world can benefit from this ancient practice. Shamanism offers abundant knowledge that can be used to develop a greater understanding of oneself and one's environment.

Shamanism in Modern Times

In today's world, shamanism has become a means to comprehend better how human energy works in harmony with our environment. It is not simply about beating drums or dancing around a fire; instead, it is an approach to healing oneself and others by connecting to the universe. Shamanism enables us to access our inner self, the spiritual realm, nature, and even our forbearers. This life path provides us with perspective and connection that can be used for personal and collective well-being.

Moreover, the current shamanic practices help those suffering from physical and mental conditions, such as depression and anxiety. Rather than masking their emotions with medications that could cause lasting harm, these healers help their patients identify their feelings. To further this healing process, shamans often perform rituals like smudging, which is the burning of herbs, to purify an individual's energy field and reconnect them with their true selves. This ultimately allows them to free themselves from lingering feelings of distress, enabling a path forward without being held back.

Ergo, shamans are not a source of harm or involved in any brainwashing, superstitious practices, or sinister cults. Instead, the term 'shaman' is derived from a Tungusic language, including Evenki and Evenk, meaning 'healer.' This hints at their ability to heal through their practice and is closely linked with the spirits of nature. As one's energy and soul align more with nature and its many forces, they become increasingly capable of healing those around them.

Searching for a shaman is easier than ever. They come in an array of styles and are found across the globe. Yet, select one well-versed in your desired tradition and willing to guide you to get the best support and direction.

People have long looked to shamans for healing, and Native American practices are only one such tradition. Many different methods of shamanic rituals are available today. As such, there are solo sessions to group gatherings in physical or virtual spaces, at home, or while traveling. No matter the setting, these ceremonies offer an opportunity to tap into bottomless inner power reserves.

Thus, shamanism can help people in today's society in several ways. It can help people to understand their problems and find solutions for them. Shamanism can also help people to overcome their problems. In addition, shamanism is a powerful tool for establishing a connection with your inner self and the universe outside of you. Likewise, it can solve issues in your personal life or interpersonal relationships. However, as mentioned, there are many different types of shamanic practices. That said, find one that fits your beliefs and personality.

2

Shamanic Beliefs

As we explore the origins of shamanism, we must also comprehend their beliefs and what roles the shaman plays in them. An exploration into why such a journey is pursued is necessary to understand this ancient practice fully. We will embark on this endeavor to gain insight into the mysteries of shamanic ways.

Communicating with the Spirit World

The shaman is a spiritual practitioner who has been present in many indigenous cultures worldwide for thousands of years. At its core, shamanism is a belief system that is founded on the idea that everything is interconnected and that spiritual and physical realms are not separate from one another. In fact, the shaman believes that spirits are all around us and can be communicated with through shamanic practices.

As a bridge between the material and spiritual realms, the shaman is revered for their talent of communing with those from beyond. From departed ancestors to gods and goddesses, they are said to be capable of reaching out and conversing with the spirits that inhabit our world. Connecting with the life force of plants and animals can provide insight and aid in healing. Moreover, shamans have used various tools and techniques to communicate with the spirit world. These can include chanting, singing, drumming, and dancing. Some shamans use hallucinogenic plants or other substances to help them enter altered states of consciousness, which can facilitate communication with the spirit world.

One of the primary ways that the shaman communicates with the spirit world is through journeying. This technique involves the shaman entering a trance-like state and traveling to other worlds or realms. The shaman is said to be able to communicate with spirits and receive guidance from them while in this state. As such, journeying can be done in various ways, but one common technique is to use a drum or other rhythmic instrument to help the shaman enter a trance state. Typically, the shaman will sit or lie down and close their eyes, allowing the drum sound to guide them into an altered state of consciousness. Once in this state, the shaman can explore other realms and communicate with spirits.

Divination is another means through which shamans get in touch with the spirit realm. This practice involves using tools such as bones, cards, or other objects to gain insight into a situation or receive guidance from the spirit world. The shaman may ask a question and then use the tool to receive an answer from the spirits. Besides that, dreams can be more than just random incoherent images and plots. Shamans believe it is a doorway through which wise and powerful messages from the spirit world can be conveyed. According to them, dream interpretation can help provide insight into pressing matters or even give guidance from the spiritual realm.

Being in communion with the spiritual realm is a gift of the spirits. It is said that the otherworldly entities choose the shaman and must undergo a stringent, rigorous training regimen to hone their talent. Through this, they develop and refine their capability to communicate with those beyond our plane of existence.

The shaman is viewed as the one who heals and speaks with the spiritual world. Through connecting with spirits, they can help those needing physical healing. By working closely with a patient, they can be guided to find the source of their ailment and then speak with otherworldly entities on their behalf to facilitate healing. In certain cultures, shamans may be invoked for more than just medical purposes; they are seen as vessels to converse with spirits regarding hunting or agriculture and perform ceremonies marking life transitions such as birth, marriage, and death.

Treating Malevolent Spirit Sickness.

Shamans are incredibly talented spiritual healers who can bring peace and harmony to those suffering from malicious spirit activity. Illnesses caused by evil spirits are common and can often be traced back to their influence. With the help of a shaman, these influences can be alleviated, allowing peace of mind and improved health.

For instance, in the case of sickness related to malevolent spirits, the shaman is called to perform a cure. Once the source of illness has been uncovered, help is requested from the shaman. A ritual is conducted to drive away the evil spirit that has taken hold of your being. Rituals can be done solo or as part of a group, with incantations, charms, and spells used in harmony to cast out the evil force.

When shamans heal an illness, they consider various factors before selecting the best action. One such factor is the harm caused to the individual, the family, or the community. Suppose an individual is possessed by an evil spirit, leading to harm to their family and others close to them. In such a scenario, the shaman may conduct a community-wide ritual to eliminate negative forces, requiring the active participation of the entire community.

Moreover, this practice involves entering a trance-like state where the shaman can communicate with spirits and send them away. In this state of spiritual communication, the shaman can request an explanation from the spirit as to why it is causing harm to its host if a problem has been left unresolved between them. For example, if the patient committed a misdeed, the issue can be settled before directing any negative energy away from the body.

Furthermore, shamans can create talismans that help ward off harmful spirits from their patients. The process of making these protective amulets involves the use of raw materials imbued with spiritual energy. Usually, a talisman made from bone or animal fur can serve as a conduit for the shaman's power, helping to keep negative energy away from the patient. Once complete, the affected individual can wear or carry the talismans to provide continued protection.

Besides that, shamans may use natural remedies to strengthen the body and prevent future malicious attacks by spirits. Prescribed remedies such as herbs, potions, and spiritual items are designed to support the immune system and restore balance to the patient's spiritual and physical well-being. Herbs, for instance, may be used to cleanse the body and spirit, purify the mind, and strengthen the body's defense mechanisms against future negative energy. Meanwhile, potions can dispel negative spirits and repel future spiritual attacks.

Shamans possess extraordinary spiritual healing skills to alleviate illnesses caused by evil spirits. These malevolent entities can be identified and exorcized using a range of rituals, incantations, and spells. By communicating with spirits in a trance-like state, shamans can remove negative energy and restore health to people suffering from malevolent spirit activity.

Vision Quests

A vision quest can be a powerful way for shamans to gain insight and wisdom from the spirit world. It is an immersive form of meditation, allowing them to tap into unseen realms, receive visions, and gain advice from supernatural entities. Different cultures and shamanic traditions offer varied approaches to the quest, each taking the participants on a unique journey of introspection and enlightenment.

To induce a trance-like state, shamans in some cultures ingest psychedelics or other substances. For others, they must fast and meditate over several days, readying their physical and mental selves for the voyage into the spiritual realm. With preparation completed, they embark on a journey of discovery, pushing the boundaries of what is real and what lies beyond.

Guided by the beat of a drum, shamans embark on a journey into the spirit world, where they encounter various spirits and entities that offer them wisdom and guidance. These ethereal beings may appear as animals, plants, ancestors, or mythical creatures. During this vision quest, the shaman receives messages through visions, sounds, and sensations that provide insight into their lives or what can be done to help others. For instance, these insights may include knowledge about healing rituals, divination techniques, and other spiritual practices. All these teachings aim to empower people with the power of nature and connection to one's inner self.

Hence, the vision quest is an essential part of shamanic practice because it allows the shaman to connect with the spirits and gain knowledge and wisdom that they can use to help others. By going on a vision quest, the shaman can gain insight into the spiritual world and bring that knowledge back to the physical world to help those in need.

Aside from that, the vision quest is a significant and profound experience for shamans. It is an opportunity to confront fears, gain an understanding of oneself, and uncover one's true path in life. This spiritual practice requires preparation, training, and guidance from a knowledgeable shaman. As such, it should not be undertaken lightly or without careful planning. Likewise, through the journey into the spirit world, the shaman can connect with their ancestors and cultural heritage. The power of this ritual makes it essential to consider all the risks involved and to enter it with intentionality and respect.

Shamanic traditions demand much of their practitioners; after years of study and practice, a vision quest can be embarked upon. For the journey to be safe and successful, the shaman must learn to enter a trance state, protect themselves from evil forces, and foster a profound connection with their spirit guides to communicate effectively.

Entering Supernatural World for Answers

Shamanic journeying is a spiritual practice that shamans of the past used to communicate with spirits. Today, it is still widely used by practitioners of many cultures across the globe. Also known as power retrieval, it requires entering into an altered state of consciousness with the help of tools such as drumming, rattling, and chanting. This journey has many emotional and physical benefits, such as healing, connection with the greater universal cycle of life and death, and connectedness with the natural world. It can be a profoundly transformational experience that brings guidance and understanding beyond our own.

However, shamanic journeys are not just a tradition of ancient cultures but are also part of modern life. People looking for guidance on their journey can contact a shamanic practitioner. For those with the will, plenty of techniques like guided visualization or meditation can be used to pursue this path independently. Whatever approach is taken, these journeys offer exciting opportunities to explore the unknown and gain valuable insight into oneself.

On the shamanic journey, shamans enter an altered state of consciousness and travel through the different levels of existence to find the missing power stolen by evil spirits. To achieve this, shamans usually use drumming to help them enter the altered state. Once they have reached the altered state of consciousness, they can travel anywhere in the supernatural world and communicate with spirits without physical bodies.

To begin this journey, a shaman must traverse the space between heaven and Earth to pinpoint the location of spiritual entities. Once this is accomplished, they must use cunning and wit to outplay them in a battle of wills. Doing so can enable them to reclaim the power previously taken from them. Not only are shamans adept at uncovering answers for others, but they also serve as conduits between us and the spiritual realm.

As such, shamans can travel to the supernatural world in search of solutions for those burdened by an evil spirit or ailment. To heal the sick, a shaman enters into a trance while clutching onto the hands of the affected individual, who soon follow their lead. In this altered state of consciousness, they may be able to uncover the past lives of both themselves and their patient. Likewise, shamans can comprehend where their souls have journeyed post-death if reincarnation is believed. This method is called 'scrying' and utilizes mirrors or other reflective surfaces to serve as gateways into another realm that holds answers to questions posed. Through scrying, shamans can find and diagnose the fundamental cause of a disease or issue, granting direction and healing.

Evoking Animal Images as Spirit Guides

Shamans are powerful spiritual guides who use their talents to help others. With the ability to shape-shift into different spirits and creatures, they are known for their close connection with animal companions. Such mystical bonds guide healing rituals, connecting the physical and spiritual realms.

As spiritual intermediaries, shamans can tap into the power of animals through spirit journeying. They are messengers who can switch between different forms in this world or the next. Shamans serve as guides and healers, bridging the divide between physical reality and divine realms. By invoking images of animals, they can access a pearl of higher wisdom and help us progress on our spiritual journey.

In traditional cultures, the shaman embodies the three facets of existence—past, present, and future. They are a healer who can see into their patients' bodies and souls, psychopomps guiding souls through death and rebirth, and an instructor teaching people how to live in harmony with their environment and each other. This connection allows them to traverse all worlds: the living world with its flora and fauna, the mortal world where our ancestors remain, and even more distant realms such as heaven or hell if those exist within your culture.

Having an "animal helper," such as a spirit animal, is the key to traversing alternate dimensions. If you find yourself in bed, feeling ill one day and then the next morning experiencing some relief yet still feeling exhausted due to your sickness, it could be a sign that something or someone has visited while you were sleeping. These spiritual forces can take many forms and offer unique insights into our realities.

By using rattles, drums, and other instruments, shamans can access the spiritual realms and call upon the animal spirits. Through the power of song or chant, they can bridge worlds and open up new horizons to explore. Different cultures have crafted various tools for such expeditions, ranging from gourds to seashells or metal bells. Native Americans often employ gourds for their rattle, making needs, yet these days some shamans opt for more modern material, like metal gourds, that can just as quickly help them on their journey.

As the shaman calls forth omens or spirit guides in the form of animal images that show up on amulets and drums, these symbols reflect the shaman and their patient. Such an image may be of a real animal, but it can also represent something beyond what we know about physical creatures. For instance, if one witnessed an eagle flying over their house during the night, followed by a dream of being chased by that same bird, this could point to a person facing specific difficulties and requiring moral support. The eagle would symbolize this person's struggle, but eagles are also renowned for their strength; they can fly high above any hindrance without requiring external support, insinuating that they will overcome any problem without relying on anyone else.

Thus, a shaman may use the form of an animal totem as a spiritual guide to give initiates power over their destinies. It can also symbolize you and your life's journey, which holds special meanings or shows significance. Animal totems can act as guardians, protectors, or even counselors on the journey to understanding yourself and the world around you.

Yet, shamanism is far more than just the practices and rituals of shamans. Through their work, healing abilities, and hunting prowess, animals in spirit form often aid them. Stories have been told of shamans transforming into animals to commune with their animal guides or using an animal's behavior as a sign from the gods that someone needs a particular cure or remedy. This special connection between shaman and beast can create powerful transformations and healing moments.

Performing Divination

Other forms of divination, including scrying, throwing bones or runes, and predicting the future, can also be done by a shaman. They can then give you advice and insight into what the future may hold by doing this.

Shamanic bones, taken from animals such as leg bones or ribs, have long been used by shamans for divination. The bones are thrown into the air or cast onto the ground. Depending on how they land, shamans interpret this as an omen to determine what may be coming up in their lives, as well as that of their clients. With this method of divination, shamans hope to gain insight and answers to their questions.

Runes are an ancient method of divination used by shamans, which can influence events in a person's life. Carved on pieces of wood or stone, they were traditionally used to record information like clan lineage and property ownership. Today, these symbols are still popularly used for their capacity to bring insight into what is happening in one's life. Though these intense symbols can be difficult to understand and master, the guidance offered by an experienced practitioner is invaluable when it comes to unlocking the power of runes. Remember that runes should be welcomed as a source of insight rather than something that controls you.

Besides that, shamans can peer into the past, prophesy about the future, and gain insight through stones. Stones are a great way to determine what is on the horizon for yourself. These mystical stones can also be incorporated into rituals of foresight or used as part of your meditative practice.

On the other hand, scrying is an ancient form of divination that requires looking into a reflective surface to uncover patterns, images, or visions. It derives its name from the English word *'descry,'* meaning to catch sight of something with the help of binoculars. When you scry, you can seek answers to questions, search for lost objects and even attempt predictions. This practice is known as *'crystal gazing'* or *'glass gazing.'*

Other forms of shamanic divination include scrying with a reflective surface, throwing runes or bones, and even predicting what is to come. Overall, shamanic divination can give you insight into your life path and spiritual journey and answers about why things are happening in particular ways. With it, you can explore and discover the mysteries of past and future events.

3

Shamanic Healing

Shamanic healing is an ancient practice with transformative power. By engaging in its teachings and rituals, people can connect more deeply with nature, restore harmony across all aspects of their lives and gain insight into their spiritual path. It provides a collaborative, holistic approach to restoring balance and well-being on many levels.

Definition

Shamanic healing has been a part of spiritual and cultural traditions for many centuries, particularly those of indigenous cultures. It is an approach to health care that considers the social, mental, physical, and spiritual aspects of one's well-being, aiming to achieve harmony between them to ensure an optimal state of health. The core belief behind shamanic healing is that illness can result from disruptions in the balance of these components, which must be restored to experience wholeness.

Connecting to the natural world is the foundation of shamanic healing, for it is understood to be the origin of life and well-being. Through rituals, ceremonies, and practices that recognize and celebrate nature's cycles and seasons, this connection can be formed. This relationship allows a shamanic healer to access an ethereal realm to work with spiritual beings such as power animals, leading to healing and equilibrium.

Shamanic healing techniques are diverse and can take many forms, but some of the most common include the following:

- **Power animal retrieval.** Shamanic healers take part in power animal retrieval, which involves traveling to the spirit world to return the spiritual ally and guide of a person who has become disconnected from it. This ancestral tradition is believed to re-establish harmony and well-being in individuals but also carries cultural significance as a reflection of their worldview. Likewise, it is seen as a way to restore balance on an individual level and at a collective level for aboriginal cultures.
- **Soul retrieval.** An age-old practice used by shamanic healers to help restore a person's soul essence, which may have become fragmented or lost due to challenging experiences. Through this spiritual journey, the individual is believed to regain a sense of wholeness and energy. Furthermore, shamans often use meditation and rituals to aid in soul recovery. By doing so, they attempt to balance the person's life and body, allowing them to reconnect with their true selves and move forward with renewed strength.

- **Extraction.** A time-honored practice used for centuries by shamans and spiritual healers to remove negative energies, entities, or thought forms from an individual's body or aura. This process frees the person from low vibrational energies causing physical, mental, or emotional illness or disharmony. Once the extraction is complete, balance and well-being are restored in the person's life.
- **Despacho ceremony.** An ancient and sacred tradition that has been practiced for centuries. It shows appreciation and gratitude for the spirit while helping manifest one's desires and promote healing. Creating a physical offering is integral to the ritual, often in a basket containing food items, flowers, and other sacred objects. Once assembled, the offering is presented to the spirit world with reverence and respect. Additionally, despacho ceremonies are imbued with unique symbolism; each item is carefully included to send specific messages or help clarify intentions or wishes.
- **Sweat lodge ceremony.** Originating from Native American cultures, this ceremony involves entering a small, enclosed structure filled with steam and heat, which is believed to bring renewal, clarity, and healing to a person's physical, emotional, and spiritual aspects. Participants often report feeling revived, rejuvenated, and cleansed after completing the ritual. Likewise, this purifying process enhances healing when a shaman guides the ceremony.

In shamanic healing, the healer collaborates with the person seeking healing. The healer helps guide them through the process, while the person is responsible for their recovery by taking steps towards personal growth and transformation. Shamanic healing is holistic in nature, as it considers all aspects of an individual's physical, emotional, mental, and spiritual when striving to achieve a balanced and healthy state. Additionally, this practice recognizes that true healing necessitates restoring the body and nourishing the mind, heart, and soul. Moreover, it embraces traditional indigenous methods such as rituals, songs, and dancing which can help to facilitate the healing journey.

Aside from that, shamanic healing is a holistic approach to health and wellness that recognizes the power of the mind-body connection. This form of healing goes beyond treating symptoms, offering an in-depth look at the source of any illness. Through its use of rituals, symbols, and traditions, it can help restore balance within the body and heal physical ailments and emotional pain. Lastly, it may assist with positive life transformations, helping people lead healthier and more fulfilling lives.

The Benefits of Shamanic Healing

As such, shamanic healing can provide many physical and spiritual benefits. From alleviating pain to giving spiritual guidance, here is a look at some of the most common advantages associated with shamanic healing:

- **Reconnect with yourself and the world.** One of the primary benefits of shamanic healing is its ability to help individuals reconnect with themselves, their spirits, and the world around them. Through shamanic ceremonies and practices, people can tap into their inner selves and access healing energy. Shamanic healing can also help restore balance in an individual's energy field and provide soul retrieval.

- **Access guidance through power animals.** Power animals are crucial in shamanic healing. These animal spirits can guide an individual in and out of life and provide insight and information about oneself. Shamanic practices such as drumming and meditation help establish a deep connection with one's power animal, offering guidance on navigating life's challenges and gaining new skills for dealing with difficult situations.
- **Discover hidden information.** Shamanic healing practices grant individuals unique access to information ordinarily out of reach. This newfound insight brings greater awareness and understanding, allowing for further personal growth and development. Those who embark on this journey are better equipped to make meaningful changes, leading to an overall improved sense of well-being.
- **Find peace and reconciliation.** Offering a unique way to gain insight and clarity, shamanic practices are often used to guide critical decisions or conflict resolution. Using rituals, drumming, and meditation opens the individual to spiritual realms, allowing them to communicate with their higher self and create inner peace. Shamanic practices also focus on clearing away any negative energy that may block someone from finding peace in their everyday life. This can lead to a deeper understanding and acceptance of oneself and others.
- **Locating lost objects or people.** By entering a trance state, practitioners can access spiritual realms and connect with their higher self or spirit guides to seek guidance on matters such as finding lost objects or people. With heightened awareness, they can often generate leads or clues that reveal the whereabouts of what was thought to be lost. Furthermore, these deep meditative states open the shaman up to the energies of the world around them, providing an intuitive understanding of what might be necessary for successful retrieval.
- **Finding answers and direction:** As an ancient spiritual practice used for centuries, shamanic healing connects individuals to their inner guidance and creates greater clarity and purpose. By using time-honored techniques such as drumming, chanting, divination, meditation, dreamwork, and journeywork, individuals can access deeper levels of consciousness to receive answers and insight into life's questions. Through this practice, individuals can gain insight into their life purpose and direction. With the help of a shamanic guide, practitioners can also find a safe and supportive environment to explore these themes further.
- **Treating various health conditions.** For centuries, shamans have employed varied strategies to heal many physical and mental ailments. Some practices involve herbs and crystals, while others include spiritual dances or chants. This holistic approach often encompasses physical, psychological, and spiritual elements to achieve total health.
- **Safe and natural healing:** Includes various methods such as traditional ritual, meditation, shamanic spirituality, and harnessing the power of nature through plants and stones. Following safety precautions and consulting with an experienced practitioner or healer before beginning your treatment plan is essential when seeking spiritual guidance. Additionally, be aware that shamanic healing is not meant to replace medical care; instead, it can be used with medical interventions for improved quality of life.**Soul retrieval.** Harnessing the power of shamanic healing, soul retrieval is a journey that can help many individuals to restore balance in their energy field. By undertaking this spiritual quest, one can reconnect with themselves and reclaim their spirit and its connection with the world. For those contemplating undergoing soul retrieval, here are some steps to consider:
    - ❖ **Find a shaman.** To begin retrieving your soul, looking for a shaman who is an experienced spiritual practitioner is essential. Such a professional can guide you through the procedure,

ensuring it is done safely and accurately. Working with an expert in this field guarantees that reconnecting with your innermost essence will be as smooth and enriching as possible. Moreover, shamans also provide valuable advice about how to keep your spirit safe in the future.

- ❖ **Guided meditation exercises.** Allow you to explore parts of yourself that may have been hidden away. As such, your shaman will ask questions about past experiences, including those before and during your birth, to gain insights into the current incarnation. This form of guided self-discovery allows you to clarify areas of your life that you may be struggling with. Likewise, it helps let go of any subconscious blocks or limiting beliefs holding you back from reaching your potential.

- ❖ **Inward journey.** Embarking on an inward journey with a shaman is essential for self-discovery, unlocking inner potential, and leading to spiritual growth. Various tools such as drumming and singing help uncover underlying issues, beliefs, or values you may have been unaware of. During the journey, the shaman helps you understand and resolve any conflicts or doubts through active reflection, allowing you to find your true purpose in life.

- ❖ **Reintroduction of missing pieces.** Chanting and meditation can bring back missing parts of yourself that have been suppressed or forgotten and re-integrate them into your being. Doing so can drastically improve physical, emotional, and mental well-being, ultimately leading to finding healing from within. Furthermore, such practices can even help discover hidden aspects of you necessary to create an authentic version of selfhood.

Plant Spirit Medicines

For centuries, shamans have employed the power of plants to heal physical and emotional ailments and restore mental and spiritual balance. In the present day, this practice is still widely applied by shamanic practitioners around the world. Here we look at some of the plants used in plant spirit medicine.

Ayahuasca

Ayahuasca is a potent Amazonian brew made from a combination of an Amazonian vine and the leaves of the Chacruna plant. For thousands of years, indigenous people have utilized this sacred mixture for spiritual healing, medicinal modalities, divination, and spiritual growth. Those who seek it are thought to gain insight and enlightenment from this powerful curative substance, which extends far beyond physical health.

When taken, ayahuasca's dimethyltryptamine (DMT) and MAO inhibitors prevent the breakdown of DMT. Subsequently, it leads to remarkable experiences, including visions, distortions in the perception of reality, and profound spiritual moments. Many who have taken it describe it as awe-inspiring and life-altering. The effects of ayahuasca are unpredictable and can last for several hours, during which time individuals experience vivid and often life-changing visions. Reports include seeing bright colors, intricate geometric patterns, and otherworldly creatures. Others report experiencing a sense of unity with the universe, heightened self-awareness, and profound insights into the nature of reality.

While ayahuasca can be a powerful spiritual tool, it has risks. Negative experiences such as anxiety, paranoia, and panic attacks have been reported. It is also important to note that ayahuasca is illegal in many countries, including the United States. Hence, using it can lead to serious legal consequences. Besides that, traditional ayahuasca ceremonies are highly ritualized and led by a shaman or curandero with extensive knowledge and experience. Without proper guidance and preparation, the use of ayahuasca can be dangerous.

Despite these risks, ayahuasca has gained popularity for spiritual and personal growth. Scientific exploration shows it may also have potential therapeutic advantages in treating depression, addiction, and PTSD. However, as with any powerful substance, ayahuasca should not be taken lightly. Those who choose to consume it must ensure they are in the presence of a knowledgeable and experienced guide aware of its legal implications.

Peyote

The arid expanses of the southwestern United States and northern Mexico are home to the humble and spineless peyote cactus. This plant is steeped in tradition, most notably its usage in Native American religious ceremonies. It is also noteworthy for its psychoactive properties, which are attributed to the alkaloid known as mescaline that it contains. Mescaline has powerful hallucinogenic effects when taken.

For hundreds of years, Native Americans in North America have sought out the psychotropic effects of peyote to take part in spiritual rituals, practice healing, and connect to the divine. Peyote is frequently consumed as a tea or chewed as dried buttons during religious ceremonies, providing participants with various hallucinatory experiences. Used for its psychoactive properties since ancient times, peyote has been an essential part of Native American culture and traditionalism.

Nowadays, peyote has gained popularity as a recreational drug, and its use has become more widespread. When consumed, mescaline produces a range of psychoactive effects, including hallucinations, changes in perception, and altered states of consciousness. The results of mescaline can be intense and last for several hours, and the experience is often described as both profound and mystical.

Despite its popularity and longstanding history, peyote carries risks that should not be overlooked. Mescaline has been known to cause many unpleasant side effects, such as nausea, vomiting, and rapid heartbeat. Moreover, the effects of consuming it can be unpredictable, leading to feelings of anxiety, paranoia, and panic in some cases. Furthermore, there is the potential for accidental poisoning due to confusion in identifying the plant correctly *(Faria, 2021)*. Lastly, even with its designation as a controlled substance, peyote is still widely used, often sold illicitly.

Overall, rich in culture and powerful in effects, peyote is a cactus containing the psychoactive compound mescaline. While its use boasts a long history among Native American cultures, it has gained popularity as a recreational drug. Those considering peyote must be aware of potential side effects and approach it with caution.

Datura

Datura is a plant that has gained notoriety for its poisonous and hallucinogenic properties. It is part of the Solanaceae family, which includes vegetables like tomatoes, peppers, and potatoes. This type of plant is native to dry climates worldwide, with habitats including desert areas in North America and Central Asia, plus certain tropical regions. Although it can be dangerous if misused, it has a long history as a medicinal aid and ceremonial accompaniment.

With its large, fragrant white or purple trumpet-shaped flowers and spiky green leaves, datura is a plant that has been used for centuries in both medicinal and spiritual practices. In traditional Native American cultures, it served as a painkiller and an avenue to connect with the spiritual realm. Other societies also used datura as an interrogation tool, using the plant as a truth serum to extract confessions from criminal suspects. Lastly, ayurvedic medicine is employed in India to cure various ailments, such as digestive and respiratory illnesses.

However, using datura carries significant risks, as the plant is highly poisonous. Dangerous levels of tropane alkaloids, which can result in delirium, delirium tremens, and unconsciousness, are present in every part of the plant. Overdose of datura can lead to death, and even in small amounts, the plant can cause serious health problems, including irregular heartbeat, high blood pressure, and respiratory failure.

Despite these risks, datura has been used for recreational purposes for its hallucinogenic effects. The plant's alkaloids produce intense and vivid hallucinations, and users report feelings of detachment, euphoria, and a distorted sense of time. Some people also report experiencing terrifying and traumatic hallucinations, which can lead to long-term psychological harm.

In addition to its toxic effects, datura is highly invasive, and its spread can be difficult to control. The plant can quickly take over an ecosystem, out-competing native species and disrupting the local flora and fauna balance. This can significantly impact the environment, making it a danger to human health and the natural world. Yet, despite its dangers, datura continues to be used for its medicinal and spiritual properties. In modern times, its use has been regulated and is only allowed under certain conditions and with proper supervision. For example, some countries allow its use for spiritual purposes in religious ceremonies, but only if the plant is used in a controlled and supervised environment.

Altogether, datura, a plant that thrives in desert climates, is renowned for its potentially fatal and mind-altering effects. For centuries, it has been used for medicinal and spiritual purposes; however, these applications come with serious risks. Death, debilitating health issues, and environmental damage are just some consequences of misusing this plant. To stay safe, always heed the advice of an experienced datura practitioner before using it in any setting.

Psilocybin Mushrooms

Psilocybin mushrooms, a type of fungus containing the psychedelic drug psilocybin, have long been revered by indigenous people across the globe for their spiritual and medicinal properties. These mushrooms are known to cause hallucinations and other effects on the human mind that have piqued curiosity among researchers and enthusiasts alike. Recently, there has been an increasing fascination with the therapeutic potential of psilocybin, leading to a renewed interest in studying the effects of these mushrooms on the human mind.

Mushrooms are a source of psilocybin, including varieties like:

- *Psilocybe cubensis* (gold top)
- *Psilocybe mexicana* (mexican)
- *Panaeolus subbalteatus* (panaeolus)

Salvia Divinorum

Salvia divinorum, commonly called *"Sage of the Diviners,"* is a psychoactive plant hailing from the Oaxaca region of Mexico. Salvinorin A's primary constituent is a potent and highly selective kappa opioid receptor agonist. This means that it uniquely affects certain brain receptors compared to what is seen with other common psychoactive substances such as LSD, marijuana, and ecstasy. The experience these effects bring forth are dramatic alterations in one's perspective, thought process, and emotions that all last for 15 to 30 minutes.

Salvinorin A's precise processes of operation have yet to be completely comprehended. Nonetheless, it is thought to alter how data is processed in the brain. Reports from some individuals describe extreme visual and auditory hallucinations, while others speak of disconnection from reality and enhanced self-reflection. The effects of salvia divinorum often elicit a feeling of traveling to other realms or having intense, dream-like experiences. This has piqued the interest of many individuals and generated curiosity about its potential for healing those suffering from depression, anxiety, and post-traumatic stress disorder. While these effects can be highly unusual, they provide an intriguing opportunity to explore alternative therapies for complex mental health issues.

Despite its potential benefits, the use of salvia divinorum carries some risks. Its potency can lead to adverse effects, including intense anxiety, paranoia, and hallucinations. Furthermore, little is known about the consequences of prolonged use of this substance on the body and mind. As such, more research must be conducted to assess its potential dangers.

Over the past few years, salvia divinorum has become increasingly popular, primarily amongst young people. This rise in usage has sparked debates regarding its potential for abuse and possible consequences. While some countries and states have prohibited selling and possessing salvia divinorum, others have limited its availability with restrictions. This psychoactive plant has been used medically and to reach spiritual heights for centuries. Its active ingredient, salvinorin A, offers a unique experience that is highly personal and can differ greatly between individuals. Although research is still required to comprehend any associated risks fully, this plant's therapeutic potential is clear. Thus, it is essential to pay attention to its use today and educate the public about its possible effects.

Kava Kava

For centuries, kava has been renowned for its soothing and anxiolytic properties. Native to the South Pacific islands, it is a species of pepper widely grown in Fiji, Tonga, and Vanuatu. Its root is used to make kava, an ancient beverage cherished for its tranquilizing effects by many indigenous cultures. Sipping on this libation is thought to improve mental well-being and create a feeling of serenity, perfect for unwinding after a long day.

Making kava starts with grounding the plant's roots to create a thick, muddy liquid. With its distinct and slightly bitter taste, this beverage is often enjoyed in social settings for celebrations or as an effective relaxing method after a long day. But the properties that make it unique come from kavalactones, the active ingredients in kava that provide sedative and anxiolytic effects. Not only can kava leave you feeling calmer, more content, and positively minded, but research has also suggested its mild pain-relieving qualities, proving helpful in treating insomnia, anxiety, and even menstrual cramps.

Research has uncovered the potential of kava to treat mental health conditions such as depression and anxiety. In some cases, the results show that it can be as effective as medication without unwanted side effects. Moreover, kava has a low risk of addiction and abuse, making it an attractive alternative for those seeking a natural remedy for mental health issues.

Besides that, the traditional drink kava has been consumed in the South Pacific islands for centuries, having been known to provide potential benefits to those suffering from anxiety and depression. However, its use should be done carefully as there are possible side effects and risks that can come with consuming large amounts of the beverage. Reports have even linked the long-term use of kava with liver toxicity and, in extreme cases, failure. Therefore, before consuming any kava, it is crucial to talk to a healthcare professional and become aware of the associated risks and possible interactions with other medications.

Medicine Wheel and Four Directions

The medicine wheel, known as the four directions, is a long-established tool for shamanism and healing. It represents balance, growth, and harmony used by indigenous people across the world for thousands of years. These four directions symbolize the physical aspects of the cosmos, along with their spiritual forces. North is associated with air; east with fire; south with water; and west with earth. Furthermore, each direction is linked to particular plants, animals, and colors, offering additional ways to access its power. By connecting with this powerful source wisely, we can discover our full spiritual potential.

Shamans can use the medicine wheel as a tool to aid in decision-making. It helps us find the answers to questions about our lives, such as:

- What should I do for work?
- Am I ready for a relationship?
- Where do I want to live?

Likewise, to explore your options thoroughly, try asking questions from different directions to see which is with you. For instance, you could question, *"What is my next step?"* and listen for responses from various directions. Pay attention to your body's sensations as you listen for answers. As such, if you hear *"apprentice with me"* from one direction and it feels right, follow that path. However, do not pursue it if it does not sit well with you for any reason, such as poor timing or other factors.

Yet, if you do not have a particular action path, trust your intuition. Listen closely to the signs you encounter and more on how this works later. Another thing you can do is evaluate what would make you happiest right now and consider how you would like your life or yourself to look differently than they currently do. The medicine wheel is an excellent tool for aiding decision-making and can also be very helpful in bouncing back from bad choices and making better decisions overall.

Examining the medicine wheel will make you aware of the energy in each direction; *north, south, east, and west*. This ancient tool can unlock hidden patterns previously not apparent or noticeable. It will help you recognize how the physical, mental, and spiritual parts intertwine in ways you may not have noticed before. When you see your life from a new perspective, you will begin to identify connections between events and relationships that have gone unnoticed.

Use this tool to make decisions daily. As you come to any choice, such as what to have for dinner or which work project you want to take up next week, reflect and ask yourself which direction best aligns with your values and life purpose. If a particular direction resonates strongly with you, pursue it. Moreover, this tool can be applied when making important decisions, such as where to live or whom to marry. As such, when joining into long-term commitments like marriage or having children, consider your dreams and goals alongside those of the people you are venturing forth with. Through rituals like medicine wheel ceremonies, you can envision the future and make informed choices about your life that could lead you closer to your desired outcomes.

Moreover, decision-making can be shaped by the four directions tool and the medicine wheel, which serve as a shamanic guide for navigating life. This tool can be highly beneficial for making decisions in life, as it helps understand different viewpoints within an issue and to anticipate the consequences before acting upon them. For instance, the eagle represents the east, representing vision and energy. When you establish a clear picture of your life, you transmit power to make it happen. Therefore, if you think negatively, that thought becomes more assertive and can become your reality; similarly, if you think positively, likewise will be what comes out of it.

Pillar 2
Spirits

Unlocking the secrets of pillar two of shamanism is an exciting journey that dives into the concept of spirits. From finding your spirit guides and angels to exploring the primordial deity and water entities, you can gain valuable insight into building a solid connection with the spiritual realm. Discovering how to communicate with spirit guides while learning the importance of water spirits helps you better understand this practice and its role in our lives.

4

Spirit Guides

Have you ever wondered how your spirit guides appear? They may appear to you as benevolent guardian angels or powerful animals such as wolves or bears. But even if these spiritual allies have never crossed your mind, you must remain aware of their presence and prioritize constantly hearing and connecting with them.

Connecting with Your Spirit Guides

Pay close attention to your intuition. Embrace it. Stay open to God's voice and the presence of those who have passed away in your lives, who love unconditionally and yearn for your contentment and well-being. Sometimes, you experience signs from your spirit guides that are subtly hinted, such as a bird crashing into the window or a song played on the radio at an opportune moment. Synchronicity also plays its part when two unrelated events occur together so that it feels like they were designed to be fused. For example, if you find yourself pondering about someone, then suddenly receive an email from them or unexpectedly come across them in person, it could signify that the other person is picking up on your thoughts.Have you been noticing these signs of unexplained occurrences in your day-to-day life? Perhaps, one of your spirit guides is trying to communicate with you. To make it easier for them, meditation can be a perfect way to create an open communication channel. By calming your mind and focusing on the here and now, you can let go of any negative thoughts or emotions that might interfere. This allows you to connect with your spirit guide and receive their messages.

As such, do the following steps to meditate effectively.

- **Step 1:** Designate a time for yourself, away from distractions like the ever-present social media. Find a period where you are awake and alert, not too tired or sleepy.
- **Step 2:** Ensure total comfort by sitting on the floor or in a chair with your feet flat. Consider folding one leg under yourself if necessary, but be sure to distribute pressure throughout your body evenly.
- **Step 3:** Make sure the position is natural and comfortable, using pillows to support your knees if sitting cross-legged is uncomfortable for you. However, keep those pillows from rising too high, as they can disrupt circulation into and out of certain areas.
- **Step 4:** Close your eyes as this process begins so you will focus inwardly on your breath or a specific mantra that resonates with you.

Connecting with your spiritual self yields a myriad of rewards. Psychic healing is an energy-based process centered around the power of intuition. Through this form of healing, you can explore your journey of self-discovery, forge a connection with your guardian angels, and uncover your life's divine mission. With the expertise of a spiritual guide, you can also utilize their divine knowledge to assist in completing any tasks or challenges you face.

For instance, if you desired to create a book with the aid of a spiritual mentor, you could utter the following words: *"I would appreciate the wisdom of my angelic guardian or any divine force present in this space right now."* Then, calmly wait for their counsel to enter your head or maybe even be written down.

Subsequently, reach out to your spirit guides and ask them for their names. By doing so, you can establish a connection with them. You could also invite them to appear in some form so that you can see and hear what they have to say; this could be through vivid dreams or drawings created by children. Request for messages which will guide your life at this moment. Furthermore, it is recommended that you take time each day to meditate and seek insights from these spiritual entities if something feels off in your physical or mental state. Be open to receiving their revelations verbally or even through writing. Moreover, certain spiritual practices like crystal healing may aid in connecting with your guides and heighten the clarity of their messages.

Your Higher Self

At first, I used to feel lost and unsure of who I was. It took me a while to come to terms with this feeling and realize that feeling disconnected from oneself or the world around us is typical. As such, trying to make sense of something without understanding the language or context can be tricky, like reading a book written in a foreign language. Without knowing the words, grammar rules, and meaning behind our reading, how can it have any real impact? Knowledge is often the key to unlocking a deeper understanding and appreciation for our lives and those around us. With this in mind, our identity is no wonder essential in defining who we are and why it matters.

Connecting to your higher self can provide clarity when making decisions and guidance on moving forward. By trusting and following your intuition, you are investing in yourself and engaging with something more significant than what can be seen in the physical world. Additionally, through meditation and stillness, you can connect more deeply to your higher self by allowing the mind to become calm and open. This opens the communication channels between you and your higher self, giving you access to wisdom from within.

Aside from that, your heart can be your best guide. It may help you make sense of an emotional and challenging situation or prepare for what is to come. Facial expressions or body language can reveal their feelings and intentions without words. Pay attention to physical sensations as well; a hint of pain, tightness, or anything else that does not feel right can alert you to the presence of danger or tell you something important needs addressing. Often, prompt action is essential to ensure nothing worse happens. To sum up, tuning into your intuition and body responses can provide invaluable insights and lead you in the right direction.

Likewise, *have you ever wondered what connecting with your higher self is like?* Drawing on your inner wisdom and tapping into it through meditation or journaling can help you gain clarity, understanding, and purpose. Your higher self knows all about you, like your strengths and weaknesses, and what brings you joy. Moreover, it is a source of unconditional love, compassion, and guidance. When asking questions like *"What do I need to know?", "How can I best serve others?"* be still and open to receiving answers in the form of thoughts or feelings in your mind or body. It can be as simple as *"I should take more time for myself"* or *"I feel frustrated when people do not listen."* This connection will provide insight into how to live an authentic life in alignment with your truth.

When hearing your inner wisdom, you need to listen closely and without judgment. Meditation and journaling are great ways to open communication channels between you and your internal guidance. One helpful step is getting in touch with your heart, letting it speak freely by tuning out the noise and focusing on your feelings. Taking even a few moments each day for self-reflection or spending time in nature can help you better understand yourself and your intuition.

Furthermore, finding inner peace and connecting with your spiritual self can be done through meditation or journaling. Meditation can be practiced as early as the first morning hour or as late as before you drift off to sleep. To find what works best for you, play around with open and closed eyes, silence, or music. Additionally, documenting your thoughts and feelings in a journal allows you to gain clarity on now and past experiences while providing an avenue to express gratitude for all the good things in life.

Meanwhile, as you take the time to pause and listen to the whisper of your inner guidance, you can gain access to an unlimited source of knowledge. This inner wisdom speaks the truth, informing you about yourself and others. When a negative thought or emotion arises in reaction to something that has occurred, it often reflects a truth within you, even if ego obscures part of the picture. For example, getting angry at someone for criticizing your physical appearance could be a sign that their words resonated with you on some level. Though such comments may have been directed with malicious intent, there is likely still an element of truth present. Embracing this newfound insight can help you develop further understanding and appreciation for yourself and others.

In general, you can access your higher self through various activities, such as meditation, prayer, journaling, and creative expression. A pivotal step to connecting with this aspect of yourself is to foster an inner dialogue and accept whatever feelings or messages come your way. Your higher self illuminates the path forward on your journey toward personal growth, joy, and transformation. By tuning into its wisdom, you can overcome fear and build resilience in life's challenges. All you need is an open heart, trust in the process, and faith that you will be led in the right direction.

Angels and Archangels

Angels are spiritual messengers that can bring relief, peace, and strength. Many cultures honor the presence of angels, including Christianity and Judaism. Members of these religions believe that certain archangels have been appointed to watch over specific areas such as health, livelihoods, and protection. Moreover, many believe angels can intercede on our behalf during struggle or hardship. With the right intentions and an open heart, connecting with the angelic realm is easier than you may think. It is often a matter of simply speaking your request aloud or asking for help in times of distress.

Understanding the distinction between angels and archangels is essential. Although both beings fall under the 'angel' heading, it is crucial to recognize that they are not interchangeable. While angels are typically described as messengers from God, archangels serve more specific missions, such as protecting individuals or providing guidance for human events. Furthermore, some religious texts designate seven archangels: *Michael, Raphael, Gabriel, Uriel, Sariel, Raguel, and Remiel.*

Thus, angels and archangels are celestial beings who serve God differently. Angels act as messengers between humans and God, while archangels have more power and are high-ranking members of heaven's army. As such, they carry out God's will on Earth and interact with humans directly to provide guidance or protection in times of crisis or despair. For instance, the archangel Michael is known to appear before people to keep them safe during dangerous situations like war zones. These divine protectors also have strong ties with humanity; providing invaluable counsel and support when needed can make a difference for individuals experiencing difficulties. This highlights how angels and archangels differ: the former are guides that help us through our daily lives, while the latter holds immense authority from heavenly realms.

Have you ever experienced the presence of an angel? Many believe that angels exist around us and can manifest in different ways. For some, it may be a dream, vision, or even a faint scent of something sweet. Others may see symbols such as birds or butterflies, which could indicate an angel is nearby. Everywhere we turn, angels may attempt to reach us, yet we may not be aware of them. To know if a messenger from above is trying to communicate, look out for strange behavior from animals or brief glimpses of light. Even if something appears normal at first glance, it could be a sign that something meaningful is happening nearby. It is also worth noting that angels are believed to arise as signs of love and protection, making paying attention to their subtle signals even more important.

Altogether, angels and archangels are powerful spiritual beings that can intervene in matters related to human life. Invoking the aid of these divine agents can provide guidance, comfort, and hope when we need it most. They are here to help if we remain open-minded, mindful, and prayerful. If we earnestly desire a deeper understanding of our place in the world or seek answers to our prayers and inquiries, they will be there with unconditional love and support. Additionally, angels are often seen as mysterious creatures responsible for miraculous events like protecting a lost child or healing from an illness that seemed incurable. These occurrences, however, often go unnoticed or even dismissed by those without faith in their power. Belief in an unseen force helping guide us is critical to understanding their presence and strength.

Ancestors

Feeling a connection to the past is something many of us can relate to. That sense of legacy and responsibility can be extreme for those with a long family history steeped in stories and traditions. *But what if you could access more than just your family tree?* Ancestors, after all, can serve as spirit guides, healing from painful experiences, resolving past issues, and offering emotional support during times of turmoil. Though asking them for help with everyday problems like chores may feel strange or intimidating initially, understanding why calling on ancestors' wisdom makes sense and how simple it is to make contact is critical. As such, it is worth considering what they might answer when you ask for their advice and the historical knowledge they could share that could benefit you in finding solutions.

Not only can ancestors help us with the everyday problems that arise in life, but they often have deeper wisdom and insight from being beyond this physical plane. They can offer counsel on issues that are far more difficult to answer or are emotional and give guidance on long-term goals or larger visions for our lives. Here we can also uncover why taking up contact with ancestors is not so strange after all. In fact, it is a form of honoring those who came before us, and turning to their experience and knowledge has been done throughout many cultures for centuries. By engaging with our ancestral guides, we may find answers, learn lessons, open ourselves up to our intuition, and live much closer to our ancestors' vision.

Understanding your ancestors' past can give you an even broader perspective on life. Looking towards the traditions and beliefs of our ancestors is also a great way to uncover the secrets of meaningful living. With access to their wisdom, you could gain insights into how they approached challenges and navigated difficult situations to make wise decisions. Additionally, honoring the memory of your ancestors can be rewarding and empowering at times when you feel lost or overwhelmed. By connecting with those who have gone before us, we can learn from their experiences and use them as a source of strength for tackling whatever life might throw.

You can ask your ancestors for help with the following:

- Discover your spiritual path and establish a connection with the divine.
- Foster meaningful relationships with people, including family members and partners.
- Prioritize physical and mental health for total well-being.
- Create financial abundance for yourself and your loved ones, pursue success in career or business ventures, and maintain strong family dynamics.

Remember, our ancestors are not just from a different place but from within us. They can offer guidance, support, and consolation; all we need to do is call upon them. To make a strong connection with an ancestor, it can be helpful to practice meditation or other relaxation techniques to become more open to the messages of your ancestor. Additionally, knowledge of your ancestors' culture, customs, and indigenous language may help create a stronger link between you and them.

However, staying in touch with our ancestors can be challenging. To help overcome this difficulty, consider asking yourself questions such as:

- How does this person view me?
- What advice would they give me about my current plans?
- What do I need from them right now?

Asking these types of questions can help us connect with our ancestors. As such, by considering how an ancestor might view us or what advice they would give, we can understand our family history and culture and how it may be relevant to our current situation.

When trying to find answers to these questions, it helps to reach within for answers that come from your own experience and knowledge. Writing down what comes up can be a powerful way to gain insight into situations and uncover solutions. Lastly, it is also wise to seek advice from others who have gone through similar experiences or may even have passed away; they may offer advice to help you navigate the challenge.

Plants

Have you ever considered having a plant as a spiritual guide? Plants can be more than just decoration; they offer an invaluable source of comfort and support, no matter what happens in your life. Even when facing the toughest questions, plants can provide healing and balance for your emotions. Plus, their calming presence can help ground you and bring clarity to your energy.

Since ancient times, plants have been revered for their healing and spiritual powers. Links between plants and spiritual practices like shamanism, centered around the belief that everything has a soul and is connected, can be traced back 30,000 years. Shamans use medicinal plants to treat physical and emotional ailments like depression and anxiety. They believe that connecting with the energy of plants through rituals can help them tap into their spirit guides, ancestors, guardian angels, animal spirit guides, and other forms of protection. Not only is this a potent form of healing. Yet, it can also bring clarity that helps guide us through life's struggles.

Connecting to your plant spirit guide is like connecting with any other spiritual mentor and goes beyond simply conversing. To create an effective connection, you must be open and receptive to the plant's energies while willing to take time from your day. Additionally, understanding the symbolic meaning of plants can help establish a strong bond with them. Embracing a ritualistic approach, such as connecting under the guidance of rituals or meditations, can further deepen the connection between you and your plant spirit guide.

In establishing a meaningful connection with your plant spirit guide, ask them vocally or mentally if they want to join you on your journey. Alternatively, visit their environment and observe them in their natural habitat. If neither of these options is appealing, take some time to think about what qualities an ideal companion should possess that could be beneficial in helping you progress in your growth and development or aiding you in the challenges presented by our lives on this planet. Additionally, remember that plants are living entities: *connecting with them starts with treating them with respect and kindness.* Showing care for the world around us is one way of developing strong relationships with other life forms.

Hence, plants are incredible living beings that have existed since the dawn. They have a deep connection to the earth, and many believe that plants possess a spirit and can be helpful to human guides. To begin working with plant spirit guides, it is essential to identify which one will work best for you.

You may already have an affinity for a specific type of plant, or you could explore your neighborhood and observe different types of trees or wildflowers in local parks or gardens. Once you have identified a specific plant, the next step is to get familiar with its unique characteristics and behavior. This will help deepen your connection and allow you access to insights and wisdom only this plant can provide.

Animals

Throughout all cultures, spirit animals have been used to connect the spiritual and physical realms. With their guidance, people can better understand who they are and their place in the world. As such, through rituals and activities, one can connect with their spirit animal to discover valuable insights about life. This part of the book will guide you in exploring this spiritual journey and unlocking the power within yourself that their spirit animal symbolizes.

People have long believed that animals are more than just physical entities and have unique abilities to reveal spiritual truths. For example, in many Native American tribes, totems or talismans are used to invoke the spirit of an animal and its traits. These can be seen to honor and pay tribute to the wisdom of these animals. With the help of these animal spirit guides, people can gain insight into their spiritual journey and personal growth. Additionally, shamans utilize not only herbs and various plants for healing but animal medicines as well. Animal medicines can come in various forms, such as extracts, parts (like fur or bones), or the whole animal.

Thinking of spirit animals often recalls Native American totems, potent symbols reflecting an animal's spirit and personality. These totems vary in interpretation among tribes. For instance, some believe that only certain animals have essences that can be used as totems. Meanwhile, others believe that all living creatures have spirits, explaining the use of various animals as symbols for human qualities such as strength or bravery. Regardless of interpretation, spirit animals can teach us about ourselves and help us connect with the natural world around us. For example, suppose your totem animal is the coyote. In that case, you adapt quickly, much like how coyotes are known for adapting to changing circumstances in their environment.

Perhaps, you may have noticed that certain animals draw you in, prompting you to ponder what deeper meanings they could be representing. Psychologists believe humans can utilize their hearts and instincts when making decisions, otherwise known as a "gut feeling," rather than relying solely on logic. A few prominent examples of animals and their related symbolism are owls which signify wisdom. Then, wolves stand for strength and leadership, while snakes represent transformation. If an animal's characteristics mirror yours, it could symbolize something about your life path or serve as a spiritual guide. To further understand the connection between yourself and animals, seek expert advice on animal symbolism and use their findings to help make better-informed decisions.

The presence of a spirit animal in your life indicates that you are connected to the spiritual realm in some way. It can symbolize strength in difficult times or guide you during personal journeys of self-exploration. Commonly, a spirit animal is associated with a particular emotion or state of being. Others believe they provide protection and wisdom to those who need it most. Additionally, it is said that each person may have more than one spirit animal associated with them at any given time. Seeing what kind of animals appear in your daily life, whether through dream sequences, artworks, or unexpected occurrences, can help you recognize the spiritual signs connecting you to all living creatures.

Linking with your animal totem can be done by looking at what it stands for in the astrological system. Astrology is a tool that allows us to gain deeper insight into ourselves and our lives based on the stars and planets. To learn more about this subject, explore the many books available on Amazon or at your local bookstore. Some people also turn to online sources such as blogs, podcasts, and webinars to access astrological information.

Deities

Developing a shamanic belief system means familiarizing yourself with its different associated deities. While there is a vast array of gods and goddesses, some are more prominent than others, such as Odin, Ra, Amaterasu, and Quetzalcoatl. Furthermore, each deity carries its powers and responsibilities, often reflecting the beliefs and values of the given culture or region. Understanding all its associated gods is essential to truly understand the construct of a shamanic belief system.

The Primordial Deity

The primordial deity is the origin of all existence. As such, its power allows for manifestation and control over all physical and metaphysical realities. This includes providing life and guidance to mortals, manipulating time and space, and creating other dimensions outside our reality. Many cultures honor this being as a divine and omnipotent figure due to their boundless capabilities, which have always been present even before recorded time. Along with this immense power comes the responsibility of maintaining balance in the universe by controlling both good and evil forces. These abilities are attributed to the primordial deity, integral to many historical and spiritual beliefs.

The Sky Deity

Across nearly every religion and culture, sky gods have been revered for their power over the elements. Moreover, the sky deity is often envisioned as an older man with long white hair perched atop a rainbow and eyes closed. This symbolizes his protective watch over the world without any interference, except when necessary. He may also be portrayed donning wings akin to those of an angel or wearing a headdress adorned with feathers like those worn by Native Americans in the battle against other tribes or nations in colonial days. In many cultures, this figure is associated with wisdom and guidance; he offers advice and protection despite not being involved directly. His knowledge is said to be vast and superior to mere mortals.

The ancient Greeks called their sky god *Zeus*, while other cultures used names like *Toran, Thor, Tāwhirimātea,* and *Indra*. In most stories involving a sky god, they are believed to be capable of controlling the weather by manipulating winds and rain. Additionally, they are usually seen as responsible for protecting people from natural disasters such as floods and storms by using mighty thunderbolts or lightning bolts. Ultimately, these gods were believed to oversee the sun's and stars' day-to-day movements across the sky.

The Sky Deity's Family

The sky god is the head of the pantheon and has a family, including:

- **Sun.** Providing light and warmth to sustain life.
- **Moon.** Illuminating the darkness, working alongside the stars as they shine brightly at night.
- **Stars.** Seen as the progeny of the sun, illuminating the night sky with their persistent glimmer.

In addition to these three major deities, many others represent different aspects of nature: wind, rain, and earth are part of this pantheon's family tree.

The Earth Mother

The Earth's mother is the world's creator and is responsible for every inhabitant. Revered as a goddess of agriculture and fertility, her rule spans plants, animals, forests, and waters. She provides her people with their daily needs so they can exist in harmony with each other and nature while leading content lives. As an expression of deep respect towards her impact on life and fertility, many cultures have celebrated the Earth mother through seasonal feasts such as Lammas or Imbolc.

The Water Spirits

Legends abound of water spirits worldwide, from kappa in Japan to nāga in India. Water spirits are seen as powerful and mysterious entities that inhabit rivers, lakes, and other bodies of water. Their demeanor towards human beings can vary depending on their type. Some are mischievous or evil, while others may be kind and benevolent.

The Ancestors

Our ancestors are an integral part of the spiritual belief system for shamans. They have passed down their wisdom and teachings through shared stories, tales, and legends over generations. Shamanism teaches that these ancestors remain close to us in human form, guiding us through life. Additionally, it is believed that the spirits of one's family, tribe, and people linger within them, granting insight into the ancestral roots that define who they are.

Altogether, ancient shamanic beliefs are based on honoring and connecting with the gods and goddesses who control the elements and influence human lives. To do this, followers of those belief systems pray to their chosen deities regularly and engage in rituals that have symbolic meanings. Knowing about these deities helps us gain insight into how the world works, and it can be a source of understanding for life's events. Additionally, to experience favorable growth, we must recognize, acknowledge, and thank those deities for their help. Honoring them gives us access to our hidden knowledge, intuition, and power.

Pillar 3
Journey

The third pillar of shamanism, the journey, is where the real work starts. We will uncover the various paths to achieving a shamanic state of consciousness, including soul flight, meditation, and rituals. Doing so gives us access to spirit guides, ancestors, and other entities in the shamanic world, which can provide unique insights and understanding of our lives and the world around us. Here we delve into the different techniques and tools shamans use to embark on their journeys and how you can use them to enhance your spiritual practice while connecting you with those unseen realms.

5

What Is a Shamanic Journey

Shamanic journeys are a type of deep meditation that offers the opportunity to explore the depths of your inner self and gain insight into yourself and situations you face. Through guided visualization, you can access your intuition and gain clarity on matters.

Soul Flight

Taking to the skies can be thrilling if it is your dream. Shamanic soul flight is an ancient practice where you leave your physical body to explore different realms. It may be done through meditation, a shamanic journey or ceremony, or even with the help of certain drugs. Through soul flight, we can gain communication with spirit helpers and discover new locations and insights. Mastering this skill requires practice, and it is best to have assistance from an experienced shaman to guide the first few flights for safety and security.

As such, embarking on the journey of soul flight requires some preparation. To gain control over the experience and to ensure a successful takeoff, one must acquire good grounding skills and be in touch with their body and mind. An excellent place to start is to find a peaceful location, perhaps without much interference, and sit comfortably in front of an altar or table with personal significance. Taking three deep breaths allows one to set their intentions for the journey ahead and focus on their inner visualizations. From here, imagine yourself soaring high above your home or neighborhood, witnessing all that lies below from a divine perspective.

Acquiring knowledge about soul flight is essential. However, that is not enough. Regular practice is necessary to experience the sensations of leaving your body. Find a trusted teacher to guide you on this journey and commit to sticking with the sessions. Even experienced shamans find it difficult during their earlier flights. So, do not be disheartened if progress is not instantaneous; take your time, practice diligently, and fly safely.

Practicing Shamanic Journeying

Shamanic journeying is an ancient practice rooted in the wisdom of indigenous cultures that enables individuals to attain knowledge and strength to heal the planet and its inhabitants. This journey is a way to gain insight into one's true self, discover authority, and access other worlds. It provides an opportunity to find accurate understanding, healing, and transformation. The shamanic journey is a path of recovery, awareness, and empowerment; it is a way to unlock the power necessary for revitalizing the earth and its people.

Going on a shamanic journey is a profound and enlightening experience. It can involve various activities such as drumming and trance dancing to enter an altered state, chanting prayers or mantras, or engaging in mindful meditation. All of these offer the individual an opportunity to receive information about their inner self and uncover hidden aspects of their life and identity. This newfound knowledge can be used for personal advancement and shared with others, creating positive change in the world. Thus, shamanic journeying is a path to empowerment and a powerful tool for awakening our true potential.

Over the years, I have been practicing shamanism, and it can be explored in many ways. It can be used as a healing tool or an initiation process to reach higher levels of power within oneself or those who accompanied you on your journey. Besides these, it can also be used as a chance to dive deeper into yourself without any predetermined goal other than gaining more knowledge through self-reflection and insight while immersed in *"the world"* beyond our physical reality.

Shamans use shamanic journeying to connect with spiritual realms, allowing them to interact with spirits and deities and heal themselves by entering an altered state of consciousness. Yet, it does not stop at shamans; anyone can learn how to do it. For thousands of years, this practice has been used by indigenous people worldwide to create bonds between their world and what they call *'the divine.'* Even today, shamans in different ceremonies across the globe are practicing shamanic journeying.

To begin your ceremony, set up a sacred space. Light candles or incense to create a ritualistic atmosphere. Place the drum on an altar or table so it is visible to all participants. Invoke each directional guardian one by one: *east (air), south (fire), west (water), and north (earth)*. Feel their unique energy as they enter from all four directions around you; visualize their presence filling the circle. Ask if any other helping spirits would like to join and if anyone needs healing work done on them at this time. Then with full awareness, embark on your spiritual journey together.

Gaining Insights Through Meditation and Rituals

Meditation is a form of training for the mind and body and is an excellent way to become more conscious of your thoughts and feelings. Incense has been an integral part of religious ceremonies for centuries, having a calming effect on both the practitioner and the environment. Not only does it create a relaxing atmosphere, but it also helps to clear away lingering negative energy while allowing positive vibrations to arise. Combining incense with meditation can be helpful to deepen concentration and focus, allowing one to benefit from its meditative effects in shorter time frames. Additionally, using incense during meditation also has spiritual and physical health benefits, such as reducing stress levels, promoting mental clarity, and relieving anxiety.

Subsequently, meditation has long been linked with improved physical and mental health, cognitive functioning, creativity, and productivity. By observing our internal state of being and listening to our thoughts, we can gain insight into ourselves and better handle life's challenges.

Likewise, practice meditation with a guide or instructor; guided meditation. With guided meditation, the power to unlock your potential lies within your mind. A skilled instructor or guide can provide you with the knowledge and guidance needed to get the most out of your practice. Numerous studies have shown that spending even a short amount of time meditating daily can significantly improve your physical, mental, and emotional health. Additionally, research suggests that guided meditation can help reduce cortisol levels in the body, thus promoting relaxation and well-being.

Rituals are also a powerful tool for self-discovery. In fact, many spiritual traditions rely on rituals to deepen their connection to something greater than themselves. Through rituals, we can encounter new perspectives or gain insight and clarity on a situation or thought process previously elusive and challenging to grasp. Additionally, they can be used as an opportunity for personal transformation by actively engaging in activities that help us explore who we are and what lies beyond our comfort zones. These practices allow us to reflect on the present moment so that we may move forward from it with greater meaning and purpose.

On the other hand, mantras are a form of meditation that can help you gain insights and clarity. Not only are they associated with religious practices, but they can also represent personal affirmations. For instance, you might constantly repeat *"I am grateful"* to remind you of gratitude. Or perhaps, you may use the mantra *"I am going after my dream job"* as a reminder of your goals. Apart from being used as affirmations and reminders, mantras can also be used to focus during yoga or mindfulness practice, allowing for deep relaxation and improved psychological health.

Hence, to unwind and practice meditation, use incense. As mentioned, incense has long been used to promote relaxation and meditation. Burning them can have numerous benefits, from calming the mind and reducing stress to increased focus. It can be used in various ways, from energizing yoga practice to helping to create an atmosphere for prayer or reflection. In fact, ancient mystics believed incense could transport prayers directly to the divine realm, or gods, for answers and guidance.

Additionally, different types of incense have their associations with different meanings; for instance, sandalwood relates to peace and tranquility, while jasmine is associated with spiritual awakening. As such, incense can also include healing properties depending on the chosen type, creating a unique ambiance. Furthermore, many kinds of incense contain natural essential oils, providing additional aromatherapeutic benefits. With so many diverse options available, there is sure to be an incense that appeals to everyone's preferences and needs.

Embodying the Practice

Staying connected to our spiritual path is essential for maintaining a sense of well-being. This book offers practical advice to help readers incorporate spirituality into their daily lives despite the various challenges, including difficulty finding resonance with a particular practice, the complexity or intensity of its demands, and limited time. The tips and guidance provided are designed to make spiritual practice a part of one's life in an accessible and sustainable manner.

Incorporating spiritual practice into our daily lives can be thorny, but there are many ways to make it work. For instance, you could commit to a short period of mindfulness each day or take a few moments before bed to reflect quietly. However, only some have the luxury of having a dedicated space for their spiritual practice. Hence, you may need to experiment with different approaches depending on your lifestyle and constraints. Furthermore, although it may take courage to be open about your beliefs, talking about them can also help build stronger connections with those around you, which is a crucial part of any spiritual journey.

Here are some ideas that might help you fully embody and integrate your chosen spiritual path into your life:

- **Do some research on your spiritual practice.** Take your spiritual practice to the next level by researching its history and origins. Delve deeper into its traditions and customs to gain an even greater understanding of it. This foundation can serve as the basis for further learning and exploration. Additionally, you could look up facts related to your spiritual practice that illustrate how they are connected, deepening your appreciation of the subject.
- **Look for a teacher or mentor.** Seeking out a teacher or mentor can be beneficial for spiritual growth. A mentor can offer wisdom, insights, and support that often comes with life experience. They can guide how to apply the teachings in everyday life. Answer any questions that might arise. Plus, help you stay motivated despite the challenges encountered on the journey. Mentors are also great resources for ideas and techniques that could make your journey smoother and more successful.
- **Find a support group.** Connecting with a like-minded community is an excellent way to seek spiritual guidance and support. Joining a support group can help you form relationships with people who share your values, such as love, and become more mindful of what matters in life. Additionally, it enables you to focus on relationships, which leads to greater well-being rather than fear. By connecting with others who hold similar beliefs, you can gain valuable wisdom and understanding. One way to connect with like-minded individuals is by joining virtual groups or attending local meetups dedicated to exploring spirituality. Virtual groups on social media platforms like Facebook provide a convenient way to interact with others who share your interests. Then, local meetups close to where you live or work can save you time and alleviate travel stress. These events offer an opportunity to build relationships with people who share your interests, allowing you to learn from each other's experiences and share advice, stories, and reflections. You can also use these gatherings as a chance to rest and relax away from the hustle and bustle of everyday life.

Making spiritual practice a daily habit will help you integrate it as a significant and essential aspect of your life. At first, you might not be able to do this, but that is okay. As you become accustomed to it, start slowly, then increase the time each day.

Embodying spiritual practices can be a powerful way to cultivate mental, emotional, and physical well-being. Every religion or spiritual ritual provides a unique set of practices that can bring harmony into one's life. For example, meditation has been an ancient practice for centuries to promote peace, clarity, and connection. Additionally, mindfulness activities have become popular tools for reducing stress and anxiety. Meanwhile, yoga helps to build strength and flexibility in the body. Integrating such spirituality into your daily routine can provide immense benefits when living a fulfilling life.

Crafting a meaningful and satisfying spiritual path is essential to your life's journey. Awareness of this importance can help guide your decisions and help you stay connected to your spirituality no matter what. Even if you do not have that connection immediately, looking after other aspects of yourself should be the first step. Besides, many struggle with feeling guilty about self-care before caring for those around them. Yet, remorse would not benefit anyone in the long run. To create an enriched experience when cultivating spirituality, explore new perspectives, and embrace various faith-related activities. Further, enrich your journey by discovering historical information and reading scripture related to your beliefs. This way, you can strengthen your understanding and appreciation of faith.

Below are some tips for getting in touch with your spirituality.

- **Take a moment to include spirituality in your daily routine.** Meditate, reflect, or pray for five minutes each day. Alternatively, consider taking a few minutes during a break or transition period for those with busier schedules to connect with your spiritual side. For example, take a few deep breaths and center yourself before starting a task, or practice mindfulness while doing a mundane activity like washing dishes. Every little moment counts towards cultivating a more spiritual mindset. Likewise, connecting with your spiritual side is invaluable, as incorporating spiritual mindfulness into your life gives greater inner peace and satisfaction.
- **Explore any religious traditions from your upbringing.** Think about the beliefs instilled in you during childhood and how others viewed these practices. Reflect on your lessons from past experiences and investigate how they impact your decisions today. Also, recognize commonalities and differences between personal beliefs and practices, with those of other people who share a similar background as you. Take time to learn about different cultures, their values, traditions, and ways of living that could be integral to understanding yourself better. Discovering your spiritual self will allow you to grow in knowledge and empathy toward others.

6

Three Shamanic Worlds

People often discuss their curiosity and desire to explore the unknown, particularly to embark on a journey into the 'lower world.' But what does that mean? Are we talking about an overseas trip or something entirely different? From a scientific perspective, this realm may not even exist. Yet there are still many who choose to pursue this mysterious quest.

In visiting such a place, a brave adventuring spirit and an imaginative approach to your travels are needed. Plus, you will uncover new sites and stories on our journey, which can be an incredible experience. Likewise, you may even find yourself learning something unexpected along the way. But first, let us explore what these mysterious realms are.

Lower World

Daydreaming and meditation can open the door to a realm often considered the 'lower world.' In this altered state, you can become an animal spirit, immerse yourself in the lower world, and explore what lies beneath the surface. Picture yourself as a spirit animal inhabiting a realm of hills and valleys, with lakes and rivers that seem oddly reminiscent of your hometown. Behold its ancient inhabitants, creatures existing since before humans ever inhabited Earth. In this hidden land, you can observe these beings engaging in activities and forming families or tribes. *What kind of food do they eat? What type of attire do they wear? How have these creatures developed a form of governance, and how does it respond to their environment?*

These questions are more than just academic musings; the answers can reveal powerful insights into the relationship between humankind and nature. As such, *do they use some technology? Can they communicate telepathically or by speaking aloud? What kind of games do they play together, and what music do they enjoy listening to? How do they craft their instruments, and if technology is employed, how does it impact them?* Through exploring such questions, you will understand more about the lower world.

For those who have never ventured to the lower world, it can be helpful to imagine descending into a cave, entering the water, or even slipping into slumber to access this mysterious realm. Awaiting your arrival, this peculiar realm is like nothing you have encountered before; it features a stunning yet barren landscape of hot and gritty terrain dotted with swirling clouds of dust and sand. There is no sign of life, with no animals or trees in sight. Not even lush greenery or fresh streams. Instead, this desolate domain is characterized by a vast expanse that provokes your senses while fueling your creativity. As you traverse its unforgiving surroundings, uncover hidden oases, rocky outcroppings, and ancient ruins that offer a glimpse into the culture and customs of the ancestors living in this realm.

Entering the lower world is much like stepping into a dream that is more vibrant and authentic than reality. As such, you are conscious of being in an environment removed from the physical realm but have access to the guidance of your ancestors. Messages and insights arise from this unique landscape, offering insight into how to navigate life's challenges. Rituals and ceremonies can bring healing and transformation on multiple levels. All of this speaks to a deeply spiritual experience that fosters growth and understanding beyond what is tangible and visible. Thus, the lower realm is a rich and enigmatic environment, allowing shamans to seek out the wisdom of the spirit world and utilize it to benefit their communities. It is believed that within these depths lies ancient knowledge used by generations of ancestors for centuries. Not only does this provide a deeper understanding of the past, but it also gives great insight into possible paths for the future. Each journey taken by a shaman into this realm can bring fresh perspectives and challenges, yielding invaluable treasures that are sure to be shared for ages.

Middle World

The middle world is a rich and expansive landscape containing the physical elements of plants and animals, weather patterns, human communities, and the more ethereal realms of spiritual energy. Shamans use this multifaceted world to service their work while making regular journeys between the upper and lower worlds. This middle world profoundly permeates human life, affecting our ability to connect and the environment. Likewise, it shapes our mindsets and informs our physical universe. A greater understanding of this deep layer of reality can bring positive life changes.

In the shamanic view, this world differs from mainstream science in that it does not distinguish between living and non-living matter or animate beings with consciousness like ourselves and other living beings without consciousness. It also does not separate humans from nature. The middle world is the physical world we inhabit and much more. For example, plants, animals, and weather systems interact with each other to create a complex web of life. Humans are part of this larger ecosystem, adding our human perspective to the mix. Looking around us can give clues about how we fit into this environment. What we see in our yards or the palms of our hands reflects and influences the interconnectedness of everything in this middle world.

Aside from that, the middle world is a complex realm of physical, mental, and spiritual energies. It incorporates the natural forces of animals, plants, weather patterns, and human-created communities and cultures. Here shamans work their magic to heal others or themselves through their bodies and minds by tapping into these energies directly. In addition to shamans, modern energy medicine practitioners believe that this middle world holds powerful forces that can be harnessed in healing practices such as Reiki, chakra balancing, qigong, acupuncture, and more. These techniques seek to restore balance and harmony within an individual's body for personal healing and to release negative or blocked energy for overall wellness.

Connections to spiritual realms, such as the upper and lower worlds, are made in the middle world. It is also a place of energetic intersection, where we can find our way to healing by interacting with its components: *plants, animals, humans and even rocks or stones*. Understanding how to work with the energies of this middle world can help us achieve greater health and happiness in our lives. The shamanic practice involves engaging with the middle world on both physical and non-physical levels so that we may gain insight through spiritual journeying and vision quests. Navigating this realm is essential to unlocking its potential for growth and transformation.

Upper World

The Upper World is believed to be a place of spiritual and divine realms, and it can be accessed through meditation and shamanic practices. Some describe it as a realm above us, beyond the physical world, while others may envision it as a dimension or alternate reality. Regardless of its description, the Upper World is where individuals can connect with higher beings. However, not only does this land offer an ethereal connection to seek guidance from entities such as teachers or wise ones. Yet, it is believed to provide access to knowledge that cannot be found elsewhere. Moreover, this higher realm contains portals that connect one's earthly life with destiny in other domains.

Likewise, the upper world is a land of magic and mystery, where you can meet and converse with a divine pantheon of gods, goddesses, and ancestors. To access the spirit realm, you must journey through dreams or meditation, enabling you to explore various planes of existence. Some are more tangible than others, but all are inhabited by beings that serve as tutors. These beings can show you how to discover your true purpose in life and help expand your knowledge of both the spiritual and earthly realms. Furthermore, they can provide essential insights into how the two intersect and influence each other.

When looking to receive wisdom and advice, the upper world is an ideal place to seek it. This realm comprises three distinct components: the sky world populated by heavenly beings, the land(s) above, home to many passed spiritual teachers and Earth itself. Interestingly, this is not just a place for guidance but also a source of powerful energy that can be tapped into. By journeying up to this higher realm, you can unlock hidden knowledge, discover ancient secrets and be aided in your work as a shaman.

Pillar 4
Connection

Pillar four of shamanism delves into connecting with the spiritual world through altered states of consciousness. This includes dreams, out-of-body experiences, astral projection, and drumming and chanting as tools to establish this connection. Lucid dreaming has also been explored as an additional form of altered state to explore this deeper connection. Additionally, many shamans believe fasting and prolonged periods of silence can further allow for opportunities to connect with the spirit world. By cultivating these techniques, you can deeply understand your shared spiritual journey.

7

Dreams

*H*ave you ever stopped to consider the mysteries of dreaming? What lies beneath our conscious minds while we are asleep? Do dreams have hidden meanings or are they simply random thoughts? These questions, and more, have perplexed us since the beginning of time. Here are some answers to the queries posed a while ago, with a few extra musings thrown in for good measure.

What Are Dreams

Dreams provide a great window into our innermost thoughts and feelings. While most dreams are experienced as incomprehensible and bizarre, many are vivid and powerful, in either black and white or color. These images may contain symbols that represent our fears, hopes, aspirations, or desires. Scientists believe that dreaming helps us process difficult emotions and experiences by making sense of the information we take during our waking life. Additionally, journaling has been used for centuries to capture a snapshot of the dreamer's inner landscape at any given moment, providing valuable insight into our subconscious minds.

When dreaming, it can be in various colors and shapes, from pastel hues to technicolor scenes. During the rapid eye movement (REM) stage of sleep, dreams occur as our brain activity is similar to its activity while awake but with certain deviations. Also, it is worth noting that this phase is fundamental for memory retention and learning processes, hence why getting optimum periods of restful sleep is essential. Furthermore, people tend to have different dreams on the same night, color or black-and-white, depending on their state of mind. All in all, there is not just one definitive way to dream; everyone experiences it differently.

Under REM sleep, your brain processes and stores information you have taken during the day while also helping you consolidate memories. You can have trouble recalling things if you do not get enough of this stage in the sleep cycle. As such, dreaming is thought to help process and regulate emotional experiences, allowing emotions and memories to be sorted into meaningful categories. This could explain why it sometimes feels like we can never fully capture a dream's details when we attempt to recount them upon waking. Rapid eye movement occurs in bursts throughout the night, with the most vivid dreaming occurring near morning.

Hence, everyone can dream, but only some can recall their dreams. While some people can vividly remember their nighttime visions, others may have no memory. Personal experiences shape dreams, so the memories will be distinct even if two people share the same dream. As such, exploring these dreamscapes can give us a better understanding of ourselves and how we interact with the world.

Out of Body Experience

An out-of-body experience, or OBE, is a phenomenon in which a person feels like they have left their physical body and are observing the world from an external point of view. During an OBE, individuals may see their body from a third-person perspective, feel like they are flying, or even travel to other realms beyond the physical world. The subjective experience of an OBE can differ from person to person, with some reporting feelings of weightlessness or tingling and others experiencing intense emotions or a sense of enlightenment.

One theory suggests that OBEs are caused by a malfunction in the brain, specifically the parietal lobe. For the integration of sensory data and the development of self-awareness, the parietal lobe is in charge. During an OBE, the parietal lobe malfunctions, creating the illusion of leaving the body. Studies that identified alterations in brain activity during OBEs support this notion. Another theory is that OBEs are extrasensory perceptions that allow people to see beyond the physical world. This theory suggests that OBEs are humans' natural ability to perceive the world beyond their physical body. Some proponents of this theory believe that OBEs result from the soul or spirit leaving the physical body and traveling to other planes of existence.

While OBEs can be transformative experiences, they can also be unsettling or dangerous for some people. If you are trying to induce one, you should be cautious and seek the right advice when approaching them. Discussing concerns with a healthcare professional is essential, as some medical conditions or medications can increase the likelihood of an OBE. Also, various means can induce an OBE, such as meditation, sleep deprivation, hypnosis, and certain drugs like ketamine or DMT. These methods are often used by individuals seeking to induce an OBE intentionally. However, it is essential to note that inducing an OBE intentionally can be risky and should only be attempted by experienced practitioners.

The subjective experience of an OBE can differ from person to person. Some individuals report feelings of weightlessness or tingling, while others experience intense emotions or a sense of enlightenment. Many people describe their OBE as a spiritual or mystical experience; some even report communication with spiritual beings or guides. In fact, OBEs are often associated with spiritual or metaphysical practices like shamanism or new-age beliefs. As such, some individuals with OBEs report a newfound sense of spirituality or a shift in their worldview. Others may feel unsettled or confused by their experience, particularly if they need a framework for understanding it.

Clairvoyant Abilities

Throughout history, clairvoyant abilities have been the source of much mystery and debate. While some believe they result from spiritual or supernatural influence, others argue that it is simply an extension of normal senses. Clairvoyance can also manifest itself in various ways, such as seeing images in the mind's eye or feeling strongly about a particular topic. Those with these gifts may be able to identify potential dangers before they occur or pinpoint the location of missing persons. In addition, some people may even claim to receive messages from the spirit world through dreams or visions. Although not everyone believes in this form of perception, many still find it fascinating.

Many clairvoyants claim that their experiences are uncontrollable and that they have little or no control over when or how they happen. They could experience unexpected epiphanies or get messages in their dreams. Others experience physical feelings like a sharp chill or tingling in their limbs. Meanwhile, some clairvoyants have even reported hearing voices or seeing visuals that seem to originate from somewhere else.

There is no one-size-fits-all technique for improving clairvoyant powers because developing these abilities is sometimes a personal experience. While some people may have a natural propensity for clairvoyance, others may need more effort to hone their skills over time. Developing clairvoyant talents could benefit from methods like energy work, visualization, and meditation. It is also helpful to contact other spiritualists or clairvoyants who can provide advice and assistance.

Moreover, it is essential to note that while clairvoyant abilities are often associated with psychics or mediums, they are not limited to these professions. Many people possess clairvoyant abilities without even realizing it, and they may experience glimpses of the unseen without consciously acknowledging them. Additionally, some clairvoyants choose not to use their powers for psychic readings or other forms of divination but to enhance their spiritual journeys or connect with loved ones who have passed on.

One common use of clairvoyant abilities is communicating with deceased loved ones. Many people who have lost someone close to them report feeling a sense of ongoing connection and may experience visions or other sensory input that they interpret as signs from their loved ones. While there is no scientific proof of an afterlife or the ability to communicate with the dead, many people find comfort in these experiences, which may offer a sense of continuity and connection even after death.

Clairvoyant abilities are a fascinating and often misunderstood aspect of the human experience. While there is no "right" way to experience clairvoyance, many people report seeing things beyond the physical realm, which can provide great comfort and insight. Whether through meditation, energy work, or simply being open to the possibilities, anyone can develop their clairvoyant abilities and gain a deeper understanding of the world around them.

Energetic Vibrations

Energetic vibrations refer to the energy movement in and around us. This energy makes up our physical and emotional states and can be impacted by external factors such as sound, light, and the energy of others. Many people believe that our energetic vibrations can also affect our perception of reality, including our experiences during out-of-body experiences.

The vibrational state often associated with OBEs can be described as a buzzing or humming sensation throughout the body. It may feel like an intense surge of energy flowing through the body, causing a tingling sensation or even full-body vibrations. This state can be extreme and overwhelming, but it is often a sign that the individual is about to enter an altered state of consciousness.

As mentioned earlier, the experience of the vibrational state during an OBE can be different for each person. Some individuals may see themselves from a third-person perspective, while others may feel like they are floating or being pulled out through their head or chest area. An individual's energetic vibration can also influence these experiences. Several things, such as our ideas, emotions, and physical state, might affect the energetic vibration of our body. If we feel low or negative, our energetic vibration may be lower, impacting our perception of ourselves during an OBE. On the other hand, if we feel positive and confident, our energetic vibration may be higher, allowing us to perceive ourselves as more empowered and secure.

In many spiritual and metaphysical practices, energetic vibration is crucial in achieving spiritual growth and connecting with higher states of consciousness. By raising our energetic vibration through techniques such as meditation, visualization, and energy healing, we can access higher states of consciousness and unlock the full potential of our spiritual selves. Also, energetic vibrations play a significant role in our experiences during out-of-body experiences. While the vibrational state during an OBE can be intense and overwhelming, it can also be a powerful tool for exploring different states of consciousness and connecting with our spiritual selves. Understanding how our energetic vibration affects our perception of reality, we can work towards raising our vibration and unlocking the full potential of our spiritual selves.

Astral Projection

Astral projection, also known as *"astral travel,"* is a phenomenon where a person feels they have left their physical body and can explore the world around them from an outside perspective. It is frequently described as a feeling of consciousness outside the body.

While the concept of astral projection may seem far-fetched, many spiritual traditions, such as Buddhism and Taoism, have explored the possibilities of astral projection for thousands of years. For instance, Hindu tradition includes the concept of the *"subtle body,"* which comprises various layers of energy or consciousness that extend beyond the physical body. Similarly, Theosophy teaches about the existence of an *"astral body,"* which can be separated from the physical body during astral projection.

Besides Buddhism and Taoism, many other spiritual traditions have explored the possibilities of astral projection, including Sufism, Kabbalah, and Hermeticism. In some cases, astral projection is viewed as a spiritual growth and enlightenment tool. Meanwhile, in others, it is seen as a means of accessing hidden knowledge or communicating with spiritual beings. Today, many people use astral projection for personal growth, spiritual exploration, relaxation, and stress relief.

One technique for achieving astral projection is deep relaxation. Many people use exercises like progressive relaxation or a body scan, which involves focusing on each part of the body, from the toes to the head, and releasing any tension. Once the body is deeply relaxed, the individual can focus on their consciousness and mental state. Visualization is another technique commonly used for astral projection. One popular method is to imagine yourself climbing a rope or a ladder out of your body or drifting upwards like a balloon. Another technique is to visualize yourself in a favorite location or alternate reality. The more vivid the visualization, the better the chance of inducing an astral projection.

During astral projection, people feel like they are flying or floating. Likewise, they may be able to interact with their environment, including the physical world or planes of existence. Some people see deceased loved ones, spirit guides, or other entities that may be present in the astral realm. These interactions can take many forms, such as conversations, receiving guidance or messages, or even receiving healing energy.

Yet, these experiences are highly subjective and can vary greatly from person to person. While some may have vivid and life-changing experiences during astral projection, others may not have any experience at all. Moreover, like any altered state of consciousness, astral projection is not without its risks. As such, many people report feeling disoriented or exhausted after the experience. Meanwhile, others have reported encountering negative entities or spirits. Hence, taking the necessary precautions before attempting astral projection, like grounding oneself before and after the practice and protecting oneself with spiritual or energetic shields, is essential.

Visions of Deceased Loved Ones

Many people struggle to find comfort and closure after the death of a loved one, and some turn to shamanic practices to help them connect with their loved ones beyond the grave. In shamanic practices, visions of deceased loved ones have shared experiences that are believed to offer guidance and healing to the living. In shamanic traditions, visions of deceased loved ones are believed to be a way of connecting with the spiritual world.

Experiences of seeing deceased loved ones can be a powerful way to reconnect with them and feel their presence. Such encounters may bridge the gap between the material and spiritual realms, providing profound insights into life and its purpose. It is believed that these visions are not random occurrences but rather intentional messages from the spirit world, where loved ones remain aware of our lives, intentions, and struggles. They offer guidance, comfort, or even warnings to help us journey. Likewise, they may provide insight into our past decisions or current situations.

Shamans interpret these messages and offer advice on integrating them into the individual's life. It may be a means of solace and resolution for some. For others, it can be a way of continuing a relationship with a loved one who has passed on.

However, not all visions of our departed loved ones are trustworthy or beneficial. Some may arise from intense grief, anguish, or other mental issues, while societal norms or media depictions could impact others. As such, approach these situations with judgment and clarity. Shamanic practices often involve visions of deceased family members providing spiritual advice and solace. Additionally, research into near-death experiences reveals that many people report having a spiritual encounter with their beloved ones when facing a life-threatening situation. Therefore, it appears that these visions can offer comfort in a dire situation regardless of culture or religion.

Each person has different experiences in intensity, frequency, and length. Although not scientifically proven, they offer comfort and solace to those who have lost loved ones, providing a sense of continuity and connection even after death. While not all visions may be genuine or beneficial, it is necessary to approach these experiences with an open mind and discernment.

Lucid Dreams

Shamanic journeys and lucid dreaming are closely linked. In fact, many shamans believe that the experience of lucid dreaming is a form of direct access to the spirit world. During a lucid dream, asking questions, receiving answers from spirit guides, and exploring unknown realms of knowledge and intuition is possible. Furthermore, lucid dreamers can also use their dreams to improve physical health or confront personal fears. All these aspects show how shamanic experiences can be enhanced with an awareness of lucid dreaming.

Besides, lucid dreaming is an incredible skill, allowing you to explore a world of limitless possibilities. With lucid dreams, you can fly to distant galaxies and experience sensations that do not exist in the physical realm. Furthermore, some have used lucid dreams as an effective tool for getting insights into their subconscious minds, such as working through challenging problems or becoming better at something through virtual practice. In addition, research suggests that lucid dreams contribute to improved mental well-being due to the sense of empowerment they generate.

Likewise, lucid dreaming offers unique opportunities for exploration and emotional healing. The activity allows us to safely process our feelings and thoughts without turning to harmful behaviors such as drug abuse or self-harm. With patience and dedication, we can dive into the mysterious realm of lucid dreams and discover new opportunities for self-exploration and personal growth. In fact, lucid dreaming has resulted in various experiences, such as overcoming nightmares or enhancing creativity. However, lucid dreaming can carry certain risks, such as sleep deprivation, false awakenings, and sleep paralysis, which may require extra knowledge and care. Lucid dreaming can also be induced through various methods, including reality checks, *mnemonic induction of lucid dreams (MILD)*, and *wake-initiated lucid dreaming (WILD)*, providing a range of options for individuals to choose from.

Mnemonic induction of lucid dreams (MILD) involves intending to remember that you are dreaming while falling asleep. This is usually done by repeating a phrase, like *"I will recognize that I am dreaming,"* repeatedly until falling asleep. The idea is that eventually, this phrase will become so ingrained in your subconscious that it will carry over into your dream, allowing you to become lucid. Meanwhile, although most people think of lucid dreams as occurring while asleep, it is possible to have a lucid dream while awake. This type of experience is the *wake-induced lucid dream (WILD)*. As such, it involves maintaining consciousness as your body falls asleep, allowing you to enter a dream state while remaining aware. For instance, this method can be done by lying still and focusing on a single thought, such as a swirling pattern, until you eventually become lucid in the dream.

Besides that, meditation can be an effective way to improve your lucid dreaming ability and overall well-being. It helps focus, relax, and be mindful in the present moment. This mindfulness enables you to be aware of your thoughts and feelings at night, allowing you to process them more efficiently so that the intrusive worries that aim to keep you awake during the night become less frequent. Additionally, meditation reduces stress levels, which are known to cause insomnia. Consequently, it may benefit individuals struggling with such sleeping problems as they will experience deeper and more restful sleep.

With lucid dreaming, you can control and bend your dream environment to your will. Whether you explore a city where animals converse or embark on an interstellar journey with an alien companion, your mind can craft any adventure imaginable. Beyond mere wonderment, dreams can also become terrifying if you find yourself face-to-face with monsters or strange dreamscapes that seem too surreal for reality. For thousands of years, various cultures have harnessed the power of lucid dreaming to uncover hidden insights into their personal lives and understanding of the universe.

Altogether, lucid dreaming allows you to explore your imagination in ways that would be impossible in the real world. Not only can you travel to distant planets and explore new and exciting places, but you can also meet characters from your dreams which can become friends or companions. Beyond this, lucid dreaming also has practical applications. For example, it can help reduce stress and increase relaxation, making it a helpful tool for those looking to manage their mental health. Additionally, lucid dreaming is surprisingly straightforward and accessible to anyone looking to get started. This makes it an attractive option for shamans seeking personal growth or insight into their spiritual practice.

8

Trance

Trance is an altered state of consciousness characterized by heightened awareness and receptivity to spiritual communication. It can be induced through meditation, hypnosis, yoga, prayer, dancing, chanting, or rhythmic music. This state of mind also offers a deeper insight into oneself and potential access to higher wisdom. By engaging in trance-like forms, often called astral projection, one can traverse the realms of divination and intuition to understand one's life path and purpose better.

Altered State of Consciousness

A subjective experience, distinct from everyday consciousness, is known as an Altered State of Consciousness (ASC). It can be heightened awareness and focus on one's internal and external experiences. Various techniques can induce ASCs, such as meditation, hypnosis, or sensory deprivation (e.g., floating in water). Certain drugs or psychedelics may also alter consciousness, although the effects vary greatly depending on the substance and dose. Understanding brainwave patterns associated with ASCs could also provide insight into their nature.

Moreover, altered states of consciousness can involve changes in a person's perception and emotions and a sense of temporal distortion. While in an ASC, individuals may experience reality differently, leading to new insights into their surroundings and fostering heightened creativity. Furthermore, recent studies have suggested that these ASCs can be therapeutically for depression or addiction.

To fully comprehend what happens in our brain during an ASC, you must understand the everyday scientific processes of our neural network. Our brains rely on electricity to send messages between neurons and activate muscles, enabled by chemicals called neurotransmitters. These neurotransmitters are small molecules produced by neurons that act as messengers and travel across synapses, narrowing gaps between neighboring cells. When these neurotransmitters bind with receptors on the receiving cell, it triggers electrical signals within the connected neuron(s). Depending on the type of receptor it binds with, it can either activate or inhibit activity in both cells' membranes, allowing them to travel through nerve networks throughout our bodies. During an altered state of consciousness (ASC), different reactions can occur in the brain due to changes in this process, such as increased levels of certain neurotransmitters influencing receptor stimulation.

Subsequently, it is believed that people in ASC have a deeper understanding of themselves and the world around them, enabling them to gain insights into some of life's most difficult questions. As such, when the mind enters a state of heightened awareness, we can often connect with the subconscious on a deeper level, unlocking new perspectives and creativity. For instance, many famous artists have used techniques to influence their consciousness to create some of their most iconic works. From the colorful paintings of Vincent van Gogh to the psychedelic sounds of the Beatles, altered states have played a major role in the creative process of many artists throughout history. Likewise, ASC has also been linked to self-reflection and a greater self-understanding. By introspecting on one's thoughts and emotions, we may address deep-seated personal issues, leading to greater self-awareness and personal growth.

Many people experience altered states of consciousness, often without being aware of it. This can happen when we are so engrossed in a movie or book that we forget where we are or during meditation when our minds wander off. Or have you ever noticed moments of clarity when time slows down and you feel connected to the world? Lots of people experience this type of altered state. The indicators of altered consciousness can include vivid imagery, heightened emotionality, absence of fear, and even feeling part of something bigger than oneself. Understanding the signs and symptoms associated with these altered conditions allows us to gain insight into our experiences and those around us. These details are detailed in the book and provide invaluable insights into new realms of self-awareness.

Drumming

Drumming has been a significant part of religious ceremonies for centuries, serving various purposes depending on the specific tradition. In shamanic rituals, drums are often used for healing, divination, and communicating with the spirit world. The use of drums can vary greatly depending on the culture, with different beats and rhythms used to evoke specific emotions or symbolize certain ideas.

In some religions, drumming is seen to connect with the divine and our inner selves, with the beating of the drum representing the heartbeat that connects us all. Certain sounds or vibrations produced by the drum can also have a special symbolism in specific religious ceremonies, such as the summoning of ancestors or deities.

Shamans use drums in ceremonies to communicate with spirits and ancestors who are not present. During shamanic ceremonies, specific spirits may be summoned to aid with healing or protection from harmful spirits.

The sound of the drum has been used in many cultures worldwide for thousands of years, often as a means of spiritual healing and connection with the divine. Drumming is believed to create an opening in the subconscious that can allow practitioners to access altered states of consciousness and gain insight into their innermost thoughts and feelings. Native American tribes traditionally used drums in ceremonial rituals to invoke powerful spirits for spiritual guidance. In modern times, drum circles are often seen as a way to connect with nature, gather good luck, and promote emotional well-being. Additionally, therapeutic drumming is beneficial for increased relaxation and relief from physical pain, mental illness, and emotional trauma.

In addition to drumming, other percussion instruments like rattles, bells, and chimes are often used in shamanic ceremonies. These instruments add texture and depth to the drum sound, often creating a sonic landscape that the shaman and participants can navigate.

Overall, the sound of the drum is a critical component of shamanic ceremonies, and it is believed to have a powerful impact on the psyche and the spirit. The steady, rhythmic beat of the drum can be a powerful tool for inducing an altered state of consciousness, connecting with the spiritual world, and accessing hidden knowledge and wisdom.

Rattles

The rattle has been a part of humanity for millennia. As such, archaeological discoveries revealed that these objects were used in ceremonial activities dating back to 3000 BCE. They were typically crafted from animal skins stretched over wooden or gourd shells with small seeds that produce sounds when shaken. Initially used for music-making, rattles were regarded as having supernatural powers. Likewise, they were believed to chase away evil spirits and attract positive energy.

In shamanistic traditions, rattles were used to induce trance states and call forth spirits during rituals. The vibrations generated by this instrument pave the way for an altered state of awareness that allows humans and spirits to bridge the gap between them. Apart from their musical and spiritual purposes, rattles were also used for other activities. For instance, shamans frequently incorporated rattles into their healing practices; some were explicitly designed for this purpose. With a rattle containing herbs, the shaman would shake it over the person's body, spreading the herbs and their healing properties on their skin. As such, the sound of shaking these rattles was believed to help drive away evil spirits who might be causing sickness in someone's life or body, making them better again.

Furthermore, rattles were used to connect to the spirit world, assisting individuals in exploring visions and gaining knowledge of their ancestors. They guide their rhythmic vibrations, and the sound produced can be meditative, helping those involved to focus on their meditations without the distraction of external noise. Additionally, rattles are often used in various religious ceremonies, such as purifying and blessing rituals. In some cultures, rattles are believed to bring luck or protection when hung over doorways or placed under beds.

Rattle-making is a traditional craft worldwide, and the process can vary widely. In Native American tribes, rattles were often made with added feathers to symbolize the connection between spirits and humans. Moreover, Latin America is known for its distinctively loud-sounding rattles. Elsewhere, in Northern Europe's Sami community, rattles are crafted from reindeer hooves. Meanwhile, Chinese culture uses bells as a type of rattle for warding off evil spirits.

To make a rattle, do the following steps:

1. Cut two pieces of leather or animal skin into circular shapes. The size and shape of your circle can vary depending on your preference.

2. Place the two pieces of leather together with the smooth sides facing inwards.
3. Using a needle and thread, stitch around the outer edge of the circle, leaving a small opening to add the filling.
4. Once you have left an opening in your circle, add the small stones, beans, or seeds into the pocket created by the leather.
5. After adding the filling, continue sewing around the outer edge of the circle until it is completely closed.
6. Cut a small piece of leather or string and stitch it to the top of the circle to create a handle.
7. OPTIONAL: Decorate your rattle, and attach any beads, feathers, or other decorative items using glue, thread, or wire.

With these steps complete, you have your unique rattle that can be used during spiritual practices or music production. Rattles can be made with various materials depending on cultural traditions. Hence, you can create a unique rattle that aligns with your preferences and practices.

Ecstatic Dancing

Ecstatic dance is a form of shamanic healing practiced for thousands of years. It involves deep introspection, physical exertion, and intense concentration, which requires gradual increases in difficulty as the practitioner continues to train. During these exercises, practitioners are encouraged to use visualization to find balance and control over their movements. Furthermore, ecstatic dancing can be used for its therapeutic benefits, allowing individuals to gain clarity in thought patterns and strengthen their connection with themselves and their environment.

In shamanic healing, ecstatic dancing can heal individuals suffering from physical or mental illness. The idea behind this method is that movement helps release negative energy from within the body, both physically and spiritually, allowing positive energy to flow freely once again. In fact, it is possible to communicate with the divine by dancing as a form of meditation. Additionally, it can aid in your recovery and increase your inner peace. Depending on what you need, you can do it by yourself or with others. Shamanistic rituals such as ecstatic dancing demand many participants. It strains your body and forces you to tune with your spirit, mind, and body.

To be a successful ecstatic dancer, having the right mindset is vital. With a combination of self-focus and concentration on others around you, it is possible to immerse yourself in the experience and find joy in movement. While it may take some time to get accustomed to this form of dance, the effort is worth it as it strengthens your physical and mental health. To improve safety, starting slowly and gradually increasing your stamina is essential; beginning with short yet intense sessions can help you reach the desired results without overexerting yourself. Ecstatic dancing is an incredible way to open up and express yourself without judgment or restrictions.

Get your body ready for more intense exercises by doing light warm-ups such as walking or stretching. Then, challenge yourself with activities like jogging in place or jumping jacks. Both exercises can help increase your heart rate and build muscle tone. Aim for three minutes of jogging in place and four minutes of jumping jacks. Additionally, it is essential to stay hydrated throughout your workout, and allowing yourself rest breaks when necessary is critical.

Ecstatic dance training often begins with learning how to breathe correctly and releasing any tension in the body. To help you do this, try this simple breathing exercise:

1. Sit or stand comfortably, close your eyes, and relax.
2. Take a few deep breaths, exhaling through your mouth after each.
3. Breathe slowly through both nostrils, filling your lungs with air before exhaling slowly through one nostril at a time.
4. Repeat the process by breathing out through both nostrils together (equalizing).
5. Do this three times per day for five minutes at a time until it becomes automatic for you.

Besides that, dancing is a captivating form of expression, emphasizing flow and emotion. It encourages movements that often feel spontaneous but comes from your internal drive. To truly tap into this art form, embrace the music while simultaneously syncing up with your partner or group. This combination goes a long way in creating an unforgettable experience. Also, as you let yourself free in the moment, let the music guide you while being aware of how each body part moves in unison with each other and the surrounding objects. Through this process, new dimensions of creative expression can be explored.

As you dance, focus on your breath and visualize your goal. For example, if you are having trouble controlling the movements of your arms and legs, focus on them instead of letting them flail about aimlessly. You may even want to imagine an invisible string attached to each limb that controls its movements; this way, you can focus on managing those strings rather than worrying about what others think of your dancing style.

However, learning to dance ecstatically is about more than just mastering the moves and techniques. As such, it is also about connecting with your own body. That said, relaxing and letting go of any worries about making mistakes is important. At the same time, proper breathing and tension release practices are essential for building up the strength and stamina required for more complex movements like spinning or jumping. With practice and patience, anyone can gain confidence in their ecstatic dancing ability.

Chanting

Chanting is an ancient practice with many varied purposes. From helping to ground oneself and find clarity of mind to connecting with spiritual guides and tapping into higher wisdom, chanting has been used for millennia. Whether used in a solitary or shared setting, this powerful tool can bring about profound changes in those who participate. In addition, using chanting as a form of meditation can greatly benefit the practitioner's well-being, allowing them to relax and connect with their inner self. With so much potential for transformation, it is no wonder chanting has stood the test of time.

By reciting mantras, one can bring positive energy into their lives and manifest the change they seek in terms of better relationships, improved health, or achieving goals. For instance, chanting "I am loved" or

"I have courage" can help boost self-esteem and reduce negative emotions such as anger and fear. Additionally, chanting can help increase resilience, decrease stress, and enhance concentration. Ultimately, this age-old practice is a powerful way to cultivate inner peace and foster meaningful connections.

Aside from that, chanting can be a powerful tool for self-transformation through its ability to unlock mental and spiritual blocks, elevate the mind into higher states of consciousness, and provide profound insights. This practice has been used by spiritual seekers around the world, from ancient cultures to modern religions. Reflective chants can help you achieve inner peace and greater clarity, improving physical health and mental well-being. As a form of meditation and prayer, chanting has been known to foster feelings of unity and connectedness with something larger than oneself. Ultimately, it is a simple but effective way to transform yourself on your path of spiritual growth.

When selecting the sounds you want to chant, you have a key responsibility. Selecting what resonates with you is about your taste and preference and which sounds speak to your consciousness the most at that moment. Remember, only you can make this choice. For example, if someone has cancer and feels exhausted, I might recommend toning instead of chanting. Binaural beats can promote relaxation by working with brainwave frequencies and calming the mind and body. As such, listening to binaural beats can be an effective way to alter the mind's neural networks to reduce stress hormones, which can then help facilitate natural healing processes within the body. Furthermore, binaural beats can be experienced through headphones at night while in bed or even during meditation sessions throughout the day for a more focused healing experience.Overall, chanting is a powerful tool for connecting with the deeper parts of our being and understanding the world around us. It allows us to access more profound levels of knowledge, tapping into otherwise inaccessible energies. Furthermore, it can align our thoughts, emotions, and intentions to manifest desired outcomes. Adding a factual component to this technique, chanting often follows established patterns or rhymes based on tradition, aiding practitioners in pursuing enlightenment and connection with nature. Finally, whatever type of chanting resonates best with you is always the right choice.

Entheogens

Entheogens have had a long-standing legacy across many cultures and religions worldwide, from Ancient Greece to Egypt, where they were known as the *"food of the gods,"* India with its Soma, China and its mushrooms, Africa with iboga root, and South America with ayahuasca. These substances induce a spiritual experience, and shamans also use them as a tool for healing practices and accessing the spirit world. Furthermore, entheogens are thought to have been used by various cultures for thousands of years now.

Shamanistic practices often incorporate entheogens to connect with other realms. Entheogens are substances that cause an altered state of consciousness (ASC), allowing users to feel different than usual, including relaxed, excited, or energized. They can be plants, fungi, or artificial chemicals, such as:

- Psilocybin mushrooms and LSD
- Mescaline found in peyote cacti
- Ayahuasca made from the vine banisteriopsis caapi and psychotria viridis

- Fly agaric mushrooms (amanita muscaria)
- Morning glory seeds containing LSA (Lysergic Acid Amide)
- Hawaiian baby wood.

These substances can trigger intense spiritual experiences where users believe they have reached a higher level of being. Likewise, entheogens use has existed throughout history for various spiritual and medicinal purposes.

Indigenous groups worldwide have been utilizing entheogens in their spiritual practices for centuries. These psychoactive substances, such as iboga root bark and peyote cactus, have powerful mind-altering effects that can bring about profound changes in consciousness. Unlike psychedelics, which often lead to confusion and disorientation, entheogens impart peace and clarity. In shamanic rituals, they are said to enable shamans to traverse into other worlds or realms beyond this one, where they can communicate with divine entities. The psychedelic experience is commonly described as an exploration of the depths of one's psyche. At the same time, an entheogenic journey could be seen as a voyage beyond the self into another reality entirely. Entheogens are also known for promoting experiences of profound insight and healing.

Meanwhile, shamans use entheogens to bridge the gap between worlds, allowing them to connect with the spiritual realm. Entheogens range from naturally derived plants and mushrooms to synthetic compounds. The benefits of these substances can vary depending on their nature, dosage, and administration. For example, some may be used as healing agents, while others are used for divination or personal exploration. Ayahuasca, in particular, is one of the most potent entheogens and has been used in South American shamanic rituals for thousands of years to acquire spiritual knowledge or communicate with spirits. However, while psychotropic drugs such as LSD, cannabis, and magic mushrooms produce mind-altering effects, they may not induce a spiritual experience and access higher realms of consciousness.

Today's indigenous people still use entheogens, which have been used in shamanic rituals for thousands of years. While these substances can be dangerous if taken in excess or by those with pre-existing mental health conditions, they can also offer a spiritual experience that may help users connect with their identity as part of nature or humanity.

Conclusion

This book aims to provide an overview of the key aspects of shamanism, including its beliefs, practices, and techniques. I have delved into the rich and fascinating world of shamanic healing, spirit guides, and the three shamanic worlds. I also explored the role of dreams and trance in shamanic practice.

In restating the book's message, I have highlighted the importance of shamanism as an ancient spiritual practice that is still relevant and effective today. This practice is based on the notion that all things have a spirit or soul and are all interconnected in the universe. The shaman's role is to facilitate communication between the physical and spiritual realms, helping individuals heal and bring balance to their lives.

Shamanism is a spiritual practice that involves an altered state of consciousness, communicating with the spirit world and healing. It involves various techniques, such as drumming or chanting, to achieve an altered state of consciousness, which can be achieved through mind-expanding herbs or psychedelic plants. The goal of shamanism is to help people connect with their inner selves and access hidden knowledge, such as knowledge of past lives or future events. Shamans exist today, they are called healers, and they use similar techniques to traditional shamans.

The word shaman originates from the Tungusic languages, and it refers to a priest or healer who uses spiritual techniques to facilitate healing and communication with spirits. Traditional shamanism is based on direct experience, being an integral part of nature, and finding meaning through spiritual development. Modern-day shamanism is spiritual in nature, but it is not religion-based. In *The 4 Pillars of Shamanism*, I provide a comprehensive guide that explores these fundamental principles and practices in detail, offering insights and practical guidance for those seeking to deepen their understanding of shamanism and put its teachings into practice.

The first pillar of shamanism is a deep connection with the natural world. This connection is seen as the foundation of shamanic practice, and it is achieved through a deep respect and reverence for the natural world and its cycles and seasons. In this chapter, we explored how indigenous cultures have maintained this connection over the centuries and the practical steps that modern practitioners can take to deepen their connection with nature.

The second pillar of shamanism is the use of ritual and ceremony. In shamanic cultures, these rituals and ceremonies are seen as powerful tools for connecting with the spirit world and promoting healing and growth. In this chapter, we explored the different forms these rituals and ceremonies take and provided practical guidance on creating meaningful rituals and ceremonies.

The third pillar of shamanism is engagement with non-ordinary reality. This refers to the realm of the spirit world, which is seen as a parallel reality that is just as real as the physical world. In this chapter, we explored the different ways in which shamans engage with this realm, including the use of meditation, visualization, and other shamanic techniques. They also provide practical guidance on developing your own shamanic practices and engaging with the spirit world in meaningful ways.

Meanwhile, the fourth and final pillar of shamanism is the application of shamanic healing techniques. These techniques are used to promote physical, emotional, and spiritual healing, and they include practices such as the use of power animals, soul retrieval, and extraction. This chapter explored these techniques in detail and provided practical guidance for personal healing and growth.

Altogether, *The Four Pillars of Shamanism* presents a comprehensive overview of the ancient spiritual practice and its enduring relevance in today's world. By emphasizing the importance of the four pillars—connection to nature, community, spirituality, and healing—in fostering a holistic and fulfilling life, I make the book's message crystal clear.

Several essential aspects of shamanism, including shamanic healing and spirit guides, were also explored. Shamanic healing involves a shaman journeying to the spiritual realm to communicate with spirits and retrieve lost soul parts. Likewise, it restores balance and healing to the individual. This powerful healing form also addresses physical ailments and mental, emotional, relational, and financial issues. Alongside these practices, spirit guides from the spiritual realm provide guidance and support to the shaman as they journey towards greater spiritual understanding and personal growth. This book also touches on the unique teachings and qualities of the upper, middle, and lower worlds that the shaman can access during their transformative journeys.

Finally, we discussed the importance of dreams and trance in shamanic practice. Dreams provide a direct connection to the spiritual realm, and the shaman can use this connection to gain insights, guidance, and healing. Trance is a state of consciousness in which the shaman can access the spiritual realm and communicate with spirits; it is a crucial aspect of shamanic practice.

In delivering on my promise, this book has provided a comprehensive overview of the critical aspects of shamanism, illuminating this ancient spiritual practice's rich and fascinating world. Through its pages, I have aimed to shed light on the beliefs, practices, and techniques central to shamanism and provide a deeper understanding of this powerful and transformative path.

The book aims to help readers find harmony and balance in their lives by connecting with the spirit world through shamanism. Also, it provides a solution for those seeking a deeper understanding of shamanism and its benefits. Through clear and accessible language, I have guided you through the complexities of this spiritual tradition and shown how its principles and practices can be integrated into modern life.

The one thing you are meant to take away from this book is the understanding that shamanism offers a path to a more fulfilling and meaningful life. By embracing the four pillars of connection to nature, community, spirituality, and healing, individuals can cultivate a deeper sense of purpose and find greater peace and happiness daily. Whether one is seeking to explore shamanism for the first time or deepen their existing spiritual practice, *The 4 Pillars of Shamanism* provides a comprehensive and inspiring guide to this rich and ancient tradition.

Glossary

Altered State of Consciousness (ASC): A state of mind different from normal awareness and consciousness, typically characterized by changes in perception, thought, emotion, and memory.

Ancestors: The people from previous generations who have preceded you biologically or culturally.

Angels: Divine beings believed to act as messengers between the divine realm and the physical world, providing comfort, guidance, and protection to people.

Archangels: High-ranking angels in many religious traditions, often associated with specific qualities or duties, such as Michael as a protector or Gabriel as a messenger.

Aura: An energy field that is said to surround and permeate a person's body, often depicted as a colorful or luminous halo.

Breathing Exercises: Techniques used to regulate and control one's breathing, often as a form of meditation or stress relief.

Burnout: the loss of motivation and fulfillment brought on by a state of physical, emotional, and mental exhaustion brought on by excessive and prolonged stress or work.

Centering: A practice of bringing one's attention and focus to the present moment and the physical sensations in the body to reduce stress and increase awareness.

Ceremony: A formal and symbolic event, often religious or spiritual, performed to mark a significant occasion or bring people together.

Connecting: The process of creating a connection or relationship between two or more things.

Connection: A relationship or link between two or more things.

Crossing Over: A term used in many spiritual and religious traditions to describe a soul's transition from one plane of existence to another, such as from the physical world to the afterlife.

Cure: A treatment or solution that alleviates or eliminates an illness or condition.

Daily Practice: A routine or routine-like behavior performed regularly and repeatedly as a form of self-improvement or spiritual growth.

Deities: Divine or supernatural beings worshiped and revered in various religious and spiritual traditions, often associated with specific qualities, powers, or domains.

Delving Deeper: The act of exploring or investigating something more thoroughly or intensively, often to gain greater understanding or knowledge.

Despair: A feeling of hopelessness and despondency, often accompanied by loss or frustration from complex or challenging circumstances.

Diagnosis: An illness, disease, or condition's identification or determination of its nature and cause, typically made by a doctor or other medical professional.

Dimension: A direction or aspect along which a phenomenon or object can vary, or a concept in physics and mathematics that refers to a physical extent or a space-time coordinate.

Divination: The practice of seeking or revealing knowledge or guidance through supernatural means, such as interpreting omens, casting lots, or consulting oracles.

Divine: Of or relating to a deity or the divine, often associated with holiness, purity, and transcendence.

Divine Beings: Creatures or entities believed to be of a divine or supernatural origin or nature.

Divine Connection: A relationship or bond with the divine or spiritual realm, often experienced as a feeling of closeness or communication with a higher power.

Earth: The physical realm of existence and the natural world, including the elements of the land, water, air, fire, and spirit.

Earth Mother: A concept in many indigenous cultures that personifies the earth as a nurturing and sustaining mother, often associated with fertility, growth, and abundance.

Empath: A person with an enhanced capacity to perceive and comprehend the emotions and feelings of others.

Endorphins: Natural, feel-good chemicals the body produces to relieve pain and create a feeling of well-being.

Euphoria: A feeling of intense happiness, often accompanied by a sense of elation and excitement.

Evil Spirit: An entity some believe is a source of negative energy and influence in the world.

Exorcism: A ritual or practice to remove an evil spirit or negative entity from a person or place.

Guides: Spiritual beings, such as angels, are believed to guide and support individuals on their spiritual journey.

Healing: The procedure of regaining physical, mental, and spiritual balance.

Healing Methods: Various techniques are used to facilitate healing, such as meditation, visualization, Reiki, and acupuncture.

Healing Sessions: One-on-one sessions with a healer, during which the person receives guidance and support for their healing journey.

Heaven: A term used to describe a realm of existence believed by some to be a place of peace, happiness, and spiritual fulfillment.

Heavenly Beings: Spiritual entities believed by some to reside in Heaven and to offer guidance and support to individuals on Earth.

Hell: A term used to describe a realm of existence believed by some to be a place of suffering and punishment.

Helping Spirits: Spiritual entities believed by some to offer guidance and support to individuals on their spiritual journey.

Higher Power: A term used to describe a divine, spiritual force or entity believed to be greater than oneself.

Higher Realms of Understanding: Realms of existence believed by some to be beyond our physical world and to hold greater knowledge and wisdom.

Higher Self: A term used to describe the spiritual aspect of a person that is believed to be their true self beyond the physical body and ego.

Illness: A physical or mental condition that impairs normal functioning and well-being.

Incantations: Words or phrases repeated to achieve a specific outcome or influence a desired result.

Incense: A substance that produces a fragrant smoke when burned and is used in various spiritual practices for its symbolic or medicinal properties.

Innate Abilities: Natural talents or skills inherent in an individual without training or education.

Inner Guide: An intuition or inner voice thought to provide people on their spiritual journey with direction and wisdom.

Inner Self: A term used to describe the true self, beyond the physical body and ego, that is believed to hold inner wisdom and guidance.

Inner Voice: A voice or inner intuition thought to provide individuals with direction and wisdom along their spiritual path.

Inner Wisdom: A term used to describe an individual's internal knowledge and understanding that can be accessed through quiet reflection and introspection.

Integrating: The process of combining and integrating different aspects of oneself, such as the physical, emotional, mental, and spiritual aspects.

Intercession: A form of prayer where a person requests guidance from a higher power, for themselves or others.

Introspection: The process of looking within oneself and examining one's thoughts, feelings, and beliefs.

Intuition: An innate capacity to comprehend something intuitively and without using conscious thought.

Journeying: A spiritual or religious rite often performed on a physical journey.

Lost Soul Parts: Fragments of a person's soul essence that has become separated.

Magic Rituals: An event intended to bring about change in the world; a ceremony involving incantations, spells, and other rituals.

Manifestation: The process whereby an idea or image comes into being; the act of embodying something in visible form; the act of becoming apparent or visible.

Mantras: The repetition of a word or sound is known as a mantra, and it can be used to improve concentration, calm the mind, and promote relaxation.

Medicine Wheel: A medicine wheel is a sacred circle used in Native American ceremonies to symbolize the four elements and directions. Furthermore, it can be a helpful tool for vision quests and meditation.

Meditation: Meditation is an integral part of many religions and spiritual practices. It involves focusing on one thing for an extended period, usually, 10 minutes, to promote relaxation, clarity, and well-being.

Message Bearers: In Native American tradition, messengers from other worlds come to earth to teach us about ourselves and our place in the universe by sharing their wisdom through stories or songs. In some cultures, these messengers are called "spirit guides" or "guardians."

Metaphysical Level: The metaphysical level refers to ideas about spirituality—beliefs about what happens after death; whether we have souls; how we connect with God; etc.—as opposed to religious beliefs like which church you go to or what ceremonies you practice (those would be on the physical level).

Mindfulness: Mindfulness is a way of paying attention that focuses on being present in your life. Mindfulness can help you be more aware of your thoughts and feelings without judging them, which may reduce stress and improve your mental health.

Modern-Day Shamanism: A contemporary form of spiritual but not religion-based shamanism. It involves using your senses to interact with your environment, finding ways to connect with others, and working with energy to help heal yourself and others.

Mystics: Mystics are people who have a strong relationship with their spiritual beliefs and seek to understand their life experiences in those terms. They often seek out others interested in exploring these ideas and are surrounded by like-minded individuals.

Occult Traditions: Occult traditions are practices that involve the supernatural or paranormal. Depending on the intent of the person using it, the occult can be used for good or evil.

Omens: An omen is an event believed to foretell future events. Omens are usually associated with a spiritual belief system and occur randomly.

Painful Experiences: Some shamanic practices may require you to participate in painful or uncomfortable activities, such as fasting or exercise, to get in touch with your body's energy centers and bring positive energy into your life.

Pilgrimage. A journey undertaken for religious or spiritual reasons.

Pillars of Shamanism: The pillars of shamanism include: *spirit communication, healing work, trance work, journeying/dreaming, and ritual ceremony/drumming.* These pillars are used together to create a holistic approach towards life balance and healing work within yourself or others needing assistance from someone trained in this healing modality.

Power Animal: An animal spirit that serves as a guide and ally.

Power Animal Retrieval: A technique where the shamanic healer retrieves a person's power animal that has separated from them.

Power Retrieval: A shamanic practice of regaining one's lost personal power or life force.

Precognition: The ability to perceive or know events or information about the future through extrasensory means.

Primordial Deity: A deity believed to exist from the beginning of time and represents the elemental forces of the universe.

Psychedelic Plants/Mushrooms: Plants or mushrooms that can induce an altered state of mind.

Psychic healing: A type of healing that involves using psychic or spiritual energy to help balance and align the individual's energy field and promote physical, mental, and emotional well-being.

Psychopomp: A being, deity, or entity that guides the souls of the deceased to the afterlife.

Psychotherapy: A form of therapy that aims to treat mental disorders by altering a patient's thoughts and behaviors.

Rattle: A musical instrument typically made of a handle and a container filled with small objects that produce a sound when shaken. It is used in various spiritual and religious practices, including shamanism.

Rattling: Shaking a rattle in a spiritual or religious context to produce sound and create specific energy.

Real Beings: Beings or entities that exist physically or spiritually and can be perceived through the senses or extrasensory means.

Realities: Different dimensions, realms, or realities that exist beyond our physical reality and can be accessed through spiritual practices or experiences.

Realms of Reality: Different levels or domains of existence beyond our physical reality can be experienced through spiritual or supernatural means.

Reflection: The act of considering or examining one's thoughts, emotions, and actions to gain insight and understanding.

Ritualized Practices: Practices or activities that have been formalized or structured as part of a spiritual or religious tradition.

Rituals: A set of actions or words performed in a specific way, often as part of a spiritual or religious tradition.

Scandinavian: Relating to the countries of Scandinavia (Norway, Sweden, and Denmark), their cultures, and their people.

Scent: A particular smell, especially a pleasant one.

Scrying: A divination technique that involves using a reflective surface, such as a crystal ball, to see visions or receive information from the spiritual realm.

Shaman: A spiritual practitioner who uses altered states of consciousness to access the spirit world and bring back information and healing to the community.

Shamanic Healing: A type of healing that involves working with spirits, energies, and elements of nature to promote physical, mental, and emotional well-being.

Shamanic Journey: A spiritual journey or meditation where a shaman accesses the spirit world to gain insight, healing, or knowledge.

Shamanic Journeying: The practice of accessing the spirit world through a journey or meditation, often guided by a shaman or a spiritual teacher.

Shamanic Practices: Techniques used in shamanism, such as drumming, chanting, or psychedelics, to achieve an ASC.

Shamanic Worlds: The worlds that shamans travel to interact with the spirits.

Shamanism: is a form of spiritual practice in which a person called a shaman enters an altered state of consciousness to communicate with and heal others.

Shape-Shifting: When someone takes on the physical characteristics of something else.

Signs: Things that represent something else, like a signpost or symbol.

Sky Deity: The deity who lives in or rules over the sky.

Soul: The eternal part of you and the force that breathes life into your body; it is composed of your positive traits and life experiences, which influence your decisions.

Soul Flight: When you leave your body into another world or state of being, like in astral projection.

Soul Growth: What happens during soul flight; is growth, development, and learning about yourself and others.

Soul Retrieval: A shamanic ritual in which a lost soul is rescued and returned safely home.

Spirit: The force that exists outside of time and space. It comprises other people's souls, animals and plants, planets, stars, and other things outside the human experience.

Spirit Allies: People or animals who have chosen to support you on your life's journey. They can appear in dreams or visions as guides or guardians.

Spirit Communication: Talking with spirits using meditation, divination tools like tarot cards or pendulums, or other methods such as channeling (which involves speaking through another person).

Spirit Guides: People who have died but still have a presence in our world; they are usually referred to as ancestors or angels in Western culture (though the definition of each varies). They are often considered intermediaries for communicating with the spirit world.

Spiritual Development: A journey towards a higher level of consciousness. It is the process by which one's awareness expands and becomes more universal. Spiritual development is achieved through meditation, yoga, prayer, and other spiritual practices.

Spiritual Guide: A person who assists another individual in their spiritual development.

Spiritual Leader: The person who leads a community or religious group; a religious leader, an inspirational figure, or simply someone who teaches others how to live more spiritually.

Spiritual Path: A path that one chooses to follow to achieve enlightenment or union with God through meditation, yoga, prayer, and other spiritual practices.

Spiritual Realm: A realm of existence outside the physical world where spirits dwell and angels are believed to reside; also known as heaven.

Stamina: The ability to continue doing something over an extended period without tiring easily; perseverance; strength of will.

Supernatural World: A nonconventional world that defies physics and scientific laws.

Sweat Lodge Ceremony: A purification ceremony that promotes physical, emotional, and spiritual healing.

Synchronicity: A phrase that describes encountering coincidences that defy logic.

The Spirit World: A place where all souls go after death; it can be accessed through meditation or other spiritual practices such as astral projection (which involves leaving one's body behind temporarily).

Trance: A state of being where you are so focused on something that you are unaware of your surroundings.

Trance State: A state in which a person becomes absorbed with an activity or idea and is withdrawn from others or their surroundings.

Visions: Seeing something that is not there, usually through drugs or meditation.

Water Spirits: Spirits that live in water, such as lakes, rivers, or oceans.

References

Aletheia. (2018, February 5). *7 types of spirit guides (& how to connect with them)*. LonerWolf. https://lonerwolf.com/spirit-guides/

Bernstein, G. (2020, February 28). *10 simple and beautiful ways to connect with your spirit guides.* Gabby Bernstein. https://gabbybernstein.com/spirit-guides/

Dreaming research papers - 894 words | Bartleby. (n.d.). Www.bartleby.com. https://www.bartleby.com/essay/Dreaming-Research-Papers-FJAF9CC44EV

Faria, M. (2021, July 12). *"Plants of the gods" and their hallucinogenic powers in neuropharmacology — A review of two books.* Surgical Neurology International. https://doi.org/10.25259/sni_560_2021

Farmer, S. D. (n.d.). *Signs from the animal world.* Unity.org. https://www.unity.org/article/signs-animal-world

Halliday, M. (n.d.). *Introduction to the medicine wheel | The Edinburgh Shamanic Centre.* Www.shamaniccentre.com. https://www.shamaniccentre.com/teachings-medicinewheel.html

Harner, M. (n.d.). *A core shamanic theory of dreams.* https://www.shamanism.org/articles/pdfs/ShamanicTheoryDreams3-11.pdf

Harner, M. (2005). *Articles on shamanism and shamanic studies: my path in shamanism by Michael Harner, from higher wisdom by Roger Walsh and Charles S. Grob.* Www.shamanism.org. https://www.shamanism.org/articles/article16page4.html

https://hraf.yale.edu/author/ajordan. (2019, March 27). *cross-culturally exploring the concept of shamanism.* Human Relations Area Files - Cultural Information for Education and Research. https://hraf.yale.edu/cross-culturally-exploring-the-concept-of-shamanism/

Jackson, J. (2018, August 15). *Shamanism - spiritual guides for indigenous peoples.* Www.linkedin.com. https://www.linkedin.com/pulse/shamanism-spiritual-guides-indigenous-peoples-julian-jackson/

Kapoor, M. (2022, December 29). *5 certain signs that your higher self is talking to you.* Mukund Kapoor's Blog. https://mukundkapoor.com/signs-that-your-higher-self-is-talking-to-you

Labate, B., Laboa, B., Mizumoto, S., Anderson, B., & Cavnar, C. (2014). The therapeutic use of ayahuasca. In *www.academia.edu*. https://www.academia.edu/27695463/The_therapeutic_use_of_ayahuasca

Mazzola, L. C. (1988). The Medicine Wheel: Center and Periphery. *The Journal of Popular Culture*, *22*(2), 63–73. https://doi.org/10.1111/j.0022-3840.1988.2202_63.x

McClenon, J. (1997). Shamanic Healing, Human Evolution, and the Origin of Religion. *Journal for the Scientific Study of Religion*, *36*(3), 345. https://doi.org/10.2307/1387852

McNamara, P., & Bulkeley, K. (2015). Dreams as a source of supernatural agent concepts. *Frontiers in Psychology*, *6*. https://doi.org/10.3389/fpsyg.2015.00283

Metzner, R. (2013). Entheogenic rituals, shamanism and green psychology. *European Journal of Ecopsychology*, *4*, 64–77. https://citeseerx.ist.psu.edu/document?repid=rep1&type=pdf&doi=284ee8a0cbefa64d1d28a98eaffc975c9863819a

Louie, M. (n.d.). *Shaman*. Michele Louie Awakening the Healer Within. https://michelelouie.com/shaman/

Oracle, L. (n.d.). *Luminous oracle*. Luminous Oracle. https://luminousoracle.com/

Plant spirit shamanism: working with plant medicine in shamanic journeys. (2022, April 27). Therapeutic Shamanism. https://www.therapeutic-shamanism.co.uk/blog/plant-medicine/

Plants of mind and spirit. (n.d.). Www.fs.usda.gov. https://www.fs.usda.gov/wildflowers/ethnobotany/Mind_and_Spirit/index.shtml

Filippo, D. S. (2006). *Angels as spiritual guides*. National Louis University Digital Commons @ NLU. https://digitalcommons.nl.edu/cgi/viewcontent.cgi?article=1054&context=faculty_publications

Shamanic healing. (n.d.). I.e. KAWA. https://www.iekawa.com/soulsessions

Shamanic journeying / psycho shamanic. (n.d.). Www.goodtherapy.org. https://www.goodtherapy.org/learn-about-therapy/types/shamanic-journeying-psycho-shamanic

Shamanism - selection. (n.d.). Encyclopedia Britannica. https://www.britannica.com/topic/shamanism/Selection

Shamanistic healing - 2028 words. (n.d.). Www.123helpme.com. https://www.123helpme.com/essay/Shamanistic-Healing-30632

Shamans. (n.d.). Nordan.daynal.org. https://nordan.daynal.org/wiki/Shamans

Thomason, T. C. (n.d.). *The role of altered states of consciousness in Native American healing.* Ecstatic Trance: Ritual Body Postures. https://www.cuyamungueinstitute.com/articles-and-news/the-role-of-altered-states-of-consciousness-in-native-american-healing/

University of Minnesota. (2006). *Shamanism.* Taking Charge of Your Health & Wellbeing. https://www.takingcharge.csh.umn.edu/shamanism

What is shamanic healing? (n.d.). Www.centreofexcellence.com. https://www.centreofexcellence.com/shamanic-healing/#:~:text=Also%20known%20as%20a%20

Williams, K. (2022). *What is a shaman? types, talents & examples.* Study.com. https://study.com/learn/lesson/what-is-a-shaman.html

THE 7 PILLARS OF MANIFESTATION

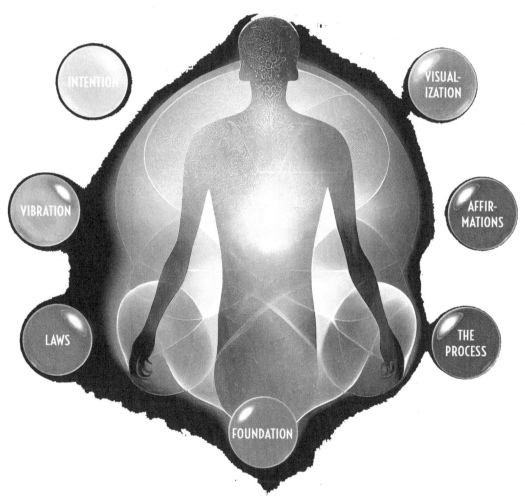

107 Techniques & Clues
to Create the Life You Want with the Power of Your Mind. Manifest Happiness,
Money, Success, and Love by Raising Your Vibration and Energy

INGRID CLARKE

Table of Contents

Introduction **391**

Pillar One: Foundation **395**
    What Is Manifestation? 395
    The Origin 396
    The Science Behind It... 397
    Becoming a Self-Fulfilling Prophecy 398

Pillar Two: Laws... **401**
    Law of Oneness... 401
    Law of Vibration 402
    Law of Correspondence.. 403
    Law of Attraction 403
    Law of Action... 404
    Law of Perpetual Transmutation of Energy 405
    Law of Cause and Effect 406
    Law of Compensation 407
    The Law of Relativity 408
    Law of Polarity 409
    Law of Rhythm 409
    Law of Gender 410

Pillar Three: Vibration **411**
    What Is Vibrational Energy?.. 411
    What Are Vibrational Beings? 412
    Connection Between Thoughts, Behaviors, and Vibrations........................ 412
    Raising Your Vibration 416

Pillar Four: Intention **425**
    Intention Manifestation 425
    Setting Intentions... 427

Pillar Five: Visualization **431**
    Power of Visualization 431

    Multi-Sensory Visualization 433

    Practicing Visualization 434

Pillar Six: Affirmations **437**

    The Power of Affirmations 437

    What Are Affirmations? 442

Pillar Seven: The Process **447**

    Identify and Clarify 447

    Ask the Universe 449

    Take Inspired Action 449

    Trust the Journey 450

    Release Attachment 450

    Be Grateful for What You Receive 451

    Watch Your Energy 452

    Let Go of Limiting Beliefs 453

Conclusion **455**

Glossary **457**

References **459**

Introduction

Something in life has you feeling overwhelmed and wanting to see change. Yet, you never lost faith that the universe was generous because beneath all your triumphs and failings lies the power of your mind. And regardless of how hard life may seem, you always find the strength and courage to push on and continue striving for something greater. Perhaps, it was because you are aware that beyond the horizon lies a dream that can be pursued, regardless of age. Or deep inside your subconscious is an abundance of knowledge, power, wisdom, and all you need to create a life far more extraordinary than what you already have. Tapping into this possibility will lead you to achieve abundance in life. Likewise, it can help you ask the universe for what you truly want and propel your path to fulfillment.

Stress is an integral part of modern life. From our jobs to our businesses, on the way to work or even home, we stress daily as a form of survival. Growing up in a Scandinavian family with pagan roots, I understand how to face and deal with various hard situations, such as chronic stress or illness, without needing medication. In fact, I have gone through a great deal of exhaustion and stress in my life. Drawing from medical, metaphysical, and occult knowledge I have gained from research, I aim to share my understanding and experiences with those seeking transformation or relief. These years of study have imparted me with profound wisdom that can help anyone going through a difficult journey find comfort and hope for the future.

It is no secret that we possess great power in our minds, and it is our right to use it to create whatever we want. All we must do is align our minds with our dreams and put in the effort to make them come true. It is neither a game nor a celestial mystery; it is reality. This is our chance to demonstrate that if we set our minds on something, visualize it thoroughly, and take the appropriate steps; we can manifest it into reality.

With incredible gifts to do whatever we desire, it can be easy to get stuck in a negative spiral. Frustration sets in when things do not turn out as expected, and life can feel like an uphill battle. But with the help of our minds, we can learn how to use these gifts for good, turning our mindset around so that it works for us rather than against us. Reading this book offers a unique solution to shifting your mentality from a place of negativity, even if you feel overwhelmed or unable to manifest the life of your dreams. It provides the essential steps to reframe your ideas and create lasting change within yourself. Likewise, in this book, you can learn how to take control of your life by understanding the seven pillars of manifestation that can influence how energy and vibrations shape reality. Additionally, it provides insight into the theories, strategies, and advice for living abundantly, joyfully, and gloriously.

Overall, this book provides a simple yet powerful and unique approach to manifestation, which starts by delving into fundamental aspects such as the practice's science, history, and definition. This pillar will help you gain insight into the concept of manifestation, regardless of your experience level. Understanding this foundation helps to equip you for success as you move on with the other pillars.

For the following pillar, we will dive deeper into the laws and principles that help open your eyes to a mental and spiritual capacity. They will teach you how to design and create your reality consciously. Plus, you will have the chance to tap into the infinite intelligence and power within yourself and the universe. As a beginner, these pillars have the information you need to start.

- **Pillar II:** Understanding the universal laws and how they impact your life.
- **Pillar III:** Delves into how to raise the vibration and manifest your desires.
- **Pillars IV and V:** Explain the power of intention and visualization.
- **Pillar VI:** Examines the impact that affirmations have on you, your relationships, and your spiritual creator.
- **Pillar VII:** Outlines a seven-step framework for creating a beautiful and extraordinary life.

I was able to discover the potential of my mind and make huge strides in life. Now, it is an honor to pass down these invaluable tools and bestow their power onto you. Through applying these methods, I've seen challenges become mere obstacles and overcome them with grace, leading to new heights in my journey. Not to mention, these very methods assist celebrities in manifesting their dreams, such as:

- Jim Carrey used the power of visualization to transform his life from a janitor to an A-list actor.
- Lady Gaga used the power of affirmation to become famous, even before people knew her name.
- Oprah Winfrey believed she would land a lead role in a movie she auditioned for at the start of her fame and fortune. She harnessed the power of clarity, universal trust, and gratitude for visualizing what she wanted and got the part.

Hence, this book offers an opportunity to manifest and reclaim control of your life. You can direct the power of your mind and build a success story unique to you, your goals, and your dreams. By exploring manifestations' common principles and practices, you will access greater pleasure, serenity, abundance, and empowerment. With these tools, you can craft your best life with healing and self-mastery as a guide. No matter where you are on your journey, this book offers a blueprint to help unlock what lies ahead.

Subsequently, the techniques and strategies you are about to read are proven to yield incredible results for people who want to tap into the healing power of manifestation. Each pillar in this book will teach you the different theories and techniques you can use in your spiritual journey to recognize your immense power to shift your life in the direction you want. I implore you to use the knowledge and strategies gained from this book to seize power. Remember, *knowledge is far more priceless when it is shared and acted upon.* Therefore, take substantial steps towards utilizing these teachings in your life; reap the rewards of realizing the greatness of realization.

Empower yourself with the knowledge you have and take action. With this, you will be closer to manifesting prosperity and abundance in your life. Aside from that, this provides easy access to information on manifestation, regardless of their physical, mental, or emotional state. And with the right mindset and perspective, you can turn things around, no matter what you face.

As you move forward with this book, please keep this in mind: *There is powerful energy already inherent to you.* You have the extraordinary capability of transforming your life using the power of your mind. Reach within yourself, tap into that energy, and use it to draw upon the universal laws. With this knowledge, you control your destiny. Likewise, you can manifest happiness, money, success, love, freedom, or whatever abundance you desire. Allow all these beautiful things to enter your life, embrace this power, and see how far it takes you.

No doubt, your life is on the cusp of a transformation as you have already taken the first step to bringing your dreams into reality—opening this book and beginning to read. Now, what happens next is entirely up to you.

Pillar One
Foundation

To manifest your goals and dreams, it is essential to construct a strong foundation. This applies to any pursuit we make as the foundation is an integral part of success. In this case, if you wish to see your dreams come true through manifestation, you need to acquire a comprehensive knowledge of its fundamentals, such as *"Why it exists?"*, *"Where its origin lies?"* and *"Why can countless people attest to its impact on their life?"* Understanding these fundamentals must be established before anything else can fall into place; hence, they form the first piece of the puzzle when entering the field of manifestation.

Once you comprehend the basics, you will realize how imperative it is to align your thoughts positively and be able to envision what you wish for, as manifestation can influence your life in unique ways. But without this foundation, you will begin your journey on rocky ground, and it will feel like such. Clarity will also be non-existent, and you will go back and forth, confused, and distracted, believing that manifestation does not work. Likewise, you will be stuck in a skeptic's mind frame, encountering feelings of stagnation, loss, and difficulty, asking yourself why it is so.

As such, this pillar will help set you up on the right foot. From the get-go, it will open your mind to the unique possibilities of manifestation. It can be a powerful tool to help you navigate challenges, opening doors that once felt sealed shut because of mistrust, lack of familiarity with the vision, or focusing on the struggle instead of the miracles of changing your outlook. Nevertheless, this pillar is here to help broaden your mental outlook and well-being.

What Is Manifestation?

According to Oprah Daily, Angelina Lombardo, a coach, and author, defines manifestation as *"making everything you want to feel and experience a reality via your thoughts, actions, beliefs, and emotions."* In other words, manifestation is the process in which you harness the power of your subconscious and align its energy with that of your goals and dreams to make them a reality. And instead of referring to the act of manifestation as 'harnessing,' think of it as a way to influence the power of your thoughts to achieve positive and empowered feelings, bringing in the energy of all you desire. Through this process, you can control your mind to create an atmosphere for these things to manifest.

Everyone can make their dreams come true. To some degree, we are constantly manifesting our reality, sometimes without even being aware. Our thoughts are potent and can help us achieve what we aspire to. Now, reflect on what is currently in your life. *How would you describe it? Is it encouraging? Difficult? Positive? Negative? Plentiful or lacking?* No matter how your life looks, know that it can always change for the better. If you are going through a tough time, try to see it as an opportunity. These challenges make us stronger and more capable of enduring hardship. Besides, manifesting is all about claiming our power. As you take action to create the life you want, ensure you are honoring your energy, owning up to any mistakes, and making choices that will allow you to move forward. It is also about the courage to choose something different if our actions are not working. Regardless, *what manifests in your life depends on your choices.*

However, remember that saying that you want something and genuinely meaning it is two different things. Many people can say they want a luxurious home or an exotic vacation, but when it comes to making these things happen, *you must be emotionally invested in them.* Feeling like there is no other option but to make your dreams a reality is what manifestation is all about. In a Google search, manifestation is defined as *something you embody*. The word embodiment could be used to describe the process of manifestation well. For manifestation to work in your life, you must feel what you intend to manifest. Believe that your manifestational dreams are meant for you to live in this lifetime, and you will stop at nothing to make them happen. As such, when you think of this innate urge to manifest your dream home or more money in your bank account, your drive and determination awaken, and things shift in your body, mind, and spirit. Then, your energy becomes infectious to the universe, and you attract abundance into your life.

The Origin

> *"All that we are is a result of what we have thought."*
>
> –*Buddha*

There are many people new to manifestation who believe that it is a relatively recent discovery. A taboo topic of magic and spirituality combined. Some have even described it as "hocus pocus witchcraft" or a journey where you create magic spells. But this is not the case. To begin your manifestation journey, you must understand its true origins. As such, you must know where it came from, how it started, and the like.

Manifestation has been around for centuries, even if it was not given the name yet. In fact, it did not become popular recently simply because someone thought it would be cool, as its origin can be traced back far before that. While the term might be new, the concept of manifestation certainly is not. Jesus speaks about manifestation many times in the bible when he talks about having unlimited power to give you what you need and wants as long as you put your trust and faith in him. For instance, 1 Corinthians 3:13 talks about how "each one's work will be made to manifest," Matthew 7:7 says, "ask, and you shall receive," and 2 Corinthians 5:7 says, "live by faith, not by sight." Many other scriptures also reference manifestation and the idea that we can manifest anything we want as long as we have faith.

What you think is powerful shapes your life and destiny. Through the practice of Hinduism, such as Kundalini yoga and the seven chakras, individuals can awaken their manifestational senses and intuition to gain insight into their true selves, allowing them to control their lives. Besides, far before we, as a human race, ever stepped foot on the earth, the concept of manifestation had already been born; *consider it a notion that has existed for ages and prevails even today.* As we grew up, we began to form our ideas and conclusions about the manifestation journey while staying within the vicinity of the original concept. Take the Law of Attraction as an example, a concept that has become familiar to many, leading to the introduction of other spiritual laws and teachings. It has been put forward that the Law of Attraction and its idea of *'like attracts like'* have persistently been at the core of how our life plays out.

So, has it only been a few decades since manifestation started existing in new-age spirituality? No, it has been many centuries since the dawn of time. By the 19th century, a Russian author named Helena Petrovna Blavatsky began introducing manifestation to the public. She wrote a book called *The Secret Doctrine*, exploring religious doctrines and speaking of our power to shape our reality. Likewise, she said that letting go of any negative thoughts and beliefs holding us back could make our dreams a reality. By pushing past these old hindrances, we can manifest anything we desire.

Thomas Troward, a 19th-century scholar and author, believed that the power of our mind could manifest what we think about into our reality. He thought whatever we immerse ourselves in, be it good or bad, would become an integral part of us. Meanwhile, his ideas toward manifestation, such as his influence on the Law of Cause and Effect, were known to have inspired the movie, *The Secret*. Troward believed that *"our mind is a center of divine operations"* and that *"the subconscious mind accepts uncritically whatever suggestion may be impressed upon it, and works out in great fidelity whatever may logically follow from the suggestion"* (n.d).

Ancient theologians and authors, who have studied spiritual and religious doctrines for many years, came to a similar conclusion about the way our minds interact with the laws of the universe; *a new-age university professor did not introduce this manifestation in our time but instead had existed for a long time.*

The Science Behind It

When we think about scientific procedures and process, scientist is passionate about experimentation. They will take an idea and mesh various substances together with a vision to form something. Yet, some scientists, like Alexander Fleming, would go on to create tangible things by mistake. In the early 1900s, Fleming was experimenting in his lab when he decided to pause his work to go on vacation. Upon his return, he noticed mold and bacteria growing in the dish he was working on because it was left slightly open. This mold became the development of penicillin, which is a common drug used today to counteract various infections.

Manifestation is like working in a laboratory of the mind. Establishing our goals and taking action to make them a reality requires a strong, unwavering faith that we can change our lives if we genuinely believe it is possible. We must have the conviction that this is possible and then take the necessary steps to make it happen. Likewise, translating thoughts into tangible, physical creations is all about doing whatever it takes to make it happen. This concept relates to taking action and pushing ourselves toward our goals. It takes hard work, stamina, complete dedication to our craft, and keeping our eye on the prize. Like Thomas Edison creating the light bulb, it took him and his team over 3,000 tries of trial and error to form the first light bulb that worked.

Many scientists have also studied the brain and its extraordinary capabilities. They have concluded that by the time we hit 20 years old, our brains have accumulated ten times more knowledge than the Encyclopedia Britannica. That means we have incredible power within us to visualize our dreams and make them a reality simply by shifting our mindset and taking consistent, inspired action toward our goals.

Becoming a Self-Fulfilling Prophecy

If we choose to, our life can be a self-fulfilling prophecy inspired by the thoughts that inhabit our minds. In all reality, our life is already inspired by these thoughts; if we do not like how our life is being formed right now, we can shift it at any moment.

Undoubtedly, there is no limit to what we can manifest by aligning our minds with the power that has been proven over time. Our capacity for creation, when used intentionally, defies all boundaries and has a timeless efficacy. Through harnessing this power of intention and thought, everything is achievable. As such, star athletes use the power of manifestation to visualize the championship before every competition. Meanwhile, celebrities use the power of affirmations to choose the life they want and the opportunities that come their way.

Using manifestation, we can become our self-fulfilling prophecy. We can prove that others need to believe in their dream life. Yet, if you do not think you will make headway on your goals based on brain research, you are right. But if you shifted your mindset and stepped into positive goal-driven energy, chances are you will amaze yourself. The things you can create simply by thinking about them will be extraordinary. And believe it or not, science has shown that success is sometimes achievable with what we have been led to believe.

For example, you go to bed in a foul mood after a heated exchange with your partner. Disappointed that no resolution was made and angered at the lack of apology from your other half, negative energy fills your being. It is no surprise that this has become a self-fulfilling prophecy as thoughts about the argument keep playing through your head. You cannot help but feel more disgruntled when you spot your partner sound asleep as if nothing had occurred. Hours later, it is time to wake up for work, and you feel like an explosion is imminent. To add fuel to the fire, there is no good morning wish from your partner, only further frustration mounting within you, as if this was not enough trouble already. Likewise, breakfast takes forever while simultaneously getting burned, and your dog decides it is time to relieve itself on the floor. As reality comes crashing down around you, you realize that you neglected laundry last night due to all the quarreling and now have nothing clean to wear, increasing the annoyance towards yourself and maybe even your partner. Your remaining patience is put on thin ice as it resonates in your mind: *"Someone else better not annoys me today!"* So, the universe says, *your wish is my command.*

Feeling overwhelmed and exhausted, you treat yourself to a coffee, only for the barista to get your order wrong. Then, someone even cuts in front of you in line, and an argument ensues. Subsequently, you make it to work only to be laid off by your boss, who informs you that your assistant called in sick. All these feel as if everything was conspiring against you, resulting in the worst day (or week) ever.

Overall, things did not go so well with your partner last night. Despite trying to resolve this, you both went to bed without common ground. That left you feeling worn out, filled with negativity, and completely unappreciative. Breaking all this down can be tough, but you must understand why these feelings arose. This negative behavior shifts the entire trajectory of how your day unfolds. Now, your brain's reticular activating system (RAS) is piqued and alert. We will discuss more how your RAS works in pillar five, so it searches for other ways to fuel your current energy. In short, the more negative energy you transfer into the universe, the more you receive in your life; it becomes a vast ripple effect of unending negativity unless you wake up one day and decide otherwise.

To manifest a favorable self-fulfilling prophecy, spreading positivity around us is essential. It always begins with three things:

- Your thoughts
- Your behavior
- Your beliefs

Believing in yourself and having an optimistic outlook can lead to a beautiful day. Have faith that you will wake up on time, motivated and beaming with positivity, and the universe will respond to your energy by providing what you desire.

The Law of Attraction is familiar to most of us, but what about the other 11 laws? In the next pillar, we will dive deeper into each one, so you can better understand how to use them for your manifestation goals. With the knowledge of the physics laws that enable manifestation, you will be well on your way to achieving success.

Pillar Two
Laws

Many of us are familiar with the notion that *"like attracts like,"* famously known as the Law of Attraction. This idea is explored in Rhonda Byrne's book *The Secret* and is also referred to in the movie of the same name. *But what about the Law of Polarity? Or the Law of Gender, or even the Law of Vibration?* Together with eight other laws, they make up the Laws of Manifestation, universal principles that align with our spiritual being and allow us to open up an energetic portal for manifestation.

Manifesting our dream life is not only a matter of understanding the Law of Attraction; it is about utilizing all twelve laws. Partnering with the universe is how we can truly become an energetic match for what we desire out of life. Knowing this means understanding how to use each law in its totality, allowing us to manifest our desired reality.

This pillar is about introducing you to the twelve universal laws, which can help us keep pushing forward despite life's challenges. Applying these laws will not magically make your life perfect, but it will bring positivity, abundance, clarity, and contentment. Understanding them will enable you to live intentionally, compassionately, and with understanding.

Law of Oneness

All living creatures are inextricably linked and part of a common cosmic symphony. Each of these breathing organisms is connected to an abundant energy source that pulses around us. Nothing happens in the universe without us, humans, birds, trees, plants, mammals, flowers, and sea animals, feeling or experiencing it. This connection is like an invisible string that binds us together in one universal force. Think of it like an energetic vibration that unites us all.

Being mindful of our intrinsic link with the world is essential to understand that anything we do, think, and feel affects all of us. When we express negativity to ourselves, it is reflected in our behavior and radiates outwards. Like the people closest to us, our pets are sensitive to this energy. This negativity has far-reaching consequences, eliciting emotions from sadness and frustration to disappointment and anxiety. Interestingly, those surrounding us may also display similar negative vibes, leaving us wondering where they might be coming from. Indeed, since everything is connected at an energetic level, it stands to reason that our energy frequency resonates with that of other living creatures in our environment.

This is the same with happy, uplifting energy. Our positivity and good vibes can be contagious. Those shared moments of joy can help make the world a better place. When we recognize this fundamental idea that we are all connected, it gives us the strength to move forward and use it as our partner on the journey. Gratitude and expression of happiness bring an energy that is both uplifting and inspiring, a feeling of oneness that we should never let go of.

Law of Vibration

The Law of Vibration works in conjunction with the Law of Attraction. Just as the first law states that we are all connected in a universally divine way, it is essential to remember that each of us and non-tangible objects vibrate on a particular vibrational frequency.

When I say non-tangible, I mean items such as desks, ceilings, and the floor, objects that are not living organisms but vibrate on a slower frequency, regardless. As humans, we are always moving and constantly on the go. Therefore, we vibrate at a higher frequency.

To manifest what we want, we need to become an energetic match for them. For example, if you desire to manifest $100,000, you must find a way to become an energetic match for that amount. If you have no idea what that looks like, you can ask yourself these questions:

- What would I be doing?
- How would I present myself?
- How would I make decisions?
- Where would I be hanging out?
- Who would I be hanging out with?
- How would I handle my emotions?

Asking the right questions can bring you closer to your goal of manifesting $100,000. To begin this process, it is essential to identify the way of being and frequency level that larger sums of money operate on. This can be a challenge if you have only been used to working with smaller sums, such as $10,000 or $50,000. So, to match this frequency and truly experience its abundance, you must learn to understand and appreciate it on its unique level. Becoming conscious of what this frequency is capable of will enable you to create the experiences necessary to manifest your desired outcome.

Law of Correspondence

Bre Brown of Modern Manifestation describes the Law of Correspondence as *"what happens around us is a direct reflection of what is happening within us" (2021).* How you feel about yourself reflects how the world perceives and reacts to you. Everything is interconnected, and your inner self directly influences your external environment.

In other words, the reality you are living now is merely a reflection. Maybe you cannot quite understand why you have not achieved as much as you had liked. But it may be due to feelings of scarcity or lack, or self-doubt and fear of failure, which take precedence over any opportunity for success. As such, fear often takes its toll on your prospects, preventing you from taking risks and pushing yourself ahead. This can lead to a cycle of never-ending scarcity and the need to always stay in survival mode. That might be difficult to accept, but do not lose hope; there is still a chance to turn things around.

The more self-aware and candid you can be with yourself, the more successful your journey of growth and change will be. Ergo, replace negative emotions towards your actions or inactions with positive affirmations and show yourself kindness so that what you experience externally reflects how you feel internally. A great way to do this is by practicing the Law of Correspondence. When you believe something good about yourself, that belief manifests into reality. Likewise, find time for self-compassion and understanding as you grow, learn, and progress through life. Granting yourself grace is not easy, but it is crucial in facilitating a healthy inner landscape that will translate positively into our external world.

Law of Attraction

Many people live by the famous law that "like attracts like," and it is all about having a clear mental picture of what you are trying to manifest. For example, if you want a car, you should create a vivid visual of the exact type of car you desire and allow yourself to experience the feeling of owning it. When you take on this mindset, believing that the item is already yours, your energy vibration will match that of owning such an item. Visualizing this in your mind will also help align your thoughts and emotions to attract whatever it is that you wish for actively. As such, focusing on positive thoughts and feelings can help draw things into your life more smoothly.

Meanwhile, radiating negative energy will likely reflect on your life. For the Law of Attraction to work in your favor, practicing positivity and maintaining good mental health is crucial. Refrain from being cruel to yourself, start noticing the good things in your life, and focus on thoughts that make you feel more optimistic about what may come. By eliminating negativity from your mind, you can open yourself up to limitless possibilities; this power should never be underestimated.

The Law of Attraction works like this: Your mental attitude directly affects your life's outcome. When you think positively, creating desirable circumstances is easier. But if you fill yourself with negativity, those same issues will be reflected in the results. Hence, *a positive outlook leads to positive results, while a negative mindset will bring about similarly dismal results.*

Remember the example I shared in pillar one? An argument before bed can leave frustration and annoyance, which will likely still be present when you wake up the following day. Even everyday tasks like making breakfast seem to take forever. Likewise, things like not having clean clothes for work or a barista messing up your coffee order can all be enough to set you off. These minor inconveniences can worsen a bad day and leave a draining feeling; this is an example of a negative ripple effect of pure frustration. Such a case is the opposite of the Law of Attraction. Instead of "like attracts like," it was more like "dislike attracts dislike." Indeed, not a pleasant experience or feeling amidst such a gloomy atmosphere.

But what could happen if you shifted your annoyance and frustration to gratefulness and humility? Chances are, after pushing through the challenge, you and your partner settle into bed feeling grateful for each other. You wake up refreshed, saying good morning to each other with a kiss. Greet your children with enthusiasm, and before long, everyone is ready for breakfast. The two of you enjoy a delicious meal together before getting on with your day and feeling renewed, knowing that you have resolved whatever had been causing friction. You head to the coffee shop and are warmly welcomed by the barista, treating you to a complimentary muffin for being an incredible customer. Upon reaching work, your boss calls you to their office and offers you a promotion that makes you feel elated. Full of cheer and enthusiasm, your assistant asked how your weekend had been while they settled into their daily routine. All these were a great start to the day.

See the difference between feeling frustrated the night before to feeling energetic, motivated, and optimistic? The Law of Attraction is a matter of simple perception. Desiring to manifest extraordinary things requires your feelings and thoughts to hold the same positive energy.

Law of Action

By taking inspired action, you can manifest your dreams and bring yourself closer to the things you want. It is a powerful tool that works hand-in-hand with the Law of Attraction. When approached positively, these two forces can produce beautiful results. However, it is important to note that they will only do something if you take action. For instance, while simply dreaming of a far-off destination is excellent, it will only amount to a little once you start taking steps toward making it happen. This could involve writing down why it is your dream vacation spot and adding it to your vision board or researching the area and budgeting for the trip. Taking action in an inspired way will help bring your vision into reality quicker than just thinking about it alone. *Yet, the Law of Action is not about taking the right action; it is about choosing to take a step, no matter what.* To be frank, we have no idea what can happen when we take action, but we know that we are taking the next step, and the outcome will be revealed to us when it is time.

Despite that, people fearing the unknown paralyze and keep them from achieving their goals. To combat this, we must take action, no matter the outcome. While it might not always lead to the desired result, it still teaches valuable lessons about perseverance and resilience. Taking small steps towards our goal can also help build courage and push past our fears. Aside from that, learning we may fail should not stop us from trying since any experience gained will benefit us in the long run. And if we successfully take action, we reap the rewards of our efforts and get closer to achieving our manifested desires. Likewise, in finding out what lies ahead, we must take the first step regardless of how scary or uncertain it may seem. Either way, it is a win-win and meant for celebration.

Alongside that, many people wrongly assume that using the Law of Attraction is enough to receive their desired outcome without effort. It appears too good to be true; if it were, as such, everybody in the world would have their wishes come true while they sit on the couch watching TV. However, this is not the case. The power of manifestation is realized when we combine positive affirmations with taking action toward our goals. When we take the time to understand this concept better, our dreams can manifest at just the right times. By combining visualization techniques with hard work and dedication, we can achieve our goals more quickly. This process can help us foster meaningful growth and transformation in our lives— something that could otherwise not be accomplished by sitting idle and hoping for something to happen.

Law of Perpetual Transmutation of Energy

By surrounding ourselves with positive energy, internally and externally, we can create a flow of uplifting emotion that radiates out into the world. This idea of positivity in motion has profound implications: when we let go of negative thinking, our internal state shifts in a way that resonates throughout the universe. On the other hand, if we focus on gratitude and happiness, these positive vibrations spread outwards and bring balance to our environment. As you intentionally cultivate an attitude of contentment and joy, you can manifest positive energy that reverberates in both personal and communal life.

For instance, the consequences are usually dire if you stay in negative energy. Likely, you may experience job loss, anxiety, unhealthy relationships, and an overall feeling that life is bleak. Subsequently, you can become overwhelmed with bills and have more bad days than good. But recognizing your negativity and taking steps to counter it through practicing gratitude can rewire your thought patterns and attract more positive experiences. Focusing on the good things in life can make joy, opportunity, contentment, and security you put forth the effort to shift your mindset away from negative thinking.

Replacing negative energy with positive and abundant feelings can be transformational. You can manifest the relationships, experiences, and resources you desire, such as a fulfilling partnership, an exciting vacation, loving friendships that offer encouragement and support, and financial security. These possibilities create a radically different atmosphere than one filled with negativity. Then, instead of fear or worry, you will experience joy, excitement, gratitude, and contentment.

Clearly, this law is about how we choose to transmute our internal energy. Learning to manifest constant positive energy can lead to a few things:

- Surrounding yourself with positive people that become your circle of influence. When you surround yourself with positive energy, your internal energy will translate into the same.
- Having better-feeling thoughts. Be kind to yourself and show self-compassion every day. Treat yourself with the love and respect you deserve so it flows back to you.
- Becoming a constant co-creator with the universe. The universe usually gives you what you want when you ask for it. Perhaps it is not in the moment, but as long as you are taking inspired action toward your goals, the universe will help make things happen.
- Constantly feeling abundant and grateful. As long as you already think abundant, despite what you do not have, the universe will conspire with you to give you more while helping you release attachment to the outcome. Feel grateful for what you have now, as gratefulness aligns with positive energy, which helps bring more abundance your way.

All these things can help transmute your energy into abundance and positivity. When your energy exhibits a flow of this caliber, you will notice that it feels easier to manifest exactly what you want rather than manifest negatively because you are transmuting negative energy within you.

With anything you learn about manifestation in this book, understand that the way you transmute your energy into the world is the way that you will manifest. Knowing this, you will find a way to shift your energy from negative to positive, so your life can drastically change for the better.

Law of Cause and Effect

Newton says, *"For every action, there is an equal and opposite reaction."* Every action you take has a certain effect on your life. This feels pretty straightforward, but in reality, many of us forget how this law can play into our lives. Nothing can really happen if we do not take a single action in our life. *Pretty simple, right?* Due to this, we cannot realistically expect to manifest what we want if we do not take a single step toward our goals.

When you entertain a scarcity mindset, it can hurt your life. This could manifest itself through feelings of lack, stress, anxiety, or worry. It is worth noting that by not doing anything to strive for your desired outcome, you still took action. Because it will still give you a result. It might not be the results you wanted, but results, nonetheless. The Law of Cause and Effect emphasizes how our choices and behaviors in the present shape our future circumstances. That's why having a proactive attitude is essential if you want financial freedom and abundance.

Once you become aware of this, the best thing to do is make the shift. Instead of getting anxious over a possible future and clouding your mind with stress and pessimism, practice positive thinking and take action for what you truly want to create. This will help you craft the life of your dreams from the steps you take based on those inspired decisions. The results of these decisions become a vast ripple effect portrayed in our lives. Many of us believe that nothing good comes from our actions, but I choose to have a different outlook. Even if things did not work out the way I expected, I still feel grateful for the lessons I have learned throughout the journey. I have taken the actions I was guided to take; therefore, the results become an energetic match and will continue aligning in the way they are meant to be.

Every action we take or do not take has a consequence; this is the belief of this law. Negative actions, such as lacking gratitude or waiting for things to come to you, will result in unfavorable reactions. As such, we would not get what we want, experience constant scarcity, or feel a lack. *So, how can you use this law to your advantage and achieve extraordinary effects?* To do this, you must understand that every action has an equal reaction and be conscious of your behavior to ensure the desired outcomes. Likewise, you must—

- Understand why you are taking the actions. If it feels inspiring, you will move forward with it and experience beautiful results because of it.
- Embrace everything, both pleasant and unpleasant; make peace with all that shapes your life's path, and appreciate every single part.
- Be clear on the results you want to achieve. When you have clarity, you will know what actions to take so the results can manifest.
- Trust yourself and the universe. The results may not be what you expected them to be, but eventually, you will understand that they are so much better.
- Surrender to what is meant to be. Release complete attachment to the outcome. Know and believe that your actions are more than enough to manifest what you desire and allow the universe to do its thing.

In short, to spark change and transformation, take the inspired actions required to invoke that change.

Law of Compensation

Have you ever heard the saying, *"what goes around comes around"*? The Law of Compensation is a universal principle that aligns with this notion: *whatever energy and actions you put into the world will be repaid with the same.* Be mindful of this when considering your actions and how they may come back to you; think positive, positive returns. When you dwell on negative actions and attitudes, it will cast a shadow on your life. As the saying goes, "Karma will get you." On the contrary, when you exude positive energy, you can expect to be rewarded for your efforts. Remember, it is all about sowing good seeds.

Helping and serving others can be rewarding, but you may find that the universe pays you back. The Law of Compensation is linked to your perceptions; taking positive steps toward fulfilling your dreams will bring back the same energy from the universe. Likewise, this law relates to your mentality. Keeping an outlook of lack or insecurity will only lead to more instances that confirm those feelings. On the contrary, having a mindset of abundance and self-love will draw forth more love and a wellspring into your life.

The actions you take determine how you are compensated. If you are ungrateful for the things you currently have, chances are you will not receive more for a while. But if you are eternally grateful for all that you have, you will receive more things to be grateful for. *See how this works?* When you think about it, it is instead a simple concept. Bottom line, *say thank you for all that you have, and the universe will say, "you are welcome."*

As Wayne Dyer famously quoted, *"When you change the way you look at things, the things you look at change."* This simple phrase exemplifies the Law of Compensation; an example demonstrated daily. If we take a moment to reframe our perspective, the objects we observe will likewise be altered. So, when you are facing hard times, finding ways to shift your outlook in your mind and reality is essential. Yet, focusing on the struggles and all the intense emotions that come with them, such as fear, stress, anxiety, disappointment, or worry, you will notice that same energy in the physical world. Perhaps, it is terrible news taking over your social media feeds, family appearing grumpy more often, or a sense of self-loathing; each can become an obstacle when attempting to tackle challenging situations and only make things worse. Somehow it feels like all these negative feelings have skyrocketed overnight, and you wonder if there is ever an end in sight. However, there is hope if you work on controlling your mindset and finding the light at the end of the tunnel.

Clearly, a reminder of The Law of Compensation is that at any moment, you have the power to change your mindset. Every 24 hours allows us to go about our day with positive actions and attitudes. However, if we do not do this and would instead view things from a pessimistic viewpoint, it is entirely up to us.

The Law of Relativity

The Law of Relativity, also referred to as the Law of Perspective, explains how everything is relative. As such, everything in your life is always happening, so you can learn, grow, and celebrate. Yet, it also greatly depends on your perspective of why things are happening. Depending on the way you perceive the situation, it can lead to either success or failure. For example, we can go through a traumatic breakup, and our minds can have two different perspectives:

1. *Why do bad things always happen to me? Why do I always attract the wrong people? What is wrong with me? Am I not lovable?* Or;
2. *What can I learn from this breakup so it does not happen again? How has it made me stronger? More confident? Resilient?*

Perspective can make a world of difference in our outlook on life. We have the choice to either remain emotionally distant, believing that we are undeserving of good fortune and abundance, or to look ahead toward the potential for self-improvement. When faced with certain situations, these experiences have likely been granted to us so that we can understand them and become more resilient if they arise again. As we progress, our journey may lead us toward becoming a better version of ourselves.

On the Law of Relativity, our perspective means more to us and our manifestations than we may realize. Suppose you desire to manifest your dream vehicle, and it does not show up when you expected it to. In that case, you can either believe that manifestation does not work and you will never get the car, or you can assume that your dream car will show up when it is meant to. Until then, you must be grateful for the car you have now and keep taking inspired action until it arrives, regardless of how long it takes.

Notice the difference in energy?

Half the population will offer a negative perspective on the situations they experience. Meanwhile, the other half will think positively and still believe that everything is possible and that there is pure potential in the world. Think about the *"glass empty or full"* analogy. *What do you believe? Is the glass half full? Or is it half empty?* Your perspective of this analogy will determine how the Law of Relativity shows up in your life.

Law of Polarity

The Law of Polarity is about understanding that everything in life comes in pairs. Negativity versus positivity, light versus darkness, white versus black, healthy versus sick, self-doubt versus confidence—everything that makes us both human and spirit has an opposite partner attached to it. When we understand this perspective, we know how to shift our minds, attitude, and behavior to see the brighter side of the not-so-great experiences we may witness, and then we have something to look forward to.

Life is full of duality; we understand this well. Consider when you are launching a business, and suddenly something happens, like a family member getting sick or your partner asking for a divorce. You can either feel like the world is ending and question whether you should pursue it or take it in stride and trust that you will learn valuable lessons about resilience, strength, and personal growth. These moments give us chances to learn how best to handle our lives no matter how difficult they become.

Some may believe they are being punished because they want to do something good, but the universe is not around for punishment. One thing remains true no matter how dark it gets; light always finds a way. This is the Law of Polarity, reminding us that no matter what happens, there is an undeniable balance in our lives. Just as we can hold the goodness that shows up in our lives, we also have the strength and the money to move through the darkness when faced with a challenge. According to the Law of Polarity, we can gain valuable insight and knowledge from our experiences while still being able to choose how we view them. Through each choice, we can make the most out of any situation and grow in different ways.

Law of Rhythm

As the seasons transition, so can you. Being mindful of the Law of Rhythm is essential for realizing your desires; all that is required is to move through life's peaks and valleys and accept what fate has in store for you. It means letting go of what you can't control and embracing those that you're unable to change.

There are a few things to remember when focusing on this law:

- Let go of the past. Feeling stuck, never moving forward, does not allow you to move in the rhythmic flow of life.

- Enjoy life exactly how the experiences are meant to play out in your life. They may not be the greatest experiences, but they are moments of lessons and growth. Trust them.
- Release negativity and find ways to move forward positively.
- Let go of the person you once were, so you can flow and align yourself with the person you are meant to become—your next-level self.

Have you ever wanted something extraordinary, like a dream job or more money in your bank account, yet it never comes to be? It could be because you are not allowing yourself to move forward abundantly. Likely, you may stop wealth and prosperity from coming your way due to limiting beliefs, and negative emotions held deep within you. Ask yourself, *"are these obstacles holding me back?"* Reflect on these a bit and see how you can make changes to live abundantly. By releasing all the negative energy, you open yourself up to more flow and a positive rhythm that helps open doors to a greater life.

Law of Gender

This law is about achieving harmony and manifesting our goals without struggle. Do not be misled by its name; it has nothing to do with gender or sex. By creating an equilibrium between masculine and feminine energy, we can find joy, peace, and tranquility. Achieving balance is the secret to unlocking a life of happiness and contentment.

For those new to understanding masculine and feminine energy, here is a simple breakdown between the two. Masculine energy is about actions making your dreams come true. Taking those bold steps, strategizing, formulating a plan of action, and setting goals all require the work of this powerful energy in your life. Through these inspired actions, you can reach the heights you have been aiming for. Meanwhile, feminine energy is a journey of trusting your emotions and embracing life. Knowing how achieving your goals will make you feel will help guide your decisions. Believe that all the things you wish for are already yours, even if they have yet to appear. Allow yourself to be open and receive them when it is time.

In human experience, you cannot have one without the other. You can embrace more masculine energy than feminine energy and vice versa. Yet, you live your life daily with both energies within you. Understanding this concept lets you know how the Law of Gender can work in your life. By creating a beautiful harmonious balance between both energies, the Law of Gender works in your life and aligns your actions so your manifestations can come to fruition.

After breaking down the meaning behind all 12 manifestation laws, comprehend how to apply them to elevate your energetic vibration. When those vibrations match up to the same level as your manifestations, it is a natural occurrence. Learning about the third pillar can be incredibly helpful in grasping and raising that vibration for a more abundant life.

Pillar Three
Vibration

Each one of us has an energetic vibration within us. As humans, we are made up of millions of cells, and these cells produce a wave of vibrational energy. Our world is filled with a constantly buzzing energy. Hear it in your heartbeat and the wind, feel it as your feet touch the ground when you walk, and sense it with every nerve ending in your body. From the unseen rhythms to what you can see, we are surrounded by vibration, an energy that pulsates through us all.

By understanding how vibrational energy works within us, we can manifest our desired abundance, love, health, and spirituality. This chapter will provide an overview of the connection between thoughts, behaviors, and vibrations that flow at the highest frequency for manifestation. Furthermore, we will discuss strategies to elevate our energetic vibration, such as thanksgiving, breathwork practices, meditation, and energy therapy. Knowing the power of our vibrational energy is crucial to achieving a life full of joy.

What Is Vibrational Energy?

Some have described vibrational energy as a *"box of emotions" (Goswami, 2021)*. Experiencing low vibrational energy leads to fear, grief, sadness, worry, stress, and disappointment. Conversely, raising your vibration allows you to recognize the feelings of happiness, peace, joy, abundance, compassion, and unconditional love. By tuning into these emotions more regularly, you can create a happier life with greater contentment.

When manifesting, vibrational energy is about tuning into a positive, energetic frequency that makes you feel excited and grateful to tap into the energy of what you want. Experiencing vibrational energy is like connecting to the Laws of Rhythm, Vibration, and Attraction. Our desire moves us; what we want to do drives our actions. We act out of choice, not necessity. Stepping into a higher vibrational frequency is as if we are choosing to turn up the music so we can no longer hear the white noise in the background that distracts us from achieving our goals. The white noise, also known as negative vibrational energy, could be limiting beliefs, negative self-talk, worry, fear, self-doubt, imposter syndrome, anxiety, lack of self-trust and confidence, and trying to do everything all on our own.

As we all know, our energetic vibration is composed mostly of pure energy, so we must be aware of how we feel. To gauge your energy at the moment, look at what you are listening to on the radio. Hearing dark and heavy tunes that have an isolating effect could signal that something is not right emotionally.

Or if you are more drawn to upbeat and optimistic songs with positive messages, it could mean you are in a celebration mode and feeling good about life. Reflect on the emotions that determine your current vibrational energy; if it is not quite where you want it to be, do not hesitate to redirect.

What Are Vibrational Beings?

Vibrational beings are not any one thing; it is all of us. Our vibrational frequency is a state of being; it is how we live. As we have stated previously, we can be a high vibrational being or operate as a low vibrational being. This depends on how we react to certain situations or experiences and the emotions that drive our reactions to those experiences.

There will be moments in our life when we may feel anxious, stressed, worried, self-doubt, or even at the worst extreme, depressed. In these moments, we are operating as a low vibrational being. We feel lost, perhaps overworked and underappreciated; therefore, our state of being is negative. Remaining in this vibration can be a deterrent that will steer us in the opposite direction of our dreams, as it can create a downward spiral of negative emotions. Without a second thought, we slip into a dark abyss, our minds soon entangled by depression. Before we know it, the feeling has deeply rooted itself within us.

When it comes to manifesting, being in a state of positivity, abundance, and gratitude is essential. Focusing on creating an uplifted, inspired, and empowered mindset is vital for our manifestations to come true. We need to be aware of the frequency we are currently vibrating at and work towards shifting it into one that resonates with these positive energies. Doing this daily can create instantaneous changes in our vibration and make our desires tangible.

Connection of Thoughts, Behaviors, and Vibrations

> "You do not manifest what you want;
> you attract what you are."
>
> *—Francesco Filippazzo*

Connecting with ourselves is simple. Having negative thoughts brings us down to low vibration. This low energy affects our behavior; before we know it, we have manifested what we did not want instead of what we did.

For instance, negative thoughts start to creep in when we lack self-confidence. We tell ourselves our goals will not be achieved and that we do not have the knowledge or experience to succeed. This leads to procrastination, feeling like an imposter, lacking action, and being unmotivated. As such, when potential clients turn down our services, it compounds these feelings of inadequacy, leading us to become less creative and less motivated toward achieving our dreams. Eventually, we may even start doubting the power of manifestation or the Law of Attraction. All of these result from low vibrational frequency; before long, we begin losing sight of our visions and dreams, forgetting who we are, and going through an identity crisis. From that, we can quickly become convinced that failure is inevitable and feeling unhappy is all we deserve.

This is an overreaching example of low vibrational energy, but you can see how deep the connection can be to our behavior, actions, and thoughts. There is a science to this, which I will explain in the following sections so you can gather a deeper understanding of our connection to the universe and ourselves.

The Science of Vibration

Vibrational frequency is a phenomenon for many people. Like other things regarding energetics—affirmations, manifestation, Law of Attraction, spirituality, and God—many people believe that it must not be accurate if you cannot see them physically. Yet, some people struggle to believe in things they cannot see with their own eyes, leading to cynicism about the world around them. This kind of thinking leads to a mistrustful worldview and gives birth to misanthropes.

However, if you were to look at this from a scientific perspective, we know that gravity exists, even if we cannot see it. *How would humans keep their feet on the ground when walking? How would we go headfirst toward the ground if we were to jump off a building? How would astronauts float in the air when they are in space without gravity holding them down?* Gravity is not a tangible product; it is a force of nature that is proven by our actions and behaviors. We cannot physically see gravity, yet, it exists.

This same belief can be brought forth when speaking about vibrational frequency. Though we cannot physically see them, vibrations have a powerful hold over us, especially when it comes to music. We groove to the rhythm of the tunes at parties and feel our favorite songs reverberate within us whenever they come on the radio. There is no denying that the energy of music captivates us completely. As we are connected to different energy sources by a certain vibrational frequency, we can be sure that our manifestations will come to fruition depending on the wavelength we are vibrating on.

Unfortunately, people often think it is not real if they do not see proof of manifestation coming true quickly. We tend to doubt the universe when our desired outcomes do not happen as expected, for example, expecting $10,000 to show up in your account by next month and concluding that manifestation does not work if it does not come through. However, this kind of thinking needs to be revised; evidence of a manifestation can be seen later for us to believe in its power. Even if what we want is not brought into our lives instantly, that is still no indication that it can never exist.

When it comes to vibration, it may seem odd at first glance. However, take electricity as an example; it is a natural force that has been around for thousands and years and is found everywhere around the globe *(Wonderopolis, 2019)*. Similarly to the idea of manifestation and gravity, although it cannot be seen with our eyes, it still counts as an absolute concept. Evidence for its realness is all around us; when we turn on our TVs, plug in our laptops to charge them, or put on our morning blender, we realize it is true. The proof that electricity exists lies within us and in science and spirituality, no matter how much we may not be able to witness its effects with sight.

In other words, we cannot physically see the vibration, but that does not mean it does not exist. Vibration is just like electricity. We cannot physically see electricity, but we can feel its energy anytime we do our daily activities. Many things we cannot see with our naked eye are incomprehensible; that is the beauty of science. All of our dreams exist on a specific vibrational frequency. As our current selves, we may not vibrate on the same level as our dreams, but that does not mean our dreams are not meant for us. Taking inspired action every day is vital to achieving our goals. When we put in the effort towards inner growth, we find ourselves resonating at a higher frequency, enabling us to bring our aspirations into physical reality.

Positive and High-frequency Vibration

To better comprehend positive and negative vibrations, start by exploring the science behind vibrational energy. This understanding will allow you to become aware of your vibration levels. In cases when it is on a negative scale, you will know what actions to take to bring it back up.

Positive manifestation operates on a high-level frequency. Many emotions are associated with this level, such as happiness, joy, peace, abundance, gratitude, acceptance, love, and courage. As you feel authentically happy, more things to feel satisfied with flow to you. When you feel peaceful, you become aware and mindful of experiences around you that help instill calm and greater harmony. In short, the more you feel grateful for what you currently have, the more the universe will give you to be grateful for.

For instance, let us say you are striving to make your dream career a reality. Feeling ecstatic and ready for the world, you purchase an outfit that will give you a professional edge in interviews. Likewise, you affirm that this dream job is on its way to you, but weeks go by, and you are still waiting for a response from potential employers. Anxiety and stress may creep in, but it is okay. Remind yourself that your ideal job will come when it is meant to happen, then shift your mindset to be positive again. Send out resumes and create connections with companies while appreciating what your current job has given you, even if it is not the role of your dreams yet. Then, one day, as if by magic, you receive a call from the employer who has captivated your attention. Regardless of its outcome, remain excited and optimistic with gratitude. This chance is to show them your enthusiasm and passion first-hand. As your energy reverberates, they offer you the job.

This example shows that you draw in what reflects your thoughts. If you are sitting around, being cynical about achieving your goals, you might find yourself in a detrimental cycle, likely to bring negative happenings. Conversely, if you take time to motivate and equip yourself and act on impetus towards attaining your objectives, you will be back on track to draw in the outcomes of your desires at a faster rate.

Hence, high-frequency vibration is a science in its own right. What you are today determines what you will attract. If your feelings and emotions are consistently balanced, optimistic, and serene, this will bring more peace, bliss, and joy into your life. However, it can be hard to remain in a positive state all the time. As human beings, we must acknowledge that moments of hardship or despair might come our way but do not have to be discouraging. When we become aware of our mental, physical, and spiritual selves, we can regain the power to transform these moments into more empowering and high-frequency vibrations.

Negative and Low-frequency Vibration

Negative vibration works like this: *The more you think, act, and behave negatively, the more negative experiences you attract into your life.* Low-frequency emotions include stress, worry, fear, anxiety, guilt, shame, pride, grief, and anger. When you feel any of these emotions, you enter a negative energetic frequency that can stop you from receiving what you want. Becoming aware of your feelings is a must to change the energy you are giving off. Taking time to be mindful of our emotions helps us shift into a positive vibe that will attract the things we desire, not what we do not. By recognizing and reorganizing our thoughts, we can move in alignment with manifesting the abundance we long for.

As such, let us assume that you want to manifest the relationship of your dreams. That said, you will need to shift away from the energetic vibrations from past harmful connections. Here is an example; say your desire is for a supportive partner. All too often, your history has been built on toxicity and destruction. Now, they have created an unconscious belief that you are not good enough or worthy of having the relationship you want. Instead of love, resentment lingers; instead of self-acceptance, a sense of unworthiness and lack of appreciation abounds. Gratitude is replaced by feeling undeserving of unconditional love, while feelings of scarcity and lack substitute abundance. All these emotions keep you firmly in the depths of low energy. And when you feel stuck in low energy, you go down a dark rabbit hole of deeper negative emotions, such as anger, doubt, worry, stress, hatred, rejection, and pride.

Fostering these negative emotions can be detrimental, leading to an increased risk of attracting people and situations with the same low vibes, which can cause further damage than you are conscious of. Acknowledging these emotions is essential, as no good will come from them aside from self-awareness and the chance to shift into a better state. Some common signs that you are stuck in a negative spiral are constantly doubting yourself, picking on yourself negatively, speaking badly about others, and continually feeling angry. Recognizing this allows you to work on improving your mental state.

Observation and Self-Awareness

Our day-to-day behavior and habits often become so entrenched that we do not notice how they affect our self-image and how we present ourselves to others. Breaking out of this cycle of negative thoughts and limited beliefs is challenging, but it is possible with a little conscious effort. Practicing self-awareness can help us to identify when unhelpful behavior patterns emerge, allowing us to make the changes necessary to alter those patterns for the better. It takes time and patience, but by being mindful of our actions, we can eventually overcome our default thought processes and develop healthier ones. With enough practice and commitment, these new behaviors will soon become second nature, helping us live more fulfilling lives where we are more at ease with ourselves.

Unfortunately, many people have spent most of their lifetime belittling themselves and embracing their limiting beliefs. These are the same people who want to change their lives and transform their mindset, but they do not know how, so they continue to run around on the hamster wheel of life, never moving forward. Yet, to make a difference, one can start taking the time to observe and practice self-awareness. As such, slow your conversations when speaking with others so you can notice the words you use. Intentionally pay attention to the way you talk to yourself by bringing these words to your conscious state of mind. Then, if your loved one is in a lousy mood, compliment them. Counteract their behavior with positive sentiments. Tell them you love them, how grateful you are for their presence in your life, and what you love about them. Surely, you will notice a shift in their energy immediately. On the other hand, the worst thing you can do in this situation is to join them in their negative energy.

In pillar six, we will go into further detail, but the bottom line is that your words can enhance or diminish somebody's life and your own. Ergo, your speech has the power to alter your destiny. Remember this as you speak to someone and yourself. Since this power is within you, it can instantly raise your vibration and others. By becoming aware and observing your energy and the energy of those around you, you can transform your mindset and others, making your environment an empowering place to be in.

Raising Your Vibration

Now that you have a deeper understanding of the differences between positive and negative vibration, there are many ways that you can implement this right away that will help you raise your vibration. Manifesting positively is about three essential things: *taking inspired action, being intentional with who you are and where you are currently, and feeling grateful for what you have.* Here are some ways to raise your vibration to a higher energetic frequency for a more abundant life.

Love

Love is amongst the highest forms of energetic vibration. Simply put, if you want to raise your vibration immediately, express love to others and yourself. Tell your loved ones how much you love them, express compassion and care for those in need, look in the mirror daily, and tell yourself how much you love and appreciate yourself.

Aside from that, you can also think of the people you love and how they bring joy to your life. A unique way of meditating and visualizing them can raise your vibration instantly. Relax in a quiet area, free from distractions. Recall their smile, laughter, and conversations with you; what they do makes you feel warm inside. Remember the last talk you had and activities like making dinner for you, calling to say hi, or even bringing chicken soup when work or illness drained your energy. Performing this exercise frequently will lift your energetic vibration quickly.

Showing affection is a simple act that can make immense changes in your life and those around you. *The more love you share, the higher your energy vibration is, and the more your outlook shifts.*

Forgiveness

To raise your vibration, forgiveness is an important one. When you are in a negative state of mind, feelings of guilt, shame, anger, annoyance, and frustration toward yourself and those around you can cause your energetic frequency to plummet. Likewise, this will only attract more negativity into your life. Although it may feel difficult, you must learn to forgive, not just for your well-being but for the well-being of others.

Of course, forgiveness does not happen overnight, as it takes time to process, analyze, and heal. Yet, writing a letter to yourself and others is proven effective when learning to forgive. You do not have to give it to the person if you choose not to; however, writing your thoughts and how you feel toward the situation rather than keeping them bottled up inside has been proven to help you effectively heal. Suppose you are in the process of forgiving yourself. In that case, you can also write a forgiveness letter to yourself apologizing for being a self-inflicted bully and beating you up instead of offering unconditional love and support. Through the process of forgiveness, you can release all the negative weight and excess baggage that is weighing you down, which in turn, makes room for positive and empowering energy.

Use Your Five Senses

Raising your vibration is about focusing on positive energy in and around you. There is abundance everywhere you look. Feeling abundant is one of the highest forms of positive energy. Learning to use all five senses will help you notice every area of abundance in your life.

- **Smell:** Take notice of the things that smell beautiful around you. The flowers, trees, coffee brewing in the morning, preparing your meals, having a glass of wine, the scent of a baby's skin, your bubble bath, the shampoo and conditioner as you lather your hair in the shower, your partner's cologne, how you smell after you first get out of the shower, the lotion you lather your body with—your nose is engulfed with scents every day. For a fun, sweet-smelling surprise, you can also walk to your favorite bakery or bake some cookies and take in how delicious they smell. Noticing simple things about our everyday life and breathing them in can help raise your vibration and experience gratitude.
- **See:** Acknowledge all the beauty around you. The way your partner smiles at you, the way they look at you, the infinite beauty of the flowers and other parts of nature, when the snow falls on the ground and glistens in the moonlight, watching a romantic movie with your loved ones, witnessing the beauty of the sunrise or sunset, reading inspiring words to start your day, reading your favorite book, the looks on your family's faces when you bring dinner to the table, their expressions when the meal is delicious—there is so much beauty around us that we can view with our naked eye.
- **Hear:** Beautiful sounds can raise our energy. Hearing your partner's voice on the phone when they call you simply because they are thinking of you, listening to your favorite song or band, hearing your dog bark when they are happy to see you, listening to an empowering podcast about personal growth, your children's laughter, the sound of a

payment notification, the unexpected call from a friend you have not heard from in a long time, a high energy song on the radio.
- **Taste:** Experiencing the kiss of your special someone, having a spoonful of your favorite ice cream or dessert, savoring a delicious home-cooked meal made by your partner, sipping on an exquisite glass of wine or cocktail, or even just taking a gulp of refreshing water—all these can excite and tantalize your taste buds. When this happens, you feel as if an energetic spark has been ignited within you.
- **Feel:** From the smoothness of your partner's skin to petting your cat when you return home, take a moment to notice the feel-good moments that happen in daily life. The loofah gliding over your body in the shower, the hot water and bubbles in a bath, and the musical rhythm as you dance to your favorite songs are all reasons to express love and gratitude. Feel the warmth of hugs from your kids every night before bed, or try gripping hands with your loved one if it has been a while since you have seen them. Do not forget how amazing it feels when someone compliments you or how great it is to make someone else feel special. Finally, take pride in completing projects, or rejoice in celebratory moments. By simply being aware of these positives around you and how they make you feel, your vibration at that moment can be raised exponentially.

Breathwork

The pace of our lives can often be overwhelming, leading to stress and anxiety. Practices like breathwork offer us a chance to find solace in the present and break away from the hustle and bustle. We often become so preoccupied with everyday tasks that we forget to prioritize living in the here and now and focus on surviving. Breathwork is a great way to pause, take a deep breath, and re-focus on the present, a guide for peace and tranquility.

Deep breathing helps you focus more on what truly matters: finding peace. Peace is a high vibe feeling. When you feel constant peace, despite what is happening around you, you vibrate at a higher frequency, allowing you to manifest more easily. There are many benefits to breathwork:

- Feeling calm
- Mindfulness
- Increases positivity
- Sense of peace
- Releases stress and anxiety
- Sense of joy and fulfillment
- Improves bodily functions, such as the heart and lungs

Meditation

Meditating is another excellent way of focusing on the present moment. It allows you to focus on the present and instills peace, joy, fulfillment, and a sense of purpose. Likewise, it helps remind you that you have a purpose on this planet and offers you abundance and prosperity. Combining breathwork while meditating is also great, as it allows you to focus more intentionally on how your body feels. Lastly, through meditation, you can dive into your emotions and understand how you are feeling.

Under pressure, meditation is a great way to alleviate this feeling and focus on finding inner peace if you are feeling anxious. Regular practice can help you identify where this anxiety stems from so you can be freed from it. Besides, meditating only takes a few minutes to raise your vibration and reap its long-term benefits. However, consistency is critical to fully experiencing these effects.

There are many ways to meditate. Some of the common ways are listed below:

- **Sitting with your legs crossed, eyes closed, and palms facing up in a receiving position.** Going for a guided meditation can be an enjoyable experience, or you may opt for the quiet practice of paying attention to your internal sensations and environmental noises. This silent meditation can help center your energy, allowing you to achieve higher vibrations without distractions. Focus solely on yourself and your surroundings and remember to note any changes.
- **Laying down on your back in a comfortable position.** Close your eyes and take a few moments to immerse yourself in the calming experience of your favorite meditation music. Let the soundwaves wash over you and drift away on a journey of relaxation. Allow yourself to relax as the music envelops you completely. On the other hand, you can choose to focus on your breathwork. Forget about anything happening around you and focus on deep breathing to find a sense of calm and peace.
- **With crystals and chakras.** Placing crystals on your heart, sacral, or solar plexus chakras can raise high vibrational energy. Clear quartz, rose quartz, citrine, and amethyst are perfect for this purpose. Intend to focus intensely while taking slow and steady breaths; you will soon feel the positive effects of crystal energy.

Gratitude

> **"You cannot feel fear or anger while feeling gratitude at the same time."**
>
> *–Tony Robbins*

Appreciating all you have in life puts out a positive energy and karma that rewards you in return. Expressing gratitude for what you possess today brings more to be thankful for in the future. Hence, being grateful for your current state is essential for achieving higher levels of joy.

To put gratitude into motion, here are a couple of exercises you can participate in:

- **Start a gratitude journal.** In being grateful, small things can be just as important as the big ones. Challenge yourself to come up with five things to be thankful for. It may seem easy, but it is surprisingly difficult for many people. For example, you could express gratitude for that morning cup of coffee made by your partner or the sun streaming in through your window and waking you up with its warm glow. But even if those things do not feel like much, they are worth reflecting on and appreciating. So, take time to focus on what makes you happy, no matter how insignificant it may seem.
- **Seize a moment to look around you and notice everything you are surrounded by.** Breathe them in and feel grateful for them. Take notice of them. Recognize the everyday wonders in life. Appreciate how amazing it is to have a partner that loves you, your children's joyous laughter, and the sheer delight of being welcomed by your pup each day. Cherish the sustenance that nourishes you—food and water. Show gratitude to those around you, like your neighbor who clears the path for you and the air that carries us all on its gentle breeze. Acknowledge each morning for letting you open your eyes to another opportunity in life. Overall, gratitude is a simple yet powerful emotion we often take for granted when fear, stress, and anxiety overtake us. Likewise, to get into a higher vibrational state of consciousness, feel grateful for who you are and what you have now.

Generosity

To lift your energetic frequency, look for ways to be more generous. Refrain from giving away all your resources but find ways to support those in need. Draw in the same energy you are radiating; if you desire financial prosperity and fertility, consider offering some of this abundance. Similarly, if you hope for a beautiful connection with a partner, focus on building positive relationships with the individuals around you.

In terms of vibrational frequency, compassion and generosity are higher. Meanwhile, scarcity and lack are not; therefore, you stay on the low vibration scale if you feel stingy with your money and your help. But if you do all that you can to offer your support and service to those around you, you feel generous, and it makes you feel good, instilling positivity in your spirit. Positivity leads to good fortune.

Diet

Eating food and consuming drinks that give you a lot of energy is essential. By creating a well-balanced diet, you consume more energy-rich food than food that does not offer you the nutrients and energy you need, such as junk food, sugar-based food, or food that contains high amounts of carbohydrates or sodium. Food such as these keeps you in a low vibrational state and produces fatigue, anxiety, bloatedness, and sleep deprivation, which can make you feel sick, lack focus and motivation, and increase stress. Hence, *the more natural, the better.*

Food and drinks that are high in energy include:

- Organic fruit and veggies (not frozen peas, strawberries, or other fruits and veggies that come from your freezer)
- Avocados
- Food that is high in protein, such as eggs and fish
- Beans and legumes
- Nuts
- Water
- Organic and natural fruit juices
- Green drinks and smoothies
- Teas

Energy Therapy

Energy therapy has proven to be effective for many, many years. These techniques combine spiritual forces of energy in and around you in order to create a hormonal balance that promotes health and well-being. There are times that we feel stuck and confused, and it seems like we are doing everything right, but our internal energy still feels off. Participating in the form of energy therapy can help balance our energy and alleviate any internal blockages that are getting in the way.

There are various types of energy therapy that you can participate in that will greatly help in raising your vibration:

- **Reiki:** With reiki, we can learn to harness our own inner strength and start the process of recovery. Through scientific research, scientists have proven that we have the power within us to heal ourselves; reiki is performed using the foundation of this belief. A professionally trained practitioner can use universal powers combined with the client's energetic frequency to help promote the body's natural ability to heal. Many people diagnosed with cancer and other illnesses have undergone reiki therapy sessions and seen positive effects.
- **Acupuncture:** Drawing from the science of Chinese medicine, acupuncture is an energy therapy designed to create balance and harmony in your body. The therapy includes puncturing the client's skin using many pin-shaped needles and strategically placing them along various meridian points in the body. Using these meridian points, acupuncture is meant to help the client's internal energy re-balance and re-calibrate so they can live healthier lives. Acupuncture can treat various issues, including headaches, back pain, joint pain, fibromyalgia, and women who are experiencing labor pains. When we experience physical pain, it is usually because our internal energy is imbalanced; therefore, it manifests into physical pain. Alleviating this pain helps you experience internal and external healing.
- **Therapeutic Touch:** Encouraged relaxation and serenity are some benefits of therapeutic touch. With it, you can improve your sleep hygiene, hasten the healing process after surgery, or reduce muscle pain. Stress and anxiety can also be managed with its help.

- **Healing Touch:** Like therapeutic touch, this energy therapy promotes harmony and helps re-calibrate your energy to experience natural healing. During a session, practitioners use their hands to connect with the client's energy and manipulate the flow within the nervous system so powerful healing can be felt.

Nature

Grounding yourself on the earth is an extraordinary way to raise your vibration. There is nothing like connecting to a natural energy source, such as taking a walk in the park or going for a hike. You get some exercise, and you change your vibration.

When connecting to nature, leaving your gadgets and artificial power sources behind is essential. Take this moment to reconnect with yourself, getting balanced in a more excellent state of consciousness. Do not let your cell phone take away your focus on the abundance and beauty that surrounds you in the present moment.

Taking a stroll or spending some moments in the backyard can make you feel better, more alive, and happier. Especially after a fight with your better half, when your kids are being difficult, or when work is stressing you out, immersing yourself in the beauty of nature can instantly shift your mood.

Yoga

Taking a consistent and mindful approach to yoga can help you nourish your body, calm your mind, and become more aware of the present moment. It is not just what happens in the external world that matters but also how you choose to react to it: yoga encourages intentional actions that prioritize health and well-being. Find inner peace through yoga; remember that the outside world does not decide your fate.

Some people will participate in yoga when they are in a low vibrational mood, such as when they feel anxious or stressed. Likewise, it can help calm their mind and give them peace and freedom from negative energy.

Moreover, yoga focuses on realigning your chakras. There are seven energy centers in our body, known as the chakras: *root chakra, crown chakra, throat chakra, heart chakra, sacral chakra, solar plexus, and third eye chakra.* Each chakra focuses on the part of the body from the inside out. For example, the heart chakra aligns your heart with a sense of purpose, love, and compassion so you feel fulfilled. The throat chakra helps open your throat so you can share your voice and message with the world. Yet, if one or all of these are out of balance, you can feel anxious, worried, closed off, stressed, and fearful, which are all part of low vibe energy. Practicing yoga moves helps realign and balance all seven chakras so you can feel more positive and raise your vibration by feeling a sense of peace, joy, harmony, and fulfillment.

Healthy Relationships

Surround yourself with people who embody positive energy, peace, happiness, fulfillment, purposefulness, intention, and gratitude; these relationships are essential for helping to increase your vibration. All of these elements add up to high vibrational energy; when you foster these qualities in those around you, your emotional frequency will be elevated too.

Jim Rohn says, *"You are the average of the five people you spend your time with the most"* (Groth, 2012). When you think about this statement, ask yourself: *Are they consistently negative? Do they curse a lot? Do they gossip or complain? Do they constantly procrastinate and feel unmotivated or uninspired? Are they prideful?*

Becoming conscious of the attitudes and behaviors you display day-to-day is necessary. If your circle is full of disempowering negativity, it could be time to reevaluate who you choose to hang around with. To raise your vibration, seek out positive, like-minded people. People with ambitions, dreams, and goals; those passionate about success. Find those authentically happy with a meaningful purpose and feeling fulfilled, as these people will bring more positive energy and help elevate your vibration.

Take a break from all the arguments with your loved ones and spend some time alone or go for a walk. That way, you can reset your energy, attitude, and mood. Conflict brings low vibrational feelings, such as anger, guilt, and shame. Shifting your mindset and changing your environment, even for a short time, can help lighten your mood and help you feel calm and peaceful. One of the most significant relationships you will ever have is your relationship with yourself. Nurturing and fostering that relationship is essential to remain healthy, fulfilled, and happy. When these emotions are a part of your life, you raise your vibration instantly.

Restore Your Surroundings

This intention is so simple yet incredibly effective. As you can see from this pillar, raising your vibration does not have to be complicated; it is the littlest steps that make a big difference.

Taking care of your surroundings is a decisive action. By taking care of the environment you live and breathe in every day, you let go of what no longer serves you and clean up your habits. Not only does this affect your physical well-being, but it also benefits your mental and spiritual health.

There are a few ways you can restore your surroundings:

- **Clean out your purse or briefcase.** This may sound simple, but it makes a world of difference. Get rid of the garbage that does not need to be there, such as the receipts you no longer need and the documents that no longer serve a purpose. Tidying up these compartments can help you feel peace and a breath of fresh air, which can help raise your vibration.
- **Clean out your wallet.** It has been said that by cleaning out your wallet, you open your wallet to receive more abundance. If you think about it, this makes sense. *How could you*

receive more money if your wallet is messy and dirty? This sends a message to the universe that you do not care about your current abundance. But by cleaning out your purse, abundance has a personal invitation to show up in your life and bank account.

- **Tidy up your home.** When your environment looks and feels unorganized and is a mess, it lowers your vibration. You feel grumpy, annoyed, frustrated, depressed, sad, and anxious. By taking a few moments daily or weekly to organize your home, especially your bedroom and office, you will mentally feel better, which helps raise your vibration.
- **Get better sleep.** 25% of our lifetime is spent in our bedroom, dreaming the night away. Having proper sleep hygiene is a crucial step in raising your vibration. When you sleep badly, you feel exhausted, tired, burned out, annoyed, grumpy, overwhelmed, lack concentration and energy, and unmotivated, which is not the right energy to start your day. Yet, implementing proper sleep hygiene makes you feel alive, excited, energetic, restored, and mentally healthy. You can practice proper sleep hygiene in the following ways: *turn off all technology at a set time, relax your mindset by reading a book or having tea before bed, put your phone on do not disturb or silent mode, meditate, say a prayer, and go to bed consistently at a reasonable hour,* ensuring you get at least eight hours sleep each night.

Now that we have discussed the importance of raising our vibration and focusing on the positive things that life offers, our next pillar will discuss the importance of setting intentions. Being intentional helps you remain focused and steadfast in your goals and dreams. When it comes to manifestation, the intention is a crucial component of success.

Pillar Four
Intention

By definition, intention means the *"purpose or attitude toward the effect of one's actions" (dictionary.com, 2019)*.

Each day, we take action on something, such as waking up to go to work or deciding what to have for dinner tonight. Likewise, we take action every day to achieve our goals, whether we like it or not. Sometimes, if we are tired when we get home, we do not feel like making dinner, but we know that we have to eat. In this case, we have three choices: *make dinner at home, order takeout, or go out.* Either way, it is our duty to make sure that we have dinner, regardless of the action behind it.

However, there is a difference between taking action and being intentional about that specific action. Using the dinner example, we can have pop and chips for dinner, which would not be healthy for our bodies. On the other hand, we can be intentional about it and make a nutritious dinner of salmon, vegetable medley, and potatoes. With the latter, it is not only healthier for our bodies, but it is also delicious.

This pillar focuses on the difference between merely taking action out of obligation and deliberately pursuing action as the pivotal step toward reaching your aspirations. By grasping this distinction, you can set your manifestation goals with purpose, insight, and pure will. When you clearly understand what you intend to do, the journey is extraordinary.

Intention Manifestation

Bob Proctor says, *"What you think about, you bring about" (2017)*. This is a perfect example of intention manifestation. Remember, when manifesting and attracting positive energy into your life, it is essential to focus on uplifting and positive thoughts rather than negative or destructive ones. As Proctor said, *"If you think negatively, you will attract negativity into your life."*

Proctor's sentiment says it all when it comes to being intentional. As such, let us assume that you want to lose weight. In terms of reaching any goal, especially weight loss, be willful as our subconscious minds often take in what we think and say. Likewise, it is essential to stay aware of the words used. Instead of telling yourself you are fat or do not want to gain weight, try to reframe those thoughts into something positive. What you ask for is what your subconscious will give you. Ergo, if you wish to avoid gaining weight, call on your mind power and focus instead on your fitness goals. That way, your subconscious will be more likely to help you achieve them rather than working against them.

Be Intentional with Your Subconscious Mind

A few things to understand about the subconscious mind when being intentional with what you are manifesting are these:

- **It loves what is familiar and dislikes what is unfamiliar.** Suppose that procrastination is usual to you, while self-motivation is not. In this case, getting out of procrastination can be an uphill battle, as your subconscious mind is hardwired to take you back to what you already know. To successfully break away from this cycle of procrastination, you must consciously encourage yourself and make self-motivation the new norm. Establishing healthy routines that excite and inspire you will also help build up your motivation so that, eventually, procrastinating becomes a thing of the past. With consistent encouragement, you will find yourself more focused on your projects and better able to fight off distractions.
- **It does not understand past or future tense; it only understands the present moment.** When setting intentions for your manifestations, remember that your subconscious interprets only what you tell. Subsequently, when you say, *"I will no longer live in scarcity or lack,"* your subconscious may think this is precisely what you want and do everything to ensure that is the case. But if you shift your words and say, *"I live in enough every single day,"* the subconscious mind will believe that you are already living in abundance and will bring more opportunities for abundance.
- **It thinks with images and words.** Referring to the weight loss example, if you tell yourself that you no longer want to be overweight, all the subconscious sees are that you desire to gain weight and will present opportunities for you to earn extra pounds. Hence, when visualizing your dreams in your mind, you must visualize them in a positive manner rather than in a negative tone, as whatever you envision, you will attract.

When being intentional with your manifestations, be mindful of the words you tell yourself and the images you think about. Anything, positive or negative, will manifest as long as you think about it. A little thought-peep can say, *"I hope I do not lose my job,"* and suddenly, you are out of a job. Manifestation requires intentionality and staying mindful. Otherwise, all your subconscious can discern is scarcity and lack. This leads to it attempting to keep you in this state, as it presumes that is your aim.

To show the power of intention when manifesting, I will share a story about a woman who desperately wanted to get married and make herself happy but unfortunately went through some miserable relationships. Intending to achieve unconditional love finally, she replaced wanting marriage with simply wanting to get engaged. So, instead of telling herself, "I want to get married," she kept saying, "I want to get engaged." Besides that, she put a picture of an engaged couple with a beautiful diamond ring on her vision board. Then, a few years later, she mentioned at the seminar has been close to walking down the aisle multiple times, yet with each attempt, the engagement fell through before marriage which happened almost ten times. This illustrates how, when it comes to manifestation, your words speak louder than you may think to your subconscious mind.

How to Become More Intentional

There are many ways to become more intentional when manifesting your dreams. Here are a few you can put into action right away:

- **Vision board.** Making a vision board is a powerful way to express your desires and determine what you want to manifest. It enables you to become purposeful in noting what you dream of. As previously mentioned, it is essential to be intentional with your thoughts and words when creating your vision board. Suppose you want to bring about an intimate marriage. From there, incorporate images and phrases describing the relationship you wish for. If you dream of having $100,000 in the bank, include visuals illustrating people who already have this amount in their accounts. There are no set rules for making a vision board; make it your own. You can design it on your computer and make it the desktop background or lock screen on all your devices and enjoy looking at it daily. Alternatively, you can use construction paper, glue, and other supplies for a more traditional approach. Another option is making a movie version of the vision board, then watching it daily to embed the words and pictures into your subconsciousness. Let go of expectations; trust that this visualization will bring about all you want.
- **Journal.** Become intentional with what you are writing about. Speak of your dreams, aspirations, and goals. Get clear on your purpose and your passions. Give your dreams life by speaking into them as though they were already happening. Jot down what your higher self is saying in your journal and assess where any blocks may stem from to help you move on past them and find freedom. Other than that, there is a journaling strategy called scripting that can aid you in honing in on precisely what it looks like to live your desired life. Write everything out in the present tense and include info such as who you are with, where you are living, and the type of food you eat, as if you were in that very moment living the life of your dreams. This method offers excellent clarity for visualizing exactly which dream life you would like yours to look like.
- **Say affirmations daily.** When you speak to yourself, make sure it is with uplifting and empowering words that are positive and in the present tense. By doing so, your subconscious will believe them and help you achieve whatever you want. For instance, if you desire to lose weight, remind yourself that you have a healthy and beautiful body. Likewise, eat nutritious meals daily that make you feel happy, lean, and gorgeous. The more positive statements you give yourself consistently, the nearer you will be to reaching your desired outcome.

Setting Intentions

Now that we have discussed how to become more intentional when manifesting your dreams, it is time to discuss how to set intentions and the importance of setting them, so you reach success.

By setting intentions, you can focus more on your goals and gain insight into what you hope to manifest. It is more than saying, "I want to have hundred thousand dollars in my bank account"; it goes beyond that. Intention-setting requires purpose, positivity, and commitment to ensure it is done correctly. To ensure your intentions are set with the right intention and vibes, it is essential to be aware of the attitude and behavior you are taking on while setting them. Additionally, having a real plan or structure for how your intentions will come to fruition can help give you direction so that you stay focused on achieving them.

Amina AlTai, a leadership and mindset coach, says, *"Intentions are an opportunity to design and take ownership of our lived experience; they are like setting the GPS for our lives" (Estrada, 2022).* By setting our intentions, we can effectively take control of our lives. It is like drawing up a roadmap to success; we can identify where we are and chart the course to our desired destination.

To set intentions successfully, you need to focus on the following information.

Know Your Destination

Get a clear vision of what you want to achieve. Ask yourself: *What is it that I want to bring into reality? A beautiful home? An amazing car? An unforgettable trip? A prosperous marriage? An incredible business?*

Whatever you desire to manifest, make it clear that you know where you are going. By setting intentions, you become purposeful with your destination. As such, instead of wishing for financial abundance, focus on what it would feel like to be financially secure. Affirm that you are already wealthy; visualize having $100,000 in your bank account, many clients, and feeling excited, blessed, and grateful. Doing this clarifies where you want to go with your wealth and sets you on the path to success.

Understand Your Why

You may be clear on what you want to manifest, *but why do you want it? What is the sentimental value you are attaching to your goals? Do you want thousands of dollars in your bank account so you can create remarkable experiences with your family and travel the world? Or is it because you want to become a philanthropist and give back to your community or favorite charity because it speaks to your heart?*

There should always be a reason behind every intentional action we set forth in our lives. When we understand these reasons, we will remain steadfast in our goals and be focused entirely on achieving them.

Focus on Who You Need to Be

Understand who the person is that has thousands of dollars in their bank account every month. *How do they dress? What do they do every single day? What are their goals and dreams? Who are they as a leader? What is their character like? How do they behave around others? Who do they surround themselves with? How do they speak? Do they speak with class, sophistication, and eloquence? How do they present themselves?*

By getting clear on the person you need to become that has manifested your dreams into reality, you know how to step into that persona. Start by releasing any blockages that keep you stuck. Focus on reducing the amount of cursing, as this type of low-vibe energy can be damaging. Analyze who you surround yourself with and look for more positive influences and networks. Re-evaluate your habits, stop procrastination, and become mindful of your choices. Once you focus more on the person you need to become rather than the person you no longer want to be, setting intentions will feel easier to accomplish.

Shift Your Mindset

Setting your sights on a target and focusing on the ways to get there starts the process of making your dreams come true. Instead of constantly striving, concentrate on being what you want. Give yourself an optimistic outlook, say positive things to yourself, convert negative ideas into supportive affirmations, be thankful for what you have already, and concentrate on what you intend to do rather than why it may not happen.

Have you ever heard the phrase, *"What if it works?"* It can be a game changer in terms of your outlook on life. Instead of worrying about failure, you can focus on optimism and possibility. By changing your mindset to this positive question, you will discover new ways to look at your dreams and goals with newfound confidence. This attitude shift is immediate and decisive, as it can help open doors previously closed due to fear.

Other than that, allow yourself to take the time to understand any limiting beliefs that keep resurfacing in your life by journaling them. Embrace a positive mindset and discover how it can help unlock potential you may not have known. See what changes can be made, and watch as they play out in your day-to-day reality. Writing them down and clarifying why they exist will help you become consciously aware of them, giving you the power to debunk them and shift your mindset to more empowering beliefs.

Be Consistent

One of the key ingredients to successfully setting intentions is to focus on consistency. Be dedicated and steadfast with your goals to accomplish them in no time. Clarity will help keep your focus and will help keep your dedication and perseverance intact.

For example, if you want to have a toned and fit body, you first need to be clear with your 'why.' Why do you want to achieve this? Is it because you want to live a healthy and active lifestyle? It is because you want to have a beach-ready body by summertime? Being clear about your goal will help you identify the specific steps you need to achieve it. That level of clarity can push you to remain consistent every day, no matter what.

Surrender Your Intentions

Being on the path of intention can be a demanding venture. When setting goals, you might feel alone, anxious, and pessimistic about bringing your dreams to fruition. Meanwhile, internal obstacles can come from doubt, procrastination, or losing enthusiasm. Not to mention convincing yourself that your manifestations would not come true because you have not seen tangible evidence yet. That said, it is noteworthy to remember that even if it feels lonely and stressful, having an optimistic mindset is always crucial.

Moreover, asking the universe for help is necessary to make your manifestations come true. Your spiritual team is always on hand to guide you through whatever journey lies ahead. Put your intentions out there and surrender them, do not cling too firmly to what you hope will happen, but keep in mind that the universe could surprise you with something different. To make sure your goals become a reality, trust the universe and let go of any attachment to the outcome; this will bring a greater sense of peace, joy, and satisfaction.

Subsequently, you must relinquish control when surrendering your intentions. So often, when we manifest, we become attached to the outcome that it becomes a block to something far greater than what we had initially envisioned. And when they do not show up as we intended, we become disappointed, upset, and stressed, which brings us into a low energetic state. By remaining focused and open and surrendering our intentions to the universe, we can feel excited knowing that the universe is partnering with us to make our dreams happen.

Overall, achieving a beautiful and abundant life starts with knowing your goals and desires. So, setting clear intentions is the key to bringing your manifestations to life. Meanwhile, visualization is an integral part of this pillar, so we will now take a deeper dive into it. Hence, in pillar five, we will be devoted to this topic discussed earlier.

Pillar Five
Visualization

During pillar four, we spoke about the importance of setting intentions so you can become clear on what you want to manifest in your life. Setting intentions gives you the freedom to be, do, and have whatever your heart desires. Furthermore, with your thoughts and intentions, you can manifest as much or little as you desire. To attract the positive energy surrounding manifestation, maintaining a high-frequency state is essential. Hence, by setting clear action steps and aligning them with your desired outcomes, you will be able to stay in the right energetic vibration for the successful materialization of your dreams and ambitions.

In making the puzzle complete, visualization is the next piece you need. Once you have set your intentions and they have been made clear to you, the next step is focusing on delivering these intentions. In pillar four, I shared that the subconscious mind only responds to the images you think about and the words you tell yourself. As such, visualization exercises will help you become consciously aware of the images and the words you think about and will help you stay on track while remaining in a positive, energetic state.

Power of Visualization

Visualization becomes essential when it comes to success as it helps you use imaginative imagery to visualize succeeding at your goals before it even happens. Likewise, it becomes powerful in its own right because it enables you to use the creative side of your brain to envision your success and feel what it would feel like before your goals come to fruition. Feeling those emotions is part of high-vibe energy, so when you can get into that state of being, what you are manifesting becomes a reality.

Envisioning is like sowing seeds in the universe. By picturing in our minds, we sow the seeds of manifestation and signal to the universe our intention. The universe takes action by nurturing and providing what the seeds need to grow—rain. To ensure they reach their fullest potential, we must act consistently every day toward achieving our dreams. When they are ready, we can harvest them, reaping an abundance of rewards from our labor.

Meanwhile, we all have dreams that keep popping up in our minds, the ones we wish to make a reality. When we focus on them, actively visualize them, and believe they can be ours, it activates our brain's Reticular Activating System (RAS). This system is made up of cells that bridge our vision and manifestation, making them just one step away from being realized. For example, if you want to manifest driving a 2023 Tesla, include a picture of the car on your vision board, and visualize yourself driving one, your brain signals to your RAS that that is what you want. From there, you will notice Teslas parked in front of your house, which you have never seen before, stopped at a red light as you cross the street, in the grocery store parking lot—everywhere you seem to look, a Tesla is staring at you in the face. Then, your friend shares that they just bought a Tesla and asks if you want to take a ride. With all that, the universe seems to be answering your call; your RAS is getting piqued as if it says, "We heard you, and here is something coming your way."

The same goes for your dream vacation. As such, imagining a dream vacation in Hawaii can be inspiring. From looking at Airbnbs to researching the islands, it is easy to picture yourself sitting on the beach in Oahu, sipping a delicious drink from a coconut shell, gazing out at the ocean and palm trees. Likely, after you do that, you start seeing ads for Hawaii popping up on social media, hearing conversations about the destination on public transportation or around the office and getting emails about flight deals; all signs you are one step closer to booking your ticket.

When your RAS is activated and aware, pay attention to the signs the universe is giving you, as your RAS's mission is to motivate and inspire you to keep pining for your dreams. Also, it brings your dreams into your physical reality to show you that you have what it takes to make them officially yours. They may not be directly a part of your life, but your RAS demonstrates that indirectly they are. That said, you need to take inspired action to make them a part of your life rather than watch people around you manifest them. Likewise, this can also happen when we visualize experiences we do not want, so remember to be mindful of how you use your RAS.

Letting Go of What No Longer Serves You

Visualization also helps with one important thing: filtering out what no longer matters. By clarifying what you want, you begin letting go of the things that do not serve you or your dreams. As such, it helps you think and dream bigger than what you can envision for your life right now; there is no limit to what you can dream about. Likewise, visualizing helps you forget what is not meant to be a part of your dream and gives you something to look forward to.

For example, you may have two passions: photography and opening a non-profit organization. Maybe when you were a child, it was your dream to travel around the world, taking pictures of magnificent places. But as you grew older, you realized that your heart and service belong in the non-profit sector, especially since you noticed so many dogs and cats running around homeless on the streets. Due to that, you dream of opening up a shelter that will give them love, attention, and care, minimizing the number of homeless pets in your city.

By using visualization exercises, such as a vision board, you can filter out what distracts you from focusing on your current dream; that is the beauty of it. Likely, your dreams can change, and that is okay. As you let go of what no longer serves you, you filter out the excess distractions that steer you away from what matters most. Likewise, you send a message to your subconscious that you are clear on what you want to manifest, and now nothing will get in your way. Lowkey, it is as if you are making a solemn vow to yourself that you are in it for the long haul, no matter what.

Multi-Sensory Visualization

Sensory visualization is a profound topic. Initially, it may feel uneasy, as if people think you are crazy, and it may feel uncomfortable. However, it will feel extraordinary once you get the hang of it.

I am sure we have all heard of the book and the movie *The Secret*. The speakers in the film talk about *like attract like*, which is associated with the Law of Attraction, just as we discussed in pillar two. If you touch and feel it in your mind, what you manifest is already yours.

There is a part in the movie where a guy is sitting in his living room, flipping through a car magazine. He comes across his dream car and visualizes that it is already his. He closes his eyes and can feel the leather seats' smooth texture. He visualizes himself cruising through the city, waving to people passing by. He can feel it when he pushes the brake pedal and shifts and accelerates the gears. He looks excited, motivated, and positive.

This scene is a perfect example of multi-sensory visualization. It is about using all five senses to visualize your manifestations, so they become a part of your physical reality.

The Power of Visualizing with Your Senses

If you dream about that vacation to Hawaii, feel your fingers clicking the buttons as you book your tickets. Visualize yourself packing your swimsuit, flip-flops, shorts, and suntan lotion. Let your excitement flow as you tell your partner that you just booked the trip to Hawaii. When you are in the air, look at the blue sky out the plane's window as you descend toward the island. Observe the palm trees cascading in the background. Listen to the pilot on the intercom telling the passengers about the weather and that you are about to land, so you must put your seatbelt on and fasten your trays upright. Feel the sun's warmth basking in your face, ready to welcome you to the island. As you land, your ears pick up the voices of the locals saying "aloha" when you pass them on the streets. Careless the luggage handles between your fingers as you pull your luggage behind you. Savour the fresh coconut water in your mouth and smell the remnants of Hawaiian rum engulfing your nostrils. Touch the door handle between your fingers as you enter your ocean view room. Enjoy the ocean in the background as you look out the panoramic windows of your hotel room or step out onto the balcony. Take pleasure from the ocean breeze in your hair, the saltwater from the ocean, and the seagulls cawing above you as you look up into the sky.

Multi-sensory visualization is a powerful component of manifestation. It is what helps your desires become tangible. The more you hear, see, feel, taste, and smell in your dreams, the faster they will come to fruition.

Practicing Visualization

Visualizing your dreams is a fun, participatory journey. It is also a collaborative journey where you learn to partner with the universe. You decide what you want, and the universe reveals the steps to make it happen.

I encourage you to engage in a visualization exercise to practice manifesting to its fullest extent. Have fun with it and allow the universe to move through you so you can receive clarity on what you want.

To effectively visualize, there are a few steps to put into action.

Journal About What You Want

Write it all down. Try not to be vague. Be as specific as possible. It is important you use all five of your senses so you can truly get a feel of what you are manifesting. It would not be as effective if you said, *"I visualize myself driving my dream car. I feel excited about it."* There is no emotional response to this statement. It feels neutral. It feels as though if you get your dream car, great. If you do not, that is okay too.

But imagine if you were to say something like this: "I am manifesting driving my 2023 Tesla. It is a beautiful cherry red and has smooth, white leather seats. I can feel my excitement as I see it at the dealership. The moment I laid my eyes on it, I knew it was the one. I can feel myself sitting on the driver's side as I cruise down the streets. I can see my partner beside me, laughing and playing with the built-in touchscreen. I feel the wind blowing through my hair as my hands are on the steering wheel. I hear my kids laughing and having a good time in the backseat. I hear them asking where we are going, and I respond with, "Anywhere the wind takes us." As I stop at a red light, I can feel the smooth velocity of the brake pedals, and I can hear the engine roaring beneath me. I am excited and grateful as we stop at a local ice cream parlor for a delicious treat. I can hear the doors close behind me as I step out of the car, and I can feel my fingers push the button to activate the alarm and lock the doors."

Sensory visualization takes manifestation to a whole new level. When writing about it, write in as much detail as possible. Feel as though your dreams have already come to fruition.

Visualize Your Emotions

How will you feel when what you are manifesting becomes a reality? You can journal about this or simply close your eyes. Allow yourself to imagine how you would feel. *Would you feel excited about manifesting your dream vacation? Would you feel at peace knowing that you have manifested thousands of dollars in residual monthly income in your business? Would you feel joyful knowing you are now married to your soulmate partner? Would you feel grateful knowing that financial abundance flows into your life daily?*

By visualizing how you would feel when you reach your goals, you can feel one step closer. They can feel instantly tangible as if they are already a part of your life. Tapping into high-vibe emotions—such as happiness, abundance, gratitude, joy, and peace—when visualizing your dreams will allow you to feel the existence of your dreams before they physically manifest into reality. The more you feel about reaching your goals, the more you become motivated, determined, and inspired to make them happen.

Step into Action Consistently

Reaching your goals is more than a one-step process or get-rich-quick scheme. For instance, creating a beach body with toned abs and lean muscle requires consistent and determined action each day. It is not a one-time job; instead needs the courage to alter habits, strength, and determination to begin reaping the rewards of hard work. Sticking to nutritional meals, exercising at the gym regularly, keeping fit and healthy, avoiding unhealthy food choices, and taking accurate measurements in your diet can become a continuous cycle of motivated behavior and a process of consistent, clarified action.

To begin, you must understand why you want to manifest having a beach-ready body. If you are not clear, you will become unmotivated, which creates a lack of consistency. Sooner or later, you will wonder why you could not reach your goals. Yet, it is because remaining consistent became a struggle; therefore, you lost motivation. Despite that, consistency seems like a manageable obstacle when you know why you desire to manifest what you want.

Make Time to Visualize

More often than not, when people complain that their manifestations did not work, it is usually because they did not give themselves time to focus on them. Given that, make time to visualize your goals every day. In the previous point, we spoke about consistency, and this is the same thing. To become effective, visualize your goals a couple of times a day. Spend 10 to 20 minutes journaling or closing your eyes and envisioning what it feels like to live your dream life. Likewise, engage your five senses to feel, hear, see, taste, and smell your dreams. Allow yourself to feel what it would feel like when your manifestations are finally a part of your life. Wake up in the morning and spend some time visualizing while having some coffee. Get into the vibes of making them happen. Allow your subconscious mind to take in your visualizations. Create imagery and words in your mind and feel like they already exist. Before you go to bed each night, visualize your dreams again. Refrain from using technology, like playing games on your phone or checking your emails. Set aside this time for you and your goals.

Now that you can grasp the power of visualization and how it can help you manifest your dreams, the next pillar will set you up for success even further. This upcoming pillar will delve into the immense power of affirmations: *the words you express, both to yourself and out loud, possess tremendous strength.*

Pillar Six
Affirmations

Throughout this book, we have spoken about how our subconscious mind controls our life and decisions. Together, the unconscious mind and subconscious mind run about 95% of our mind *(Freud, 1915)*, so when we think about this, we wonder what is going on in the back of our mind to make us feel negative.

Affirmations are powerful in reframing our minds to believe more empowering beliefs. There is no doubt that your mind is a powerful tool. The words we tell ourselves can control our minds so strongly, thus affecting our behavior and decision-making.

This pillar will help you understand how powerful affirmations can be in your life. We will be discussing a few things:

- The importance of the thoughts and words we think and say.
- The importance of becoming self-aware of our words to ourselves and others.
- The importance of the words we say to the universe.
- The power of affirmations and how to write them effectively.

Understanding these key points, you will begin developing awareness of your actions, behaviors, and thoughts. Additionally, you will learn to notice what you are saying, how you are saying things, and how it emotionally affects yourself and others.

To manifest what you want, creating and practicing affirmations consistently will help you combat negative thoughts that disempower you. As such, they will help train and condition your mind for more positive beliefs so that, moving forward, you continue to empower yourself rather than tear yourself down.

The Power of Affirmations

Knowing how to transform your life starts with being mindful of the words the ones you say to yourself and those you share with others. Often, it is easy to overlook the power of such words when directed internally, so it can be surprising how much negativity we tell ourselves without even being aware of it. But awareness of our comments makes positive changes as our outlook is reflected in our lives.

Sometimes, we have moments when we feel like our lives are not going right and say things like, *"my life sucks."* But it is important to remember that the universe is listening, and it may take your words as affirmation that you want your situation to stay the same. You can feel frustrated at why nothing is changing even though you are trying to make a difference. To break out of this cycle, we need to be conscious of how much power our words have on our overall lifestyle.

For example, you could tell yourself, *"I am the Queen (King) of Procrastination"* every day. Although you may say this jokingly, your subconscious mind does not know the difference between a joke and truth; therefore, it will take your statement literally. From that, you constantly procrastinate when you try to work on a project with a deadline. As such, when you sit in front of the computer to work on the task that needs to be done, you find yourself playing game after game on your phone; hence, it seems that you have become exactly what you have repeatedly told yourself.

Ergo, pay attention to the words you say to yourself, as they have a powerful effect on your subconscious. Instead of using negative words, opt for positive ones. This way, you will shift your mindset and energy frequency to a higher vibration. In high-vibe energy, your positive manifestations start showing up in reality; *it is not 'magic,' but science.* And as you try speaking positively to yourself, you will experience its rewards.

Thoughts and Words Create Your Reality

The reality that you live in today is a reflection of your thoughts and beliefs. Hearing this can be challenging and upsetting but allow me to explain further. Every single aspect of your life has been shaped by the mental processes that you have gone through.

Think about it, *when we have negative feelings toward ourselves, what happens?* — we believe them. Our subconscious mind does not know the difference between positive and negative. It only knows of the present moment; therefore, it will believe whatever you tell it. If you tell yourself, *"I am not beautiful, and I will never find a good relationship,"* any relationship the universe brings you will not feel good enough. Your partner could treat you like royalty, but in your mind, you are thinking: *"Why are they even with me? I am not worth it. There are many other beautiful people they could be with. Why me?"* Due to this belief, your confidence and self-esteem are non-existent. Then the worst thing that could ever happen to you at this moment happens—they break up with you. In your mind, the breakup just affirmed that you are not beautiful, and you will never find a good relationship; otherwise, they would not have ended it.

Suppose you flip the situation around and think, *"I am so much to offer in a relationship. I am attractive, smart, and intelligent. My partner will love me for who I am".* Chances are that you will meet someone who cherishes you, and you give it your all. Interesting conversations flow naturally between the two of you, they express admiration for your beauty, and you feel confident taking their words as truth. This blossoming romance sees your self-love increase each day, and you are thankful for finding a partner who truly knows how to treat you right.

Norman Vincent Pale once said, *"Change your thoughts, and you change your world" (Zach, 2012)*. Realizing that our beliefs shape our reality, it pays to be attentive to our words in our internal dialogue and find ways to turn disempowering ones into more positive statements. Our belief system is shaped by the time we are between zero and seven; what our parents say or do not say, how they behave, and the experiences they create for us become part of who we are. Thus, those same patterns may imprint on your psyche if you hear them speak negative thoughts or live out lack-based stories. Fortunately, with awareness and a new empowering mindset, we can break away from limiting thought patterns and create a completely different world. In short, choose better thoughts, and you will change your life.

Words You Say to Yourself

Let us face it; *we are often our own worst bullies.* In grade school, someone in your class threatened you with their intimidating behavior, bullying everyone they could find and putting everyone down. Unfortunately, you may have become a target of their aggressive tendencies, leading to derogatory names, physical bullying, and hurtful rumors. Childhood felt unbearable due to the bully's oppressive acts, leaving behind issues like depression, anxiety, and low self-esteem that you had to carry into adulthood. You believed whatever untruths were spoken against you due to this inevitable cycle of torment.

> *"You are a loser."*
> *"You suck."*
> *"No one will ever like you."*
> *"Your dreams are stupid."*
> *"You are ugly."*
> *"You are trying too hard. Stop being so desperate."*
> *"You are helpless."*

These words take a huge hit on your self-esteem. Many years later, you still believe these words, and your life is evidence that these statements are true. Now, imagine this is one bully from outside of you that made you feel this way. *What happens when you realize that there is an inner bully inside of you?* One that is stronger and more intimidating. As such, *do you know that self-talk has more impact than what someone who has gone from our lives might tell us?* It sinks right in if you look in the mirror and tell yourself you are not up to par and are not beautiful. However, if we express our uniqueness and loveliness to ourselves, we may initially be reluctant to believe it, but eventually, we do come around. Strangely enough, negative ideas are accepted more quickly than positive ones; negative thinking enters our minds easily due to our conditioning since childhood.

Look at the media; it portrays negativity every single day. Yet, cannot help but pay attention to them since it is all anyone ever talks about. Oddly enough, we rarely see uplifting stories covered by the media. When this was discussed, someone commented, *"Negativity makes the news, but positivity does not."* Taking this statement into account, the words you say to yourself matter. To manifest everything you want, you must start with the words you say to yourself. Our negative thoughts can get in the way; they are conditioned to do so regardless because they are what we are used to, but the trick is to become aware of them and shift them immediately. Rather than hang onto the belief that manifestation does not work, shift this and tell yourself better thoughts.

As I mentioned earlier, Tony Robbins quote, *"You cannot feel fear or anger while feeling gratitude at the same time" (2014)*. In other words, it is impossible to have negative thoughts and positive thoughts at the same time. You cannot say, *"I hate myself, but I love myself."* It just does not work. In fact, it sounds a bit silly when you say this statement out loud.

Since your thoughts and words create your reality, find a way to change your perception. A world-renowned hypnotherapist, Marisa Peer, says, *"Tell yourself a better lie" (2022)*. I want you to know something as I refer to this statement: *The negative anecdotes you tell yourself are false.* They are a lie you convey to protect from potential harm. Yet, your subconscious believes the negativity and stores it in the back of your mind to protect you. In this instance, this is where telling yourself a better lie comes in handy. As you shift your self-inflicting words, you may not believe them right now, but rather than tell yourself lies that are full of negativity and shame that block you from receiving what you want, you might as well shift your perspective and tell yourself an optimistic lie. At least it is full of empowerment and inspiration, and you will believe it to be true in time.

Words You Say to Others

There is a famous quote by Maya Angelou, *"People will forget what you said, people will forget what you did, but people will never forget how you made them feel" (Gallo, 2014)*. But with all due respect to Maya Angelou, I disagree with this statement. *Yes, people may not remember exactly what you said, but these words make them feel the way they do.* If you are having a conversation with someone and you are constantly degrading them and tearing them down, telling them that *"their ideas are stupid"* and *"no one will ever go for them,"* you can be sure that their subconscious mind will remember what you said and store these words for later use to help protect them from potential opportunities where this belief can rise. Your words will make them feel like they do not have anything good to offer the world, and they will experience sadness, worry, stress, anxiety, and, in extreme cases, depression. Subconsciously, they will remember your words for many, many years to come.

So, do your words matter to others? *Absolutely.* The words you say to others can either do two things:

- Make them feel good
- Tear them down

Paying attention to how we communicate is essential, not just with ourselves but also with others. A single derogatory remark can be damaging, eroding someone's self-worth and uniqueness. So, taking the time to consider our words is an invaluable practice that will help us cultivate meaningful and respectful relationships.

To help explain this further, here is a bit of a harsh example. *Full disclaimer, it is a trigger warning.* Referring to the bullying example in the previous section, we can all agree that some bullies are downright mean. They will say anything as a means to tear their victim apart. According to MedPage Today, Shannon Firth has said that teen suicide has jumped 29% within the past decade (2022). Adolescents who experience bullying double the likely cause of attempted suicide *(Hinduja & Patchin, 2019)*, which makes suicide the second leading cause of death for people 10 to 34 years old *(National Institute of Mental Health, 2022)*.

Our words can greatly impact how someone else feels; they can give strength or make somebody feel destroyed. That is why we need to be careful and think before we speak instead of acting impulsively. Unfortunately, it is too common to act first and reflect later; conversations like this can get us into trouble. And so I am sharing this example to demonstrate how powerful our words can be, especially when the other person may be emotionally vulnerable. Hence, take precautions in what we say so that the message we want to express is conveyed in a way that will empower the recipient rather than cause harm.

To be mindful, we can do a few things:

- **Take a deep breath before speaking.** When entering a heated discussion with someone close to you, take a deep breath. Before your words become a detriment to another's subconscious and self-esteem, take a few deep breaths before saying your following sentence. Taking the extra time will help you calm down and help make the conversation go smoother. This is called emotional intelligence.
- **Step away if needed.** To refrain from saying something you do not mean and needing to ask for forgiveness later, leave the room for a few moments. Go for a walk, step outside for some fresh air, retreat to your bedroom—take a moment to collect your thoughts. Doing so will calm your emotions, so you return to a neutral state of mind and then have a more constructive conversation.
- **Do not allow your emotions to drive your conversations.** Getting angry can make us say things to others we may later regret. That is why speaking from a place of neutrality rather than an emotional state is essential, as apologies and forgiveness become almost inevitable otherwise. Keeping a level head when engaging in conversation is critical to having productive discussions.

Words You Say to the Universe

As our words have extraordinary power to affect ourselves and others, they also send a message to the universe, stating our intentions.

> *"Every thought, feeling, word, and action you put forth is a memo to the universe."*
> –*Dr. Debra Reble*

Giving voice to negative thoughts and words can send subtle yet powerful messages to the universe. When you are running a business and, in a state of frustration, express an unwelcome wish like "I wish I did not have these clients anymore," even though it may be an emotional reaction, the universe will take it literally. Suddenly and almost as if by magic, your clients cancel their contracts, or their circumstances change, making it impossible to work with you. Likely, the universe grants your wish; you no longer have to deal with those clients. In response to your plea, you have been given what you asked for; your request has been heard.

> **"Unspoken and spoken words are among the most powerful energetic forces we have for co-creating our reality."**
>
> *–Dr. Rebel*

Whether you like it or not, you collaborate with the universe every day. Anything you think about, the universe hears. All you say, the universe listens. Your thoughts and words become your unspoken and spoken intention. They become the plans you co-create with the universe. You state the intention, whether positive or negative, and the universe does its job to comply with your request.

So, the next time you think or say something, consider that it may materialize into reality. Complaining about your job to everyone is not expressing gratitude or love. Love is one of the most powerful forces in the universe, and when you show love and appreciation, you receive more of those feelings back into your life. Just as hate or negativity brings the same energy back to you, it is indispensable to recognize how your words and actions reflect your relationship with the universe. You might be sending out messages that do not align with what you want in return; remain conscious of adjusting your attitude and behavior when conversing with the universe.

What Are Affirmations?

Affirmations are uplifting and empowering affirmations that, if said regularly, can bring about significant life changes. With words of encouragement, they help to battle and question negative thoughts. Using such powerful affirmations, one can change their existing limiting beliefs into more optimistic thought processes. For instance, start your day off with an empowering conversation of self-affirmations. Look in the mirror and focus on your strengths, accomplishments, and anything that puts a smile on your face. Choose words to warm your heart and set yourself up for success each morning. Practice repeating these positive affirmations, as they can lift you and brighten up even the toughest days.

Moreover, affirmations can be a great way to boost your abundance and self-love. When you recite positive statements to yourself, you start believing them and feel more confident. Despite this, many people are still uncertain if these affirmations help. And so, if your attempts at affirmations did not work out, the underlying reason could be one of two things:

- You are not saying the appropriate ones for your situation (we will discuss this in more detail in the next section).
- You are not allowing yourself to believe what you are saying because your negative thoughts and beliefs are taking precedence over the positive shifts; therefore, they feel stronger than changing your mind.

If this is how you have felt about affirmations in the past, knowing how to write them to transform your life will give you the confidence to have a breakthrough.

How to Write Affirmations

As we discuss this section, I want you to remember something: *your thoughts have the power to become self-fulfilling prophecies.* This is not magic; it is based on scientific research and studies demonstrating evidence that what we think, we become. Hence, what we think of becomes our reality.

When we question ourselves and ask, *"What if I fail?"* our minds can easily conjure up many ways to demonstrate why we are not succeeding. This evidence can be persuasive, making us believe that our thoughts about ourselves are true. Remarkably, these negative ideas come unbidden into our heads without us meaning them to. They become part of us due to being conditioned subconsciously to think they are facts. As we contemplate our musings, our subliminal mind duly searches for data near us to persuade us of their integrity.

However, what if we turn our thoughts around, such as not settling into negative thought patterns without conscious effort but intentionally choosing to amplify and cultivate uplifting ones? Likely, since our words and thoughts shape our life experiences, choosing to use language will bring you closer to your goals. Besides, affirmations are a powerful tool and can bring about invaluable change.

To write an affirmation statement that speaks to you and resonates with what you are currently struggling with, it is best to remember the areas you would like to change. An affirmation's effectiveness happens when you can focus on one issue at a time. By doing this, your subconscious can take note of it, and the universe can work to help bring the truth of the statement to your life. Below are a few points to keep in mind when creating your affirmations.

Focus on One Key Area

Any negative thought you can turn into a positive one. But it is important to focus on one area that you struggle with at a time. Once you have overcome it, you can move on to another issue. For example, *do you have a fear of public speaking? Do you desire to have an amazing relationship with a loving partner? Do you want to love yourself deeply and unconditionally? Do you struggle with losing weight?* Choose an area that you are deeply passionate about changing. When you know what that is, your subconscious mind will be open to changing it, and you will feel motivated to take consistent action. Your subconscious mind is conditioned to focus on only one area at a time, so make it count. As you believe what you are saying, you can add another affirmation for a different area of your life.

Choose a Realistic Goal

This is a vital aspect of affirmations. Not believing in what you say to yourself, your life will not change how you would like it to. Perhaps, it will feel like a never-ending journey; eventually, you may quit because you feel affirmations do not work. Yet, keep in mind that you must choose affirmations that work for your circumstances. For example, if you want to earn more money and currently make less than $1000, refrain from affirming that you want to make $100,000. Although this goal seems *"nice to have,"* it would not feel real. In your mind, it will feel like, *"Yeah, right. No way this can ever happen."* But if you affirm that you want to make $5,000, that will feel more achievable, and you will likely reach your goal in no time. So, if $100,000 is your ultimate goal, you can work your way up the ladder by starting with a simpler yet empowering goal with which your mind can get on board.

Release the Negative

For your affirmations to be effective, find a way to let go of the negative jargon that shows up in your mind. Journaling helps you do this. Think about how you want to feel and the outcome you want to get out of saying affirmations, and take notice of the negative statements that show up to combat your positivity.

> *"You are not good enough."*
> *"You are crazy to think your life can change."*
> *"That will never happen."*
> *"Stop lying to yourself."*
> *"Your life will always stay the same."*

Once you have written down all the negative statements, you can combat them with a positive comment. For example, *"I live a beautiful and abundant life every day,"* *"I have the power to change my life anytime I want,"* *"I am more than enough,"* and *"My life is being transformed every single day."* By reinforcing positive statements, you combat the negative, by, in the words of Marisa Peer, telling yourself a better lie.

Speak in Present Tense

In pillar four, we discussed that the subconscious mind only knows present-tense statements. Hence it does not know the difference between positive or negative and past and future. So, when creating your affirmations, speak in the present tense. Instead of saying, *"I will own my dream home,"* expressing something like *"My dream home is on its way to me"* will enforce a positive reaction. Likewise, writing your affirmations in the present tense becomes a self-fulfilling prophecy, as if you are tricking your mind into believing that you already have what you are manifesting. Thus, it will conspire with the universe to ensure it tangibly shows up.

Be Emotionally Connected

Creating affirmations to ensure a change in your life can be highly effective, but they only work if you have an emotional attachment. For instance, if you want to become a better public speaker, you can say, *"I am a confident speaker who wows my audience every time I step up on stage."* Feeling yourself saying these words can feel very exciting and motivating. Maybe it puts a smile on your face every time you visualize yourself on stage. However, not feeling emotionally attached to your affirmations will make them feel vague and unbelievable. Likewise, you will not feel motivated to continue. Your inner bully might even get in the way. Whereas, if you say an affirmation that brings meaning to your life when you think about it, it is bound to come to fruition.

Writing affirmations to help transform your life can be fun, empowering, and exciting. They are proven to help get you out of bed in the morning, ready to start your day with high-vibe energy. When you feel abundant, grateful, and full of joy, you see your manifestations come true. The final pillar is tying everything you have learned in this book to feel like your manifestation journey has succeeded.

Pillar Seven
The Process

Pillar seven, the last leg of the journey, is where we tie everything together. Everything that we have spoken about will all make sense.

It is one thing to think about manifesting your goals; it is another to put your efforts into action. So many of us get so pumped and motivated to change our lives, but when it comes to taking action, our goals seem to go to the back of our mind, and before we know it, our life remains the same. Usually, this happens because the hustle and bustle of day-to-day activities get in the way of our goals that do not feel achievable; therefore, we lose motivation. Think about new year's resolutions. On December 31, feeling excited, motivated, and energized, most of the world creates new year's resolutions. Then, as of January 1, they are ready to get rocking and make it their best year. Yet, a couple of months into the year, they are back to square one. They are no longer pumped, excited, or fueled with positive energy; instead, they are trying to keep their head above water, surviving through day-to-day obstacles. Then December 31 rolls around again, and the cycle repeats.

Certainly, you can say as many affirmations as you would like and get your mind on track, but your life will stay the same without any physical effort. The manifestation journey is a give-and-take energy; *you take action, and the rewards follow.* One key thing for success is a realistic strategy that is easy to follow and will keep you inspired. Often, when manifesting, we do not think about the steps to put in place, and at the end of the day, we are left with no rewards to reap.

On this pillar, the content will help keep you motivated and excited to begin your manifesting journey. The steps are easy to follow and will give you the clarity you need to keep going. As said throughout this book, the hardest thing is to remain consistent, especially when something needs to be fixed. Yet, this pillar will help alleviate your stress and worry and motivate you to continue working toward your goals.

Identify and Clarify

To manifest, you need to know what you want to manifest. Clarity and transparency are what will make the dream work. But when there is no clarity, there is no dream. *Sounds simple, right?*

Write down a list of things that you want. It can be anything. Allow yourself to dream truly. *What is it that you want to manifest? Your dream home? Is there a vacation you have wanted to take for years? Do you wish for a family of your own?* Dreaming of having a loving partner to grow old with? Or do you want more clients in your business? Whatever it is, get crystal clear on your desires. Understand why you want them. Allow yourself to be emotionally connected to them; this will keep you motivated and help you persevere.

As such, do not just say, *"I want to manifest my dream home because it sounds nice,"* as this statement does not sound motivating. Instead, say something like this, *"I want to manifest my dream home because I am excited to watch my children play in the backyard. I am excited to cook delicious meals in my state-of-the-art kitchen, host holiday dinners, and have hot cocoa by the fireplace. My dream home is where I will grow old with my partner while having sleepovers with our grandchildren. We will cuddle in bed, watch funny movies, and snack on popcorn. This dream home is where everyone calls it their home away from home."* With this statement, you will feel more excited to think about and inspired to achieve it. Thus, setting yourself up for success from the beginning of your manifestation journey is how you perceive your experience from the get-go and will determine your outcome.

On the other hand, *have you been trying to get clear about what you want for a while and have yet to be successful?* Not a problem. Asking yourself *why questions* will help; it is called the **Seven Levels Deep Exercise**. This exercise will help you gain clarity and should take a few minutes to complete. You can do it with as many of your desires as possible.

Here is how it was done: Start with one question and then answer it in your journal. Chances are, the first question will sound a bit vague and empty, but the trick is to keep expanding your answers as you continue asking yourself questions. Around the seventh question is when you will receive deep clarity about why you want to manifest something.

Take a look at how to do the exercise with our ideal home as an example.

1. ***Why do you want to manifest your dream home?***

   I have wanted to manifest it for a while; it would be awesome to have it.

2. ***Why would having your dream home be awesome?***

   For most of my life, I have only been renting the homes I have lived in, so I would love to have a place I can call my own.

3. ***Why does having your home matter to you?***

   Having my own home feels like success to me. I would love to give my family the home they deserve, where we can live in it for a long time and create remarkable memories.

4. ***Why does this matter to you?***

   I would love to see my children raised on a property they can call their own. I am excited to watch them run around and play with their friends in the backyard. I am excited to see them bring friends for movie nights and sleepovers. I am looking forward to hosting Christmas for my family and decorating my house with a ton of festive decor. I am excited to cook dinner with my partner in the state-of-the-art kitchen we designed while having a glass of wine. Afterward, we cuddle on our oversized, white leather sectional with a fluffy blanket as we watch a movie on our 60-inch wall-mounted plasma TV. We tuck our kids into bed and then enjoy the rest of the evening together, basking in our love and feeling grateful for a place we can call home.

The statements went from, *"I want to own a home because I think it would be awesome to have"* to *"I want to own a home because of the extraordinary experiences and memories we can create as a family."* Ergo, identifying what you want to manifest and getting clear on why you want to manifest it does not have to be rocket science. All that should matter if your manifestations are heart-centered and unique. And when you feel emotionally connected to what you want, the power returns to you.

Ask the Universe

The universe has your back, no matter what. Once you know what you want to manifest and why you want it, reach out to the universe. Ask for guidance from your spiritual team. You are always co-creating your life with them, so you must communicate with them consistently. And as a verse in the bible says, *"ask, and you shall receive."* However, if you do not ask, how can you receive anything? Sure, the universe can guess what you want, but if you are not clear with them from the beginning, it may give you something you did not expect or desire.

There are many ways you can communicate with the universe:

- Prayer
- Journaling (you can keep a spiritual journal, which contains your conversations with the universe)
- Meditation
- Visualization exercises
- Affirmations
- Manifestation rituals

Choose a way that resonates with you and be consistent with it. When you have clarity, you can share your thoughts with the universe and ask them to bring them to you, which will work to make it happen. Then, as you receive what you are asking for, you must also express gratitude to the universe for helping you bring it to fruition. Yet, being ungrateful, the universe may work slower to bring you other things. In essence, *why would they continue helping someone who is not grateful for what they receive?*

Take Inspired Action

If you want your manifestations to come to fruition, you must take action. Take steps toward achieving your goals. They do not have to be big steps; they can be small daily. For example, if you want to launch your first business and get clients, you must do more than sit around waiting for clients to come to you. First, identify why you want to launch your business. Then, you must conspire with the universe, tell your spiritual team what you want, and ask for it. Once that is done, you must create a website, launch your social media pages, and tell your audience what you are doing.

Staying motivated during the process and having fun are essential. However, procrastination will occur if you find that things are starting to feel tedious or lonely. That said, it is helpful to have affirmations ready as they will keep you on track. Plus, having a daily to-do list can help you stay on top of your commitments without becoming overwhelmed. Now, this checklist will help keep you inspired and on track to achieving your goals that day. As long as you hold yourself accountable for achieving your daily tasks, what you are manifesting will show up before you know it.

Trust the Journey

To truly conspire with the universe, you need to trust its guidance. Throughout your journey, there may be times you will feel like giving up because things are not working as quickly as you would like them to. This will feel frustrating, and you may feel disappointed and upset and believe that trying to manifest was a waste of time, and says, *"Nothing has happened yet, so clearly manifestation does not work."* With that said, the universe hears you loud and clear. Now, they are going to show you evidence of why you believe manifesting does not work and would not give you anything at all. And once again, you have proved that you could never achieve success.

This may sound all too familiar. Yet, here is something you need to know: *Even though it does not seem like anything is working, something is happening beneath the surface.* When we plant a seed, it takes a while for it to sprout. We nurture and care for the seed daily but cannot physically see it growing. Little do we know underneath the soil, the seed is growing inch by inch. Every time we nurture it, it grows even more until one day, when it is time, tiny leaf peaks through the dirt and out into the open.

Therefore, have faith in the process; your request to the universe has been heard, and you have its support to help nurture your seed until it blooms. If you struggle with complex or negative thoughts, remember your affirmations and say them until you feel content. Being in this tranquil state allows for further progress on your journey.

Release Attachment

As humans, we crave control in every aspect of our lives. If we somehow lose it, we feel defeated as we are not used to not getting our way one way or another.

Throughout the manifestation journey, it is effortless to get ahead of ourselves and hold a tight leash on the results. We want our dreams to show up in our physical reality so badly that we forget to have fun and enjoy the process. However, by not relinquishing control, you do not allow the universe to co-create with you. Due to that, it cannot work its magic in your life and show you the next steps if you have a tight grasp on the whole project. And so, you must learn to let go. Release attachment to the outcome and fully trust the universe and the plans they have for you.

Moreover, we all yearn to achieve our goals as quickly as possible, but sometimes this can leave us disappointed and discouraged if we do not get the desired outcome. Yet, by releasing expectations and trusting that whatever happens is for the best, we may find that our situation turns out better than we imagined. Taking the time to appreciate and enjoy the journey towards those goals rather than speeding through will ensure a much more fulfilling experience in life.

Be Grateful for What You Receive

Ego and pride get in the way of your manifestation journey. However, always express gratitude whenever you have reached your goal or are one step closer. Show appreciation to the universe for helping you move closer to calling in your manifestations. As such, if ego gets in the way, thinking that you succeeded alone and had no help from the universe or anyone else, you step back into low-vibe energy and forget about trusting the process. When that happens, it would not be surprising that things stop flowing your way.

Simply put, when you are grateful for what you currently have, the universe will give you more things to be thankful for. On the contrary, by allowing your pride to control your receiving, the universe will do what it can to keep you humble. Usually, that means pausing all abundance until gratitude becomes a part of your life again.

Overall, gratitude is one of the strongest emotions for effective manifestation. Think of it as being more grateful means receiving more. And to tap into a more grateful heart, here are some ways you can do:

- **Priming.** Every morning, you can do a priming meditation to set your day up for success. This exercise offers huge benefits as it gets you to think about all the things you are grateful for. They can be big or small. The first book you have published, meeting your partner, celebrating an anniversary, the birth of your children, the first day you got your new pet, the time you bumped into an old friend at a coffee shop, the time your partner surprised you with your dream vacation, the day you fell in love, the moment you visited Italy for the first time and sat in the Sistine Chapel—if you think about it, there are many things you can prime your heart to feel grateful for every morning.
- **Journaling.** Very similar to the priming exercise, but instead, you write down what you are grateful for. You can do journaling in the morning and evening if you wish. I encourage you to start small; begin with five or ten things. You can gradually increase to 20 or 30 and make your way up. Some of the most successful people in the world can think of over 100 things to be grateful for every day.

- **Focus on what you have now.** Be grateful for it. It could be watching your children grow up. The way your partner makes your coffee and brings it to you in bed every morning. The friends that call you regularly to see how you are doing. A steady paying job that helps you pay the bills every month. A successful business brings in residual income and amazing clients every month. The clients who have already chosen to work with you. The car that brings you to work every single day. A warm house to keep you and your family safe and protected. The abundance of food you eat daily. When you acknowledge all you have now, the universe will continue bringing in more goodness.

Watch Your Energy

As you know, the Law of Attraction states, "like attracts like." Hence, take care of your energy during your manifestation journey, as you will receive the same energy you are showcasing to the universe. For instance, if you are always angry, frustrated, and annoyed that things are not working your way, the same energy will come flooding back to you. It will be evidence that manifestation does not work, your life will still feel like a mess, and it will feel like everyone you have ever loved is conspiring against you. You will feel like a victim, not a champion.

However, if you choose enlightenment, abundance, and gratitude instead, you will receive the same back tenfold. It will feel like your life is finally clicking into place; you will meet extraordinary people, your creativity will skyrocket, and you will feel motivated and inspired every day. Your life begins to transform because you are paying attention to your energy. Positive and negativity are like an energetic force field that tries to pull you in at any chance. Whatever you decide to gravitate toward will be up to you, but it will depend on how your energy is feeling.

If you are in a funk and you want to shift your energy instantly, here are some helpful tips:

- **Put on some dance music and move to the rhythm.** Dancing releases endorphins and gets your adrenaline pumping, which helps bring you into an immediate state of joy.
- **Watch a comedy.** Funny movies or shows bring out the laughter in you. Smiling (laughter) releases dopamine, endorphins, and serotonin, known as happy drugs.
- **Meditate.** Meditating will help you feel calm and relaxed when stressed and worried. Likewise, take a few deep breaths and say your affirmations while you are smiling.
- **Smile.** No doubt, smiling makes you instantly happy, especially if the person you are smiling at smiles back at you. In this situation, it feels like instant gratification and being authentically happy changes your life.
- **Sit up straight.** Your posture plays a big part in how you feel in every moment. If you are always slouching, you feel mentally, emotionally, and physically exhausted and wish for the day to be over. Besides that, it might even make you feel sad or alone. Being mindful of your posture can brighten your mood right away. Sitting up straight rather than arch-

ing your back makes you feel alive, alert, and motivated. Plus, it promotes a healthy spine, so it becomes a win-win.
- **Go for a walk.** Grounding yourself in Mother Nature can certainly put you in high-vibe energy. As such, it promotes calm and stillness and helps bring peace to your mind, body, and spirit.

Let Go of Limiting Beliefs

When you have not received your desired results, ask yourself why. Perhaps, it could be because you are still holding onto some negativity blocking you and keeping you stuck. And with such negativity, you must clear the path so positivity can start flowing your way. Remember, *abundance cannot flow on a busy road*; you need to remove the resistance, so it does not get stuck trying to get to you.

There are a few steps to take to fully clear any negative distractions:

- **Acknowledgment.** Understand why limiting beliefs are a part of your life in the first place. *Are they protecting you from potential harm?* When you allow yourself to understand, you create a deeper relationship with yourself that is full of love and happiness.
- **Forgiveness.** Free yourself and others from instilling limiting beliefs in you. Let go of the past so it no longer harms your present or future.
- **Accountability.** *Do not play the victim; play victor.* Hold yourself accountable for adopting these limiting beliefs and negative thoughts, and forgive yourself for holding onto them for so long.
- **Embrace.** As you hold yourself accountable, embrace and accept all parts of you. Understand that your limiting beliefs may not leave your life for good, but feel grateful that they are around to demonstrate your resilience and determination.
- **Shift.** Reframe the negative thoughts. Create new and empowering beliefs that will uplift you and keep you humble.

Another thing you can do is to write yourself a letter. We spoke about this exercise briefly in pillar three. Following these steps, write a letter acknowledging why the limiting beliefs are lingering and express gratitude to them for keeping you safe up to this point. Make a promise to yourself that you will strive for a better life because that is who you are. Vow to yourself that you will do everything in your power to release the resistance that keeps you stuck so you can transform your life and habits into empowering ones that keep you motivated.

By following this process, you are guaranteed to manifest your dreams. It will take some time, so it is important to remember to trust the process and to call on the universe for guidance. Even if things are not showing up right away, that is okay. Allow things to flow and learn to balance your energy so you can feel abundant, prosperous, and authentically happy. When you can stay in this state, what you are manifesting comes to fruition effortlessly.

Conclusion

You have reached the end of the book. Congratulations! I hope you are proud of yourself for accomplishing this part of your journey.

We have covered many aspects to help you start your manifestation journey on the right path. I trust that you will take these pillars and develop your understanding of the subject matter in a way that relates to you and your situation.

The only way for us to learn is to grow, and by reaching the end of this book, you have grown on a deeper level, mentally, physically, and spiritually. Not everyone seeks to better themselves consistently, but by reading this book and applying the knowledge to your own life, you have taken the next step toward personal and professional growth.

We have covered many topics to help enlighten you on your path:

- **The origin and science behind manifestation.** By understanding this, you can get behind what it truly means to manifest your dreams.
- **The 12 spiritual laws of the universe.** By now, you understand that manifestation is not simply about the Law of Attraction. That is only one law out of twelve. I encourage you to use these laws to get what you truly desire out of life. Notice how they play into your life, see which ones resonate with you, and then focus on them.
- **The importance of vibrating at a higher frequency.** The higher the energetic frequency you vibrate daily, the easier it is to manifest anything you want. Understanding how vibrating on a certain energetic frequency affects your life by changing extraordinarily.
- **The importance of gratitude** and how feeling grateful can change the trajectory of your life.
- **Why healthy relationships are essential and how they connect** to your manifestation journey with yourself and others.
- **Setting intentions for your goals is vital** so you know where you are going and how to get there.
- **Taking inspired action consistently** can improve your life (it is not just about the big steps!).
- **Why learning to co-create with the universe** can transform your life immediately.
- **The importance of visualizing your dreams** and how visualization techniques can help shift your subconscious mind into believing your dreams are possible.

- **The power of the words** you say to yourself, others, and the universe. Change your words, and you change your life!
- **How to create empowering affirmations** that can set you up for success.
- **Getting clear on the process** while having fun, watching your energy, and trusting the journey.

I intend to help you through a challenging phase in your life by writing this book. Maybe you are struggling financially or feeling stuck in a job you hate. Perhaps you wish to find a beautiful relationship or take that vacation you have longed for several years. Whatever you are currently going through, I have done my part by providing incredible solutions in this book that are guaranteed to change your life. I have shared a blueprint of what it takes to drastically change your life. Now it is up to you to take the next step: take action. Once you do, there is no doubt your life will transform, but without inspired action, your life will stay the same.

If you know someone who could also benefit from reading this book—your parents, friends, coworkers, cousins, siblings, your children's friend's parents—anyone that you know that is also struggling and would like to get their life back on track, I trust that you will share this book with them. This book can benefit anyone ready to make a drastic change in their life: Those prepared to go after their dreams and manifest them into reality. It is never too late to say yes to yourself and your dreams. Sharing this book with our loved ones, you help them experience freedom and healing.

Lastly, I encourage you to apply the knowledge you have learned on these pages to your life. If there is one thing I would like you to take away from this book, it would be this: You have the innate power in your mind to create extraordinary things. What we lack is the action that keeps us motivated and inspired. Applying this knowledge eliminates inaction and promotes inspired action. Action that makes us excited to get out of bed in the morning, with a smile on our face and pep in our step. Your manifestation journey begins the moment your thoughts form—create them wisely, and you will one day live the dream life you have envisioned.

Glossary

Affirmations: Positive and empowering statements, words, or phrases that are known to set you up for success; affirmations can be anything related to wealth, business, relationships, health, wellness, or spirituality. Usually begins in the form of an "I Am" statement.

Consistency: Taking action regularly to build a stable habit while focusing on your well-being.

Emotional Intelligence: Understanding how to regulate your emotions and balance them in the middle of certain situations so the outcome does not appear negative.

Emotional Regulation: Balancing your emotions so they do not affect your decision-making.

Gratitude: Demonstrating thankfulness in receipt of a gift, help, or service; acknowledging one's efforts and showing appreciation for how they have impacted your life.

Intention: A heart-based plan that focuses on a goal or outcome.

Inspired Action: Setting yourself up for success by knowing and fully understanding why you want to manifest something and using those reasons to keep you motivated in reaching success.

Journaling: Writing down your sentiments, thoughts, and feelings in a notebook on a particular subject to understand the root cause of an issue.

Law of Attraction: A philosophy dating back centuries that helps us understand the interconnection between our thoughts, actions, and behaviors.

Limiting Beliefs: A state of mind in your subconscious that, when perceived, can cause a negative impact on your life that results in feeling stuck, unmotivated, confused, and never moving forward.

Manifestation: The scientific process of visualizing something in your mind and turning it into a tangible person, place, or thing.

Meditation: A creative art form that helps you calm your mind, relax your body, and bring peace to your well-being. It can be in the form of music, sounds, or voice activation.

Multi-Sensory Visualization: Utilizing all five senses (see, hear, taste, touch, smell) to effectively visualize succeeding at your goal before it happens.

New Age Spirituality: A mixture of divine beliefs, both in a religious and spiritual context. People who follow new-age spirituality do not believe in one thing; they study different religions and engage in various spiritual practices.

Present Moment: Being aware and acknowledging what you have in your current surroundings; taking a moment to check in with yourself and your energy without getting distracted by technology and social media.

Releasing Attachment: Surrendering, having faith in the unknown and letting go so you can be open to an unexpected outcome.

Pseudoscience: A collection of practices disguised as part of scientific studies but don't appear to be factual or true.

Spirituality: Divinity; the belief that a greater power guides your path. Not based on religion; based on a cluster of beliefs.

Subconscious Mind: The facility in your mind that stores memories, experiences, and other information; often referred to as the mind's warehouse and makes up about 95% of the mind's capacity together with the unconscious mind.

Surrender: Having faith in the process and fully trusting the journey without a logical understanding of what will happen.

The Universe: A group of spiritual beings or entities who co-create with you to help transform your life.

Vibrational Being: A state of being; the energy you perceive in the universe.

Vibrational Frequency: The speed at which a human's energy is calculated. If you radiate negative energy—such as frustration, anger, and worry—your vibrational frequency is low. Meanwhile, your vibrational frequency is higher if you radiate positive energy—such as happiness, gratitude, joy, peace, and enlightenment.

Vision Board: A creative form of visualization. It can include magazine clippings, printed images and words, and colorful and unique ideas of how you want your life to be, a powerful manifestation technique.

Visualization: A manifestation technique that helps us think in imagery and words to clarify what we want.

References

Bob Proctor. (2017, April 27). AZ Quotes. https://www.azquotes.com/quote/805850

Borbala. (2017a, June 26). *5 ways to raise your vibration and have more positive energy (part 1).* Follow Your Own Rhythm. https://www.followyourownrhythm.com/blog-1/2017/6/18/5-ways-to-raise-your-vibration-and-have-more-positive-energy

Borbala. (2017b, July 10). *10 toxic habits that are lowering your vibration (part 2).* Follow Your Own Rhythm. https://www.followyourownrhythm.com/blog-1/2017/6/18/5bsh1ryhitjsknubf47tnv1grtc6nq

Bradley, J. (2018, March 15). *Sensory visualization — A clear path to manifestation.* Medium. https://medium.com/@judestur/sensory-visualization-a-clear-path-to-manifestation-9461d8c01514

Brown, B. (2021a, October 4). *Law of Action | The 12 universal laws of manifestation.* Modern Manifestation. https://www.themodernmanifestation.com/post/law-of-action

Brown, B. (2021b, October 18). *Law of correspondence | The 12 universal laws of manifestation.* Modern Manifestation. https://www.themodernmanifestation.com/post/law-of-correspondence

Brown, B. (2021c, November 15). *Law of cause and effect | The 12 universal laws of manifestation.* Modern Manifestation. https://www.themodernmanifestation.com/post/law-of-cause-and-effect

Brown, B. (2021d, November 29). *Law of compensation | The 12 universal laws of manifestation.* Modern Manifestation. https://www.themodernmanifestation.com/post/law-of-compensation

Brown, B. (2021e, December 26). *Law of perpetual transmutation of energy | The 12 universal laws of manifestation.* Modern Manifestation. https://www.themodernmanifestation.com/post/law-of-perpetual-transmutation-of-energy

Brown, B. (2022a, January 23). *Law of relativity | The 12 universal laws of manifestation.* Modern Manifestation. https://www.themodernmanifestation.com/post/law-of-relativity

Brown, B. (2022b, February 6). *Law of rhythm | The 12 universal laws of manifestation.* Modern Manifestation. https://www.themodernmanifestation.com/post/law-of-rhythm#:~:text=let

Butterworth, E. (n.d). *New thought pioneers: Thomas Troward.* Truthunity.net. https://www.truthunity.net/courses/mark-hicks/background-of-new-thought/thomas-troward

Bullying, cyberbullying, & suicide statistics. (2020). Megan Meier Foundation. https://www.meganmeierfoundation.org/statistics

Cannon, M. (2015, December 14). *10 accidental scientific discoveries and breakthroughs.* InterFocus. https://www.mynewlab.com/blog/accidental-scientific-discoveries-and-breakthroughs/

Cronkleton, E. (2022, June 27). *Energy therapy: What to know.* Medical News Today. https://www.medicalnewstoday.com/articles/energy-therapy#uses

Davis, T. (2020, September 15). *What is manifestation? Science-based ways to manifest.* Psychology Today. https://www.psychologytoday.com/us/blog/click-here-happiness/202009/what-is-manifestation-science-based-ways-manifest

Davis, T. (n.d). *Manifestation: Definition, meaning, and how to do it.* Berkeley Well-Being Institute. https://www.berkeleywellbeing.com/manifestation.html

Duda. (2017, August 30). *What does Buddhism have to do with the law of attraction?* Little School Of Buddhism. https://littleschoolofbuddhism.kickassmuse.com/buddhism-law-attraction

Edison's Lightbulb. (2014, March 8). The Franklin Institute. https://www.fi.edu/history-resources/edisons-lightbulb#:~:text=In%20the%20period%20from%201878

Estrada, J. (2022, June 29). *Setting intentions are a "part practical, part magic" wellness practice, experts say.* The Zoe Report. https://www.thezoereport.com/wellness/how-to-set-intentions-for-manifestation

Filippazzo, F. (2021, January 4). *The Law of attraction: Energy, frequency and vibrations!* Medium. https://medium.com/know-thyself-heal-thyself/the-law-of-attraction-energy-frequency-and-vibrations-1d3fc438bbc1

Firth, S. (2022, October 12). *Teen suicides jump 29% over the past decade, report finds.* Medpage Today. https://www.medpagetoday.com/psychiatry/generalpsychiatry/101188

Forrest, L. (2007, November 28). *We are vibrational beings.* Lynne Forrest and Conscious Living Media. https://www.lynneforrest.com/spiritual-principles/vibrational-frequency/2007/11/we-are-vibrational-beings/

Freud's model of the human mind. (n.d). Journal Psych. https://journalpsyche.org/understanding-the-human-mind/

Gallo, C. (2014, May 31). *The Maya Angelou quote that will radically improve your business.* Forbes. https://www.forbes.com/sites/carminegallo/2014/05/31/the-maya-angelou-quote-that-will-radically-improve-your-business/?sh=5137d154118b

Goswami, P. (2021, September 28). *Vibrational energy and 9 ways to implement into your workplace culture.* Vantage Fit. https://www.vantagefit.io/blog/vibrational-energy/

Grasso, H. (2022, July 17). *The power of intention: 10 steps to manifesting your reality.* Gaia. https://www.gaia.com/article/the-power-of-manifestitation-10-steps-to-manifesting-your-reality

Groth, A. (2012, July 24). *You're the average of the five people you spend the most time with.* Business Insider. https://www.businessinsider.com/jim-rohn-youre-the-average-of-the-five-people-you-spend-the-most-time-with-2012-7

Guerin, N. (2015, July 20). *7 steps to manifest anything you want -- including money.* HuffPost. https://www.huffpost.com/entry/7-steps-to-manifest-anyth_b_7806936

Hay, L. (2014, November 26). *The power of affirmations.* Louise Hay. https://www.louisehay.com/the-power-of-affirmations/

Healthwise Staff. (2022a, January 3). *Healing Touch.* Myhealth.alberta.ca. https://myhealth.alberta.ca/Health/Pages/conditions.aspx?hwid=aa104487spec&lang=en-ca#acl6879

Healthwise Staff. (2022b, January 3). *Therapeutic Touch.* Myhealth.alberta.ca. https://myhealth.alberta.ca/Health/Pages/conditions.aspx?hwid=ag2078spec#:~:text=Therapeutic%20touch%20is%20based%20on

Hinduja, S. & Patchin, J. (2019, May 29). *School bullying rates increase by 35% from 2016 to 2019.* Cyberbullying Research Center. https://cyberbullying.org/school-bullying-rates-increase-by-35-from-2016-to-2019

Hurst, K. (2018, April 6). *The 12 spiritual laws of the universe and what they mean.* The Law of Attraction. https://thelawofattraction.com/12-spiritual-laws-universe/

Hurst, K. (2019, June 5). *Law of attraction history: The origins of the law of attraction uncovered.* The Law of Attraction. https://thelawofattraction.com/history-law-attraction-uncovered/

Intention definition & meaning. Dictionary.com. (2019). https://www.dictionary.com/browse/intention

Intermountain. (n.d). *Why it matters how you talk to yourself.* SelectHealth. https://selecthealth.org/blog/2019/05/why-it-matters-how-you-talk-to-yourself

Irven, J. (n.d). *19 ways to raise your vibration.* Sustainable Bliss Collective. https://www.sustainablyblissco.com/journal/raising-your-vibration

John, H. (2019, September 25). *British Science Festival: 7 ways dancing can improve your life.* British Science Association. https://www.britishscienceassociation.org/blogs/bsa-blog/7-ways-dancing-can-improve-your-life#:~:text=Dance%20has%20been%20scientifically%20proven

Lieber. A. (2022, July 16). *The 7 major chakras: What you need to know and how to work with them.* DailyOM. https://www.dailyom.com/journal/the-7-major-chakras-what-you-need-to-know-and-how-to-work-with-them

Lopez, C. (2020, January 31). *The science behind good vibrations.* Balance. https://balance.media/good-vibrations/

Kurt, E. (2018, October 16). *2 high vibe drinks that will raise your vibration.* The Elegant Life. https://theelegantlife.com/manifesting-confidence/raise-your-vibration/

Mayo Clinic Staff. (2022, April 30). *Acupuncture.* Mayo Clinic. https://www.mayoclinic.org/tests-procedures/acupuncture/about/pac-20392763

McGinley, K. (2019, September 18). *How to Raise Your Emotional & Spiritual Vibration.* The Chopra Center. https://chopra.com/articles/a-complete-guide-to-raise-your-vibration

McLeod, S. (2015). *Freud and the unconscious mind.* Simply Psychology. https://www.simplypsychology.org/unconscious-mind.html

Mind Tools Content Team. (n.d). *Using affirmations.* Mind Tools. https://www.mindtools.com/air49f4/using-affirmations

Moe, K. (2021, June 4). *5 visualization techniques to help you reach your goals.* Better Up. https://www.betterup.com/blog/visualization

Molitor, M. (2019, October 5). *The power of your brain | The 95-5% rule.* Linkedin. https://www.linkedin.com/pulse/95-5-rule-michele-molitor-cpcc-pcc-rtt-c-hyp?trk=portfolio_article-card_title

Mullins, E. (2008, August). *The process of the law of attraction and the 3rd law, Law of Allowing.* University of Wisconsin-Stout. http://www2.uwstout.edu/content/lib/thesis/2008/2008mullinse.pdf

Peer, M. (2022). *Tell Yourself a Better Lie: Use the power of Rapid Transformational Therapy to edit your story and rewrite your life.* RTT Press.

Potter, P. (2013, May 1). *Energy therapies in advanced practice oncology: An evidence-informed practice approach.* Journal of the Advanced Practitioner in Oncology 4(3): 139–151. https://www.ncbi.nlm.nih.gov/pmc/articles/PMC4093427/

Reble, D. (2017, January 19). *Words are powerful intentions to the universe.* Debra Reble. https://www.debrareble.com/words-powerful-intentions-universe/

Robbins, T. (n.d). *How the law of polarity can transform your life.* Tony Robbins. https://www.tonyrobbins.com/ask-tony/polarity/#:~:text=What%20is%20the%20law%20of

Robbins, T. (2014, October 31). *Tony Robbins quote.* Facebook. https://www.facebook.com/TonyRobbins/posts/the-antidote-to-fear-is-gratitude-the-antidote-to-anger-is-gratitude-you-cant-fe/10152793591744060/

Rollins, S. (2020, October 2). *The power of visualization: Improve your skill by training your mind.* Esports Healthcare. https://esportshealthcare.com/power-of-visualization/#:~:text=that%20way%20again.-

Rose, B. (2021, September). *The vibrational frequencies of the human body.* Research Gate. https://www.researchgate.net/publication/354326235_The_Vibrational_Frequencies_of_the_Human_Body

Scott, E. (2022, November 7). *What is the law of attraction?* Verywell Mind. https://www.verywellmind.com/understanding-and-using-the-law-of-attraction-3144808

Shahnawaz, G. (2021, July 8). *How yoga raises our vibration.* My Name is Ghanwa. https://www.mynameisghanwa.com/post/how-yoga-raises-our-vibration

Smith, S. (2023, January 24) *What does the bible say about manifestation?* Openbible.info. https://www.openbible.info/topics/manifestation

Spiritual Counseling Training: Intention manifestation. (n.d). Universal Class. https://www.universalclass.com/articles/spirituality/spiritual-counseling-training-intention-manifestation.htm#:~:text=What%20is%20intention%20manifestation%3F

Stanborough, R. (2020, November 13). *What is vibrational energy? Definition, benefits & more.* Heathline. https://www.healthline.com/health/vibrational-energy

Suicide. (2022, June). National Institute of Mental Health. https://www.nimh.nih.gov/health/statistics/suicide

Taleszia. (2018, April 14). *Top 10 foods for raising your vibration.* Happy Earth People. https://happyearthpeople.com/2018/04/14/top-10-foods-for-raising-your-vibration/

Vibrational energy - an overview,. (2013). ScienceDirect. https://www.sciencedirect.com/topics/chemistry/vibrational-energy

Vilhauer, J. (2020, September 27). *How your thinking creates your reality* | Psychology Today. https://www.psychologytoday.com/us/blog/living-forward/202009/how-your-thinking-creates-your-reality

Wayne Dyer Quotes. (n.d.). BrainyQuote. https://www.brainyquote.com/quotes/wayne_dyer_384143

Who discovered electricity? (2019, May 11). Wonderopolis. https://www.wonderopolis.org/wonder/who-discovered-electricity

Wilinski, A. (2017, January 30). *Choose wisely: How our words impact others.* Brain Injury Services. https://braininjurysvcs.org/choose-wisely-how-our-words-impact-others/

Wolchover, N. & Leggett, J. (2021, December 22). *Top 10 inventions that changed the world.* Live Science. https://www.livescience.com/33749-top-10-inventions-changed-world.html

Wong, K. (2023, January 18). *What is the law of vibration and how to use it.* The Millenial Grind. https://millennial-grind.com/how-to-use-the-law-of-vibration-to-manifest/

World Smile Day - How smiling affects your brain. (2017, October 6). Aultman. https://aultman.org/blog/caring-for-you/world-smile-day-how-smiling-affects-your-brain/#/

Zach. (2012, March 9). *"Change your thoughts, and you change your world...".* Zach Mercurio. https://www.zachmercurio.com/2012/03/change-your-thoughts-and-you-change-your-world/#:~:text=Norman%20Vincent%20Peale%20once%20wrote

Zapata, K. (2022, July 22). *Exactly how to manifest anything you want or desire.* Oprah Daily. https://www.oprahdaily.com/life/a30244004/how-to-manifest-anything/

Made in the USA
Columbia, SC
18 August 2024